Courage & Cancer

A Breast Cancer Diary:
A Journey from Cancer to Cure

Marilyn R. Moody

RHACHE PUBLISHERS, LTD., GARDINER, NY

Marilyn R. Moody

Courage & Cancer

A Breast Cancer Diary:
A Journey from Cancer to Cure

Rhache Publishers, Ltd., Gardiner, NY

Courage & Cancer: A Breast Cancer Diary—A Journey From Cancer to Cure by Marilyn R. Moody

Cover Design by Carolyn Hutchings Edlund
Book Design by Rhache Publishers, Ltd.
Production services provided by Richard H. Adin, Freelance Editorial Services, 9 Orchard Drive, Gardiner, NY 12525 (914) 883–5884
Editor: Meredith Kennedy
Author photograph by Don Thompson, © 1996 Rhache Publishers, Ltd. All rights reserved.

Published in the United States of America
Printed in the United States of America.
0 9 8 7 6 5 4 3 2 1

 Rhache Publishers, Ltd.
9 Orchard Drive • Gardiner, NY 12525–5710
(914) 883–5884 • (914) 883–7169

ISBN 1–887288–01–5

Library of Congress Cataloging-in-Publication Data

Moody, Marilyn R., 1946–
    Courage & cancer : a breast cancer diary : a journey from cancer to cure / Marilyn R. Moody.
        p.   cm.
    Includes bibliographical references and index.
    ISBN 1-887288-01-5 (pbk.)
    1. Moody, Marilyn R., 1946–Health. 2. Breast–Cancer–Patients–California–Biography. I. Title. II. Title: Courage and cancer
RC280 . B8M59   1996
362.1'9699449'0092–dc20
    [B]   96-819
                                                                    CIP

This book is a gift of love.

It is dedicated to

Rita Pelrine
Without you this book would not exist,
And to my Breast Cancer Sisters everywhere.
We are "Many faces, one family."*

A special dedication

In loving memory of
Wendy Frankel
who gave me so much support and inspiration.

*saying from the Church of Religious Science, Huntington Beach, CA

Foreword

Foreword by
Grace Smith, Ph.D.

---

*"I have witnessed the fortitude with which women sustain
the most overwhelming reverse of fortune. Those disasters
which break down the spirit of a man, and prostrate him in
the dust, seem to call forth all the energies of the softer sex,
and give such intrepidity and elevation to their character;
at times it approaches to sublimity."*
Washington Irving (1783-1859)

Throughout history, women have been referred to as the "weaker" sex, but in my opinion, women are survivors and unsung heroes whose daily acts of courage are often disregarded or devalued. As a result, I pay close attention when I learn of a woman's narrative about her own personal journey.

I have never met Marilyn Moody face-to-face. The first time we touched was during an online writer's forum where she had posted a message asking for advice about the book she was writing. I offered to read her manuscript because I was interested in its topic—breast cancer. For the past seven years, I have been discouraged about my own state of health and the C-word. In 1988, after years of error-free mammograms, a suspicious reading occurred. My physician suggested that I think immediately about a double mastectomy as a preventive measure.

At the time, I was 43 years old, in a high-pressure job with a boss who lacked integrity. I was racing to complete the dissertation for my doctoral degree, and I was in the middle of physical therapy for a partially herniated lumbar disc. Adding to these stresses was the realization that my long-term marriage was disintegrating. My most mindful family member, my daughter, was away on a college field study in Europe, and my 17 year old son wanted to stay out of the anguish between his parents. I felt absolutely powerless with no resources to turn to for help.

When the shock from my physician's words had worn off, I found myself in the throes of depression with the feeling that my life was totally on hold until my health issue could be resolved. And then, I decided to look for another physician who would look at my condition holistically. Within two months, I found him in a neighboring state, and I'm happy to report that today, I still have both of my breasts. My condition has not improved, but it has not worsened either, and I've learned to live with the knowing that any day can bring the news that I, too, will have a mastectomy, and probably, a double one, at that.

When I offered to read Marilyn's manuscript, it was for two reasons. As a published author who teaches writing at the university level, I wanted to lend any assistance I could. Good writing, in my experience, is hard work. More selfishly, though, I wanted to see for myself how another woman was able to handle the ups and downs of a mastectomy and follow-up chemical treatment. I've often wondered whether I'd have the courage to embark upon such a journey and whether life would ever normalize again.

What I learned during the process of knowing Marilyn is that her book is written straight from the heart of an ordinary, yet truly extraordinary woman. The famous author, Victor Hugo, once said, "No one knows like a woman how to say things which are at once gentle and deep." And that's Marilyn—gentle and deep, like a see-saw between fear and courage, between health and illness, between wholeness and surgery, and between laughter and tears.

Begun as a diary to track her feelings, Marilyn's book illustrates her range of moods, thinking, and reactions to her experience of dealing with breast cancer. Running parallel to the treatment are her efforts to manage her life and to resume where she left off before cancer. Nowhere during her journey through the process of diagnosis, surgery, recovery, and adjustment does she refer to her actions as heroic. But that oversight doesn't surprise me.

As an urban university teacher, I'm aware of the grit and determination my adult learners have displayed in their lives. My experience is that most people do not regard themselves as courageous. They just move on, doing the little steps that enable them to take bigger steps and finally, giant steps to their goals. They don't get the Medal of Honor or the Bronze Star for bravery, but they continue to move forward, despite the odds or the obstacles, to get to the dream or to reach the hope upon which they cling for the moment. Yet it is these unsung heroes, these "Marilyns," who illustrate the human condition and picture life as it is—replete with relationships, tales from the heart, hope, tenderness, encouragement, and paths to inner peace. It is these uncelebrated individuals who most move us and inspire us, for they are most like us—just plain folks who are on a similar pilgrimage in what we call life.

Marilyn's story, as you will see, is truly about a woman of distinguished valor, a woman whose courage to beat cancer, to resume her normal day-to-day activities, and to set goals for the future may be more than any of us think we are capable of doing when the C-word or any other major calamity strikes at our very being. Marilyn's account is about her own human condition, but it could be about our life, too. We can identify with her in the worst of moments and in the best of them because Marilyn's story could be our story.

Marilyn's is the kind of book most of us like best—a true story about an ordinary person who finds meaning in her life. Why? It reminds us that problems are given to us so we can solve them. It prompts us to strive, to conquer, and to sustain hope. It causes us to stop and reflect—what messages may be waiting for us in our own lives? And most of all, it shows us that reaching out for support creates courage in ourselves and in others we know and love.

Grace Smith, Ph.D.
Friend

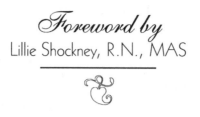

Foreword by
Lillie Shockney, R.N., MAS

This is one of the most inspiring books you will ever read about a woman's courageous battle and successful victory with breast cancer. Marilyn Moody has dealt with many crises in her life, many of which were challenging and devastating, but none quite as wrenching as this one. As it is for so many women, she was surprised to discover that she had breast cancer. It caught her off balance and in a situation that she had never faced before—a situation that depended on her treatment choices, her attitude, her self-determination—and her support systems could leave her not just without a breast but without her life ahead of her.

Medical researchers say that the most feared disease to a woman is breast cancer. It's no wonder; the incidence of breast cancer has continued to grow in numbers over the last decade. What was once a disease which primarily struck women in their 60s and 70s, now strikes at almost any age once a women has passed her 25th birthday. A disease whose frequency was once only 1 in 50 women, was 1 in 9 in 1993 and was 1 in 8 in 1994.

Breast cancer doesn't discriminate. Women of all races, colors, religions, and cultures have been touched by this known killer. It lacks charm, wit, and personality. It arrives in a woman's breast and, once having quietly established residency there, will grow undetected until mammography finds it or the woman herself discovers it while doing a self breast exam. Once it is detectable by one of these means it has usually been growing there for several years.

The best weapon against breast cancer is early detection. That's why self breast exams and the mammogram are so very important. And if a woman with no known risk factors thinks that she is immune from getting this disease, she better think again. Why? Because 70% of the women diagnosed each year also have no known risk factors.

In 1994, more than 180,000 women were diagnosed with breast cancer. Marilyn Moody became one of these women. And more than 46,000 additional women died from the complications of this disease. That means that every 3 minutes another woman is told that she has breast cancer and every 11 minutes a victim dies of the catastrophic effects this killer causes.

Though it is a disease feared by women, they are not the only ones affected by this type of cancer. About 1,000 men a year are also diagnosed with breast cancer, but that is not the issue here. What is important to recognize is that when a woman is diagnosed with breast cancer it affects her and everyone who loves and cares about her. The impact such a diagnosis has on a woman, her lover, siblings, parents, and friends can be so emotionally devastating that it cripples everyone for a period of time.

When a woman is diagnosed as having breast cancer, her first reaction usually is one of fear of succumbing to this disease and dying. While dealing with those feelings, she must also focus on the probable impact of her treatment. The cultural significance of breasts is instilled at an early age. They are symbolic of many things, including femininity, sexuality, and motherhood. Regardless of her size, a bosomy silhouette in the mirror remains very important to a woman. The fear of losing her breasts is very powerful. Some women are willing to sacrifice their own lives for the preservation of their breasts by foregoing treatment.

A breast cancer diagnosis requires decision-making about the treatment plan and care necessary to help her become a breast cancer survivor. Two decades ago, no decisions were made by the patient. The doctor assumed much of the responsibility and the patient had to live with those choices. A woman's right to participate in her medical care for cancer treatment is an important and positive step made by healthcare providers, although it can add anxiety to the patient during a time when she is already overwhelmed with information. Treatment options have dramatically improved over the last two decades. A woman may opt to have a lumpectomy with radiation rather than having a complete mastectomy. She may be advised to have chemotherapy, sometimes experimental. She must also make decisions about whether or not to have her breast reconstructed and which surgical option to choose. Each decision requires careful thought and places an additional burden on the woman. She questions the adequacy of her information in making good choices for herself both medically and psychologically.

Family and friends also suffer. Fear of losing the woman they love can paralyze some men, leaving them unable to effectively provide emotional support. With breast cancer striking younger, premenopausal women, more family members than ever before are directly impacted by this disease. The parents of a woman diagnosed with breast cancer are oftentimes devastated by the news. Although their instincts tell them to "bring her home to be nurtured back to good health," they realize that their "baby" has a life and family of her own. If the woman also is a mother herself, she has real fears of leaving her children if the disease cannot be controlled. She will also worry that she may be one of the 3 – 4% of women with breast cancer to genetically pass this disease on.

This story is about my dear friend, Marilyn Moody, who was diagnosed with breast cancer in 1994. She became one of those 180,000 women referenced above. You will learn how she discovered that she had breast cancer, what treatment options she was offered and chose, and how she and her family and friends, together, weathered out the storm giving her the ability and fortitude to successfully become a breast cancer survivor. She carries you through her breast cancer crisis by sharing with you her every emotion, from the day she learned of her diagnosis, through, and beyond the completion of her treatment. She shares with you her innermost thoughts and emotions through journal writings and letters written to her dear friend Rita, as well as to others, who became her support system. Her story is inspiring for other women facing this same crisis. She describes her efforts to amass complete medical information permitting her direct participation in the decision-making process for her care. She sought out other breast cancer survivors to learn from them what to expect and how to cope with various aspects of treatment. And Marilyn demonstrates the benefit of keeping a positive attitude and open communication with the people she loves, and who also love her so very much.

Presently, based on research studies conducted throughout the United States, there are more than 1.2 million women who are breast cancer survivors. There are also an additional 1 million women who have breast cancer but don't know it yet. As a breast cancer survivor or friend of one, you will find comfort in knowing that the thoughts that you are experiencing or have experienced are shared by others like yourself. You will appreciate and come away inspired by Marilyn's courage, sense of humor, and determination to beat this disease. And remember. . . you could be among the 1 million unknowing women in the US who have breast cancer, but don't know it yet.

Lillie Shockney, R.N., MAS
Friend, Breast Cancer Survivor, and
Author of "Joining the Club—The Reality of Breast Cancer"

Author's Note

These letters to others, and the notes to myself, were written beginning in May 1994. The majority were written to Rita, my best friend, who lives just outside of Boston, Massachusetts.

May 1994 was a busy and memorable month in my life. The 12th of May was my last day at my old assignment with my employer of the past fourteen years. It was also the day that my HMO's Physician's Assistant told me that my routine, bi-annual mammogram showed a suspicious lump. She scheduled me for a biopsy on May 20th.

On Friday the 13th, I started my new job within our large agency. At the age of 47 I was making a quantum leap in my career path. For the prior eighteen years my main workload consisted of administering welfare benefits or supervising case carrying staff. I was now focusing on computers versus people. The switch was made impulsively. As I saw it, and as my agency would probably call it, this would be an excellent "growth opportunity." As of the 13th my new title became "Systems Coordinator." I was one of a team of five systems "experts" for approximately 3,500 employees, and even the word "systems" intimidated me. My knowledge of PC's, at that point, was basically how to use one as an electronic typewriter.

The story, written in these letters, is my introduction to the world of breast cancer and to personal computers. Both subjects were about to expand my horizons. In a few months time I did make some headway into the desired growth spurt. And, in that same time, my life became one similar to that of a roller coaster ride. But, what I discovered on the way restored my faith in my fellow man. I also believe that my experiences through this journey helped me to become a better person.

Throughout all of it I had Rita keeping me centered. She's the one who had a "free subscription" to these almost daily letters. She was my therapist. She's the one I could simultaneously laugh and cry with.

Rita also had a suspicious lump at the same time that I did. Hers was fortunately determined to be a cyst. We went through this cancer experience together, one day and one step at a time. Rita has been my best friend for the past thirty years and she truly is my "bosom buddy."

Marilyn R. Moody
January 1, Saturday

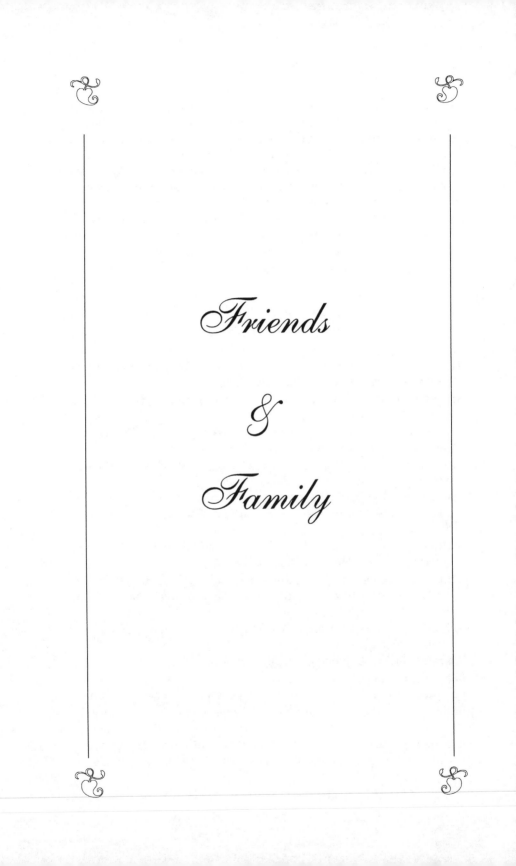

Friends

&

Family

I realize that in my letters and journal entries I have written about many people who were in my life this past year. Since the people in my life are all new to you, I would like to take the time to introduce you to them, and to give you a brief explanation of our relationships. Without this list of characters you may become confused. I have listed people alphabetically so that as you read, and perhaps question who someone is, you can come back to this section and become acquainted with each. At times I have listed two people together, because this is how I think of them. Also, in my letters I misspelled some names and this is my opportunity to note the corrections. In case I might have overlooked anyone—please forgive me. It is my pleasure to introduce the following:

Some of the names in these letters have been changed
to respect the privacy of loved ones.

Allen—a country dancer and long time friend. We have dated occasionally over the years of our friendship.

Amanda—a new girlfriend of my oldest son, Arthur. She is the mother of Kaytlin.

Amy—an online acquaintance and a member of our online cancer group. She lives in New York.

Ann—a fairly new friend who I have become very close to. She has recently become a country dancer too.

Art—my third ex-husband, who I was married to for ten years. We remain close friends. He lives in Northern California with his fiancee.

Arthur—my oldest son, and he was also my roommate at the time I was diagnosed. He is the father of Dani.

Arthur & Darleen—my first ex-husband and his wife. He is the natural father of my two sons, Arthur and Eric. They live in New Hampshire.

Ashley—the younger sister of Art, and daughter of Laura. She is my former sister in law.

Barbara—a dear, and long time, dance friend.

Betinia—my special chemo nurse.

Bev—a breast cancer sister at work who has a good sense of humor.

Blaine—an online acquaintance who I had the opportunity to meet in person.

Bonnie & Joyce—Bonnie is a member of our online cancer group. She lives in Southern California. Joyce is a close friend of Bonnie's.

Brian—my son Arthur's best friend.

Bridget—my very wonderful daughter-in-law who is married to my son Eric. She is the mother of Tyler.

Bruce—a co-worker and later my new supervisor.

Bud —my very much loved and appreciated big brother. He lives in Northern California with his wife Lynn. He is Erica's father.

Caitlin (Kaytlin)—the three year old daughter of Amanda.

Catherine—the Physcian's Assistant who was with me for the biopsy, mastectomy and later follow-up.

Chau—a former employee at my prior work assignment.

Cheryl—my breast cancer sister from our online cancer group. She lives in Georgia.

Chris—a co-worker and work friend for twenty-five years.

Clara—an employee of Rita's in Massachusetts.

Crystal—the wife of one of my co-workers. She is a Social Worker who facilitates a breast cancer group in my area.

Dani—my four year old granddaughter, and the daughter of my oldest son, Arthur. Dani lives in the mountains of Southern California with her mother.

Danielle—a very dear friend who was a former employee at my prior work assignment.

Deanna—an online breast cancer sister from our cancer group. She lives in Oklahoma.

Don—the man I could never seem to catch. He is also a dancer and someone I have dated sporadically, before and after my cancer diagnosis. We remain very good friends.

Dot—my sweet aunt, and the wife of my Uncle George.

Elaine—my longest friendship since childhood. She resides in Massachusetts.

Eric—my youngest son who is married to Bridget. During my chemotherapy treatment period they gave me a second grandson, Tyler.

Erica—my lovely niece who was living in Boston when I was diagnosed. She later moved back home to Northern California. Erica is the daughter of Bud and Lynn.

George—my uncle who lived in Southern California with Aunt Dot. He passed away during the time of my chemotherapy treatments.

Grace—an online friend who I have never met face to face. She offered to review this manuscript in it's early stage. Grace lives in Michigan and she also wrote one of the forewords for this book.

Dr. Gruber—my primary Surgeon. She performed the mastectomy and I see her on an on-going basis for follow-up.

Jack—Rita's fiancé who lives with her in Massachusetts. They also own a home in New Hampshire.

Jacqui—a co-worker and a breast cancer sister. She joined our online cancer group.

Jane—the founder of our online cancer group. She is also a breast cancer sister and resides in Michigan.

Janette—an online acquaintance who offered to review the manuscript in it's early stage. She resides in Oklahoma.

Jeanne—the County nurse who I saw when I was released to return to work after the mastectomy.

Jerry & Gloria—my wonderful neighbors.

Jessica—my breast cancer sister at work and a very good friend.

Jill—a breast cancer sister and member of our online cancer group. She resides in the Southern California mountains.

Joan—Art's older sister who lives in Massachusetts, but she visits her mother, Laura and sister, Ashley here in Southern California. She was my former sister-in-law and is a breast cancer sister.

Joe—a country dancer and long time acquaintance.

John—one of my former work managers and now a friend.

Jon—a friend who lives in Northern California. He is the best friend of my fourth ex-husband, Rob.

Joyce—a co-worker at my former work assignment and a dear lady.

Juanita—a co-worker and long time acquaintance.

Justin—a former boyfriend.

Karen—my supervisor for a short time on the new assignment to Systems Division.

Karen & Bob—long time dance friends.

Ken—a member of our online cancer group. He lives in Pennsylvania.

Kris—a member of our online cancer group. She lives in Massachusetts.

Laura—my former mother-in-law from my third marriage and a good friend. She is the mother of Art, Joan and Ashley.

Lillie—one of my first breast cancer sisters who I met online, a dear friend and the author of one of the forewords for this book. She resides in Maryland.

Linda—a former co-worker and friend.

Linda—Rita's other best friend who lives in Massachusetts. She lost a younger sister to breast cancer.

Lisa—Rita's daughter who lives in New England.

Lois—my neighbor here in Southern California who is also a Massachusetts native.

L.S. (Linda) & Nancy—long time, very close friends who live in North Carolina.

Lynn—the best sister-in-law that I could ever have hoped for. She lives in Northern California with my brother Bud and is Erica's mother.

Marvette—our Systems Division secretary and a friend.

Mary—a breast cancer sister and an online cancer group member. She lives in Virginia.

Mary Beth—a breast cancer sister that I met through my Plastic Surgeon, Dr. Trung.

Michelle—Assistant Minister at my church.

Mike—a member of our online cancer group. He lives in Virginia.

Newton—a co-worker who's wife is a breast cancer sister.

Nick—my three year old grandson and the son of my daughter Tamsin.

Dr. Nielsen—my oncologist who I will continue to see every six months.

Pat & Betty—twins who country dance and who have a family history of breast cancer.

Paul—a dear friend, sometimes a dance partner and a former boyfriend.

Peggy—a breast cancer sister and member of our online cancer group. She lives in Southern California.

Phu—a co-worker and a computer whiz.

Ray—my temporary dance partner.

Regina—my long time and wonderful hairdresser.

Reid (Reed)—Brian's brother and a friend, and later the roommate, of my son Arthur.

Rich—my publisher at Rhache.

Rick—co-worker and long time friend who has a very quick sense of humor.

Rick—an online friend who lives in my area. We have never met face to face, but we continue our online friendship.

Rita—my best friend who lives in Massachusetts and the one who read these letters first. She is Jack's fiancee and Lisa's mother.

Rob & Sherry—my fourth ex-husband and his current wife. We were married for only one year, but we remain friends.

Sandi—my current work manager.

Shannon—my former work manager and now a friend.

Sharon—one of my first breast cancer sisters that I met online. She is now a member of our online cancer group. Sharon first introduced me to the name "breast cancer sisters." She lives in Pennsylvania.

Stephen—the man I met online who later became my boyfriend. He lives in Northern California.

Stephen Parkhill—an online acquaintance and author.

Sue—one of my first online breast cancer sisters. She lives in San Diego.

Tamsin—my daughter, and friend. She is the mother of Nick.

Teharu—my daughter Tamsin's boyfriend.

Dr. Tioleco-Cheng—my Family Practitioner who I will always be grateful to since she sent me for my routine mammograms on time.

Dr. Trung—my Plastic Surgeon who performed the reconstruction surgery.

Tyler—my newborn grandson and the son of my youngest son, Eric and my daughter-in-law, Bridget.

Warren—a very nice man that I first met online, and later met in person. We remain in touch.

Wendy—my breast cancer sister who I met in our online cancer group. We became very close in a short period of time. Wendy lived in New York City.

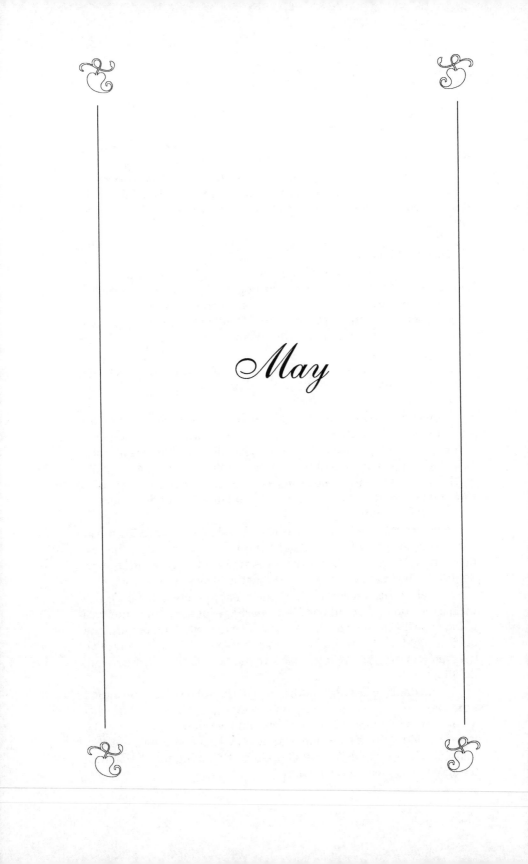

May

May 16, Monday

Hi. It's me again,

I know you're going to get sick of this, but I have Word Perfect 5.1 installed. I plan on using it to write you letters from now on. I'll be able to save them so that when we are old ladies we can publish a book, or something.

This was my second day on the new job. Everyone was cracking up when I told them about my getting the PC home, and setting it up on my own on Saturday. And then, of course, these technical people had to go and ask me questions regarding this "machine." Naturally I did not know the answers. When I was asked how many megabytes of RAM it had, I was stumped and said, "Don't ask me hard questions yet." Of course I've since looked it up, and just for the record I have *four*.

My current roommate at work, Phu (for the next two weeks any-way), explained how to install this word processing program. I am so proud, because I did it and this letter is proof.

He has been so helpful. Everyone in there has been so patient with me. I feel guilty because I have to keep asking questions. Phu was ex-plaining something to me today. I finally said to him, "Please talk baby talk to me." I feel like I'm in pre-school and they are all at a graduate level. Tomorrow I will be attending a computer school, and hopefully, learning how to do "Windows." (And you know I *don't* do windows, ovens or refrigerators!)

When I got home from work Eric and Bridget were here. They had been to the doctor, and they listened to the baby's heartbeat for the first time. The kids are so thrilled. In six weeks they will have an ultrasound done, but they don't want to know what the baby's sex is.

Danielle called me tonight. Originally she was going to take me to the hospital on Friday, but I had left a message for her that Arthur was going to do it. She filled me in on everything that was happening at my old job. I told her I was so glad I was out of there. Of course after I've been on this new job awhile I may wish I was there but, I strongly doubt it.

I went dancing last night and, as usual, I had an exceptionally good time except for a joke made by one of my dance partner's which I thought was in poor taste. When I told him about the surgery for the lump he said, "My dear, I don't know how to tell you this, but that lump is called a nipple." I didn't appreciate this humor at all, and I thought it was pretty insensitive.

Well, I have a busy week coming up. I will be glad when Friday is over and also, when next week comes and the biopsy results are in.

I think I am going to enjoy my new job immensely, once I learn it. And, now you can get all these great typed letters from me instead of phone calls. I'll save the money from the phone calls to pay off my VISA for this "machine."

All's well here. It's late and I still have a few more minor things to do to the PC before I get a shower and crawl into bed. (I refuse to become totally addicted to a computer like some of the men I've known.)

Bye. Love you,

$\mathcal{M}$ay 17, Tuesday

Hi,

This one should be quick and easy. I had to write because my "photographer" friend just called. He is really having a tough time between juggling his ex-girlfriend, his two jobs, and trying to keep his studio operating. I don't envy him one bit.

We talked a long time. I told him that between my current, questionable health concerns and my new job, which is so different for me, that I have too much going on right now to be involved with anyone. Besides, he isn't ready to be in another relationship either. We've agreed to just be friends.

I feel good that he called, and that I could express my feelings to him, and tell him where I'm at right now regarding not wanting an involvement.

Oh, he did say that he will call me Friday night to see how I'm doing after the surgery. And, naturally we talked about computers. He is in the market to buy one also. Rita, I *have* to learn this job. I feel as though there is so much that I don't know. I am so used to having answers for people, and being an "expert" in whatever position I am in. In this one I feel like I know so little. Maybe I should have paid more attention to Rob and Paul, and learned what they knew about computers.

I'll be glad when the biopsy is over and the results are in.

Love you!

$\mathcal{M}$ay 18, Wednesday

Dear Rita:

I hope you don't mind but, I'm trying to learn how to set up page numbers and I will constantly be trying something new, so you are my guinea pig. See, I can write you, instead of calling so often, and be practicing things that I need to learn. This Word Perfect 5.1 is only a small part of what I must learn, and it'll be practiced on you.

Actually, I finished my first project at work. They gave me a very easy one. It took me two and a half days, and was nothing compared to what the other Coordinators have assigned to them. The funny part is that Phu helped me do a big part of it. I would have been totally lost without him. All it was, was the smallest section in the handbook for our e-mail system. The project was to rewrite it with new conventions.

This means we are redoing the tab sets, fonts, margins, and other things like that. It's a totally different format per the new Manager's requirements. I've got other sections to do too. They aren't all that short, but they are the easy ones compared to everyone else's.

I tested all the instructions in the section on our e-mail system to make sure the keystrokes are correct. Then I passed out copies to the other Coordinators, and my boss, to review and comment on. Tomorrow I start the next one, after I've tested one that another Coordinator has completed. It's a long one and some of the instructions have errors. They are having me test all the sections since I don't know how to operate the various segments. In other words I'll be learning the office system, and finding the errors at the same time.

Boring, huh? Actually, so far I'm enjoying it, but I want to know how to do all of it right **NOW**.

I had my pre-op appointment with Catherine, the Physician's Assistant today. She's young and quite pleasant. And, then I had a chest x-ray, an EKG, an interview with the anesthesiologist, and a blood test. All of this was to pre-admit me for the biopsy on Friday.

I'm trying really hard to cut down on my spending so I can pay off this PC. I'm actually washing cotton clothes that I normally would take to the dry cleaners. I even pumped my own gas today. (This is a biggie for me.) And, I had my car washed on a week day instead of on the week-end in order to save a dollar. Of course you must have noticed that I haven't called you all week either. Instead of calls you are getting these "terrific" letters.

I will be so glad when I get the results of the biopsy and know for sure that I don't have cancer. My next desire is to learn this new job so that when people call me with questions I won't have to run to my co-workers for the answers.

Enough for tonight.

Love,

May 20, Friday

Rita:

I got your card yesterday. It's really pretty. I put it here at my work-station.

It's five o'clock in the morning and I've been awake since three. It took me forever to fall asleep last night so I've only had about four hours sleep. I guess I'll be sleeping real good at the hospital. (**I want to get this over with!**) I know the surgery isn't going to be so painful. It's just that I know I will be anxious waiting for the results. Deep inside I know that I *do not* have cancer, but there's that little doubt that maybe I'm wrong and that's what keeps bothering me. When I talk to Danielle, Ann, and Barbara about this I keep a positive attitude, **but** still I admit to you that I am worried.

Tonight, or I should say last night, I went to a free mini-type computer class. It was at the store where I bought the PC. The class was very interesting and I learned about hardware, and more about the different kinds of software. I know that I need to upgrade this machine already. This probably won't make sense to you, and I know you could care less, but I got 4MB of RAM and I can see that I need at least 8MB. Normally there is a service charge, but the store will do it free if I bring in the computer soon. The reason they'll do it free is that the salesman was aware of the possibility that I might be using it to telecommute and that I would have to have our e-mail system installed. To add our e-mail system requires at least another 4MB. Also, I know that some of the programs I'll be installing in the future will involve more RAM. The other Coordinators tell me that upgrading is a continuous process when a person gets heavily involved in computers. ($$$)

All I read anymore is computer magazines and books. I want to absorb as much of this as soon as I can. I feel bad at work when I do, and say stuff, and ask questions which are dumb. (Of course, at the time I don't know how stupid I'm being.) Then a day or two later I'll read something and realize how ignorant my co-workers must think I am. But, I'll catch up. It may take me awhile, but I know I have it in me to do this.

Today I went with one of the Coordinators to do a one on one train-ing with a new secretary in our agency. She needed to learn the very basics of our AOS (e-mail) system. The training is called "Quickstart" and it takes the place of the actual classroom training which she will be getting in a couple of months. Anyway she was really bright and it went real well. He said she was the exception. Afterwards I studied the Quickstart steps most of the day. I feel 80% ready to start doing it. Doing this training is going to be a part of my job soon. I also work the "Help" desk and answer users' questions when they call us in a panic. At the end of the training he gave the secretary our phone numbers. This secretary called me twice during the afternoon with questions. The first one was easy and I was able to help her. At five o'clock she called and I was lost. No one was available except my boss, so Karen handled it for me. As it turned out it was an easy problem too, but I still didn't know the answer.

A friend of mine, that I used to work with when I was in Quality Control, just got promoted. Rick will be coming to Systems to fill the vacant Coordinator position on the mainframe team. I am so glad. First of all, I really like him. He's got a fantastic sense of humor. We get along good. He's "wicked" intelligent and ever so "quick." But, the best part is that I won't be the only new kid on the block!

Well, I guess I'll play some Blackjack on the PC. Now I have to get some Backgammon software so I will have "someone" to play against.

I'm hungry as usual.

Bye. Love you,

May 20, Friday

Hi,

I'm home and the biopsy went really well. I'm just having some minor discomfort. It's not so bad. I know you said you'd call, but I don't have the results yet. They'll give them to me next Friday, the 27th, and then I'll call you.

I got to the hospital before eight o'clock in the morning. They checked me in and gave me two Valium. At ten o'clock I was taken to the x-ray department for a zillion uncomfortable mammograms. The radiologist gave me a local. I was so doped up. When they finally lined up some kind of a little circle template over the area where the lump was, they injected a wire thing (like a "fish hook") and some dye. It took about two hours to get everything done in the x-ray department. I guess it was because of the lump being in such an awkward place. The operating room staff called to ask where I was, and what was going on. At noon I went in to surgery.

In the operating room I was hooked up to an IV that had a drug in it to make me sleepy, and they also put another local anesthetic into my left breast. The surgery lasted one hour and twenty minutes, and I slept through most of it. Once in awhile I sort of woke up enough to hear some of what was going on, but I never felt anything, which was just fine with me. After that I went somewhere and slept until three, when they woke me up to do the hospital type things they do. I was still groggy, but I had to go to the bathroom really bad.

Around three-thirty they unhooked the IV. At that point I was wide awake and thirsty. They gave me some water, and some decaff and I watched TV. I was ready to go home about four o'clock. Arthur came for me a little after five and he was amazed that I was up and dressed, and in such good shape.

I came home and had a huge can of soup and toast. (I have to eat light for twenty-four hours and no showers for the same time period.) Arthur's at the store right now getting me some frozen yogurt. What a great son.

Don, the "photographer" just called to see how I was. I am so glad I am over my crush on him. His news is the same old story. He and his ex-girlfriend have gone back together again since he called me last. I'm glad I talked to him and let him know that I was no longer interested in a relationship with him. I don't think he knows what he wants. But, then do I?

I hope for his sake that it works out this time. He is obviously crazy about her and he wants it to work. Why else would he keep going back with her? How many times has it been, — that he's told me about?

Tomorrow I plan on just hanging out around here. The apartment is dirty, but I'm not cleaning it. I'll probably spend the day plowing through the stack of computer books I've got.

I hate for you to waste the call tomorrow. I wish I could just fax this to you now. If you get a PC with a fax/modem (which this machine has) we could fax our letters to each other's PCs.

Bye. Love,

May 21, Saturday

Rita,

Don't you just love all these letters? I should be writing "Dear Diary." But, guess what? I feel human again. I just took a shower and shampooed my hair. And, I had to remove the dressing. This was my first look, and yuck. I am really cut up, not to mention that the whole left side of my breast is purple. All in all though I feel better than I had expected. There was some pain last night, but not enough to keep me awake. I got up today and did three loads of laundry, cleaned the apartment and the patio, ironed, and even went to the beach for two hours. Tonight I cooked a huge dinner. I also backed up my computer's hard drive onto thirty-three diskettes. (I knew you'd be interested.) Of course I've been doing most everything a lot slower than my normal speed, and with some caution. I am trying to favor my left side a little.

I got two videos to watch tonight. (I'm not totally becoming a computer nerd here.) I finally got the "Joy Luck Club."

My friend Barbara called and I told her about the on-going saga of the "photographer." You know I really would rather be without a man at this point than settle for some of the single guys I keep running into lately. See, I am making progress in my personal life.

I hope I get a nice long letter from you soon as I really don't know what is going on with you. I mean is everything okay? You and Jack? Money? Do you still want me this summer? (Especially after my phone calls and these letters.) When they tell me that I don't have cancer on Friday I'm going to buy the plane tickets for August. I don't care if they are on sale or not. They will be my celebration from all this anxiety.

Okay, enough. I want to check out a few more things on this PC and then it's movie night for me.

Bye. Love you,

May 22, Sunday

HAPPY BIRTHDAY L.S.!

I hope this letter arrives in time to wish you the best. I know it's in a few days and I may be pushing my luck. This will probably be one of your better birthdays though since you are closer to your family and friends. I wish I could be there with you, too, to celebrate.

You said I haven't been writing. Maybe now that I have a PC I can remedy that. Letter writing is definitely much easier with this machine.

What's the news here? Well, lots as usual. The big one is my health. A month ago I had my every other year mammogram and they found something suspicious and called me in the next week for further x-rays. The "whatever" was in a bad place, near my left chest wall and muscle.

I was called in to my General Practitioner's office the following week so she could tell me that I was being referred to a specialist. The specialist had both my 1992, and my current mammograms. Then, she explained why it was necessary to operate. In 1992 there was something small. It had grown since then, and they felt it was best to remove it for a biopsy.

I had the biopsy last Friday. Naturally there's no dancing for me this week-end. I go back next Friday to get the results. I don't believe I have cancer, but I want to hear them say it so I can stop thinking about it.

While all this was going on I also had major changes at work. Wouldn't you know it? If it doesn't rain, but it pours, or whatever that saying is. Three weeks ago the Systems Program Manager was looking for any Program Assistant to rotate to Systems as a Coordinator. I put in a memo on the spur of the moment. I did say that I had only a very basic knowledge of our agency's computer Systems and programs. But, I stressed that I learn quickly, and that I was analytical and logical. I got the assignment through default. No one else put in a memo. My last day at the Work Program was the day I got the news of the scheduled surgery. I had to go back to my old office after hearing the news from the doctor. When I got back to work there was a party for me which my staff had planned as a farewell. They had a camera and a camcorder going. I'm sure I looked like someone in a state of shock. That's how I felt after leaving the doctor's office anyway. They had tons of food, and decorations. It was all so overwhelming, but I handled it okay. (At least I think I did.) They were a fantastic group of people to work with. I am going to miss them.

The next day I had to tell my new boss that I needed time off for a half day pre-op appointment for a surgery planned on my Friday flex, and that I would need time off the next week for a follow-up appointment. I didn't tell her what the surgery was about. (Nice way to start a new job, huh?) My new boss, Karen, is such a sweetheart though. I like her a lot.

Anyway, I have been on my new job one week. The day after I started I went to a computer store and blew up my VISA buying a home computer system. I have so much to learn. The other Coordinators have years on me in experience and knowledge. In the evenings I no longer read love stories. I am either playing on the PC or reading books and magazines about computers. I feel so incompetent compared to my co-workers. But, **I will catch up.**

My love life just isn't. I dated about half a dozen different men once, twice or three times each since the broken engagement almost six months ago. I've decided that I do not have the time or energy right now to try to find "Mr. Right," and that I prefer being alone. (I know all this must be coming as a surprise to you.) I am still dancing when I can, and I'm so busy with family and grand-kids that I don't know where I would fit a man into my life right now anyway.

I love being a grandmother, and I look forward to my third grand-child from Eric and Bridget in November.

Is this enough news for one very over due letter?

Have a wonderful birthday. I love you and Nancy lots.

Bye,

May 22, Sunday

Rita:

I know you are going to like this letter because it is going to be short.

I was taking a shower and thinking about the day, and I thought of something, and I said, "I have to remember to tell Rita." So here goes.

Arthur and I went up to the mountains today. The weather was beautiful. The drive was perfect. Even though Arthur and I live together we don't spend a lot of time in each other's company. On the way up and back (about three hours total) we had the chance to do a lot of talking. It was wonderful. He is serious about going back to school to get his degree. He may start in the fall. I, too, have thought about going back to school and finally finishing my bachelor's degree. I am not as ambitious as him though, and I may wait until I feel I've gotten a good handle on this new job.

He and I talked about a lot of things. It was a kind of deep talking at a different level for us. You know, I really am proud of him, and the way he has matured, and the way he thinks and acts. He is a wonderful son, a super dad, and an all around good person. I like him!

Dani, Arthur and I had so much fun at Lake Arrowhead. We bought bread to feed the ducks and we did a lot of walking. Dani was really wound up. I got her a pink (had to be pink) ball and some "Barney" hair ties.

I guess this letter got longer than I expected.

Danielle just called to see how I was. She said that when she had her biopsy done it was not like this. She got the results the same day while she was still at the clinic.

I'm tired. It's time to hit the computer books before I go to bed.

Bye. Love you,

May 24, Tuesday

Hi,

I was so glad to get this letter and the pictures from you. Is that your dining room with a sitting area now? What happened to the oriental screen? And where were the other pictures taken?

My General Practitioner, Dr. Cheng, called me at work yesterday to see how the surgery went. I told her it was okay. She wanted to know the results. I explained that I wouldn't know until Friday morning, and that the suspense was unnerving to say the least. She said she would try to get the results sooner than Friday and call me back. Well,

I haven't heard from her so I don't know what to think. The way I see it is, if she calls me back it's good news. If I don't hear from her, then what can I say?

I am just loving my new job even though I have so much to learn. Last night I tried to do something with this home machine There was a misunderstanding from something Phu said to me yesterday. I spent over an hour doing what I thought he said to do. Finally I realized it just could not be right, so I canceled it. When I went in to work today and told him my problem he started laughing. Phu had used the wrong terminology and apologized. Any computer literate person would have understood, but since I take things "literally," and I'm not computer literate yet, I followed his exact wording. Well, I redid it tonight and it took me about two minutes.

I feel good because I am able to converse better with the people I work with. What with all the reading I'm doing in the evenings, and all the trial and error that I am experiencing with my hands-on attempts at home, I am making some progress.

Tonight I stayed after work with my boss, Karen and my Manager, Sandi. I shared my experience from last night with them. Then they told me some of their old, PC "war stories" with their home computers

The people in Systems are so nice. They are intelligent, funny, and easygoing. This is such a change from where I just left. There are no angry clients. I don't have to be the boss. I'm not running from one end of the building to the other ten million times a day.

I have two meetings tomorrow. Also, this week on Thursday or Friday I will be going out to one of the districts to do my first Quickstart training with a new employee. I'm also working on my second project for the new format of the current e-mail system handbook. I know this has got to be boring for you, but for me it is so interesting. It's new and a real challenge.

Oh, I got the weirdest piece of mail forwarded to me today from my old office. It was one of those chain letters, a "do or die" type thing. (And, getting it this week was especially creepy.) It was addressed only to "Marilyn M" at the PO Box for the Work Program. I didn't recognize the handwriting, but it was mailed from Santa Ana, and post marked on May 14th. With all my years with the agency I've never had anything like this happen before. It had to be someone who had my old business card in order to have the PO address. I have my suspicions as to who did this, but like with the phone calls I have no proof. Is this crazy or what?

Well, I'm trying out a new font on this letter and I'm curious as to how it'll look once it's printed.

Keep practicing your Spanish. It's good that we both continue to learn new things, no matter what the subject. Hopefully it'll help us keep our minds sharper, longer. Now where did I put my glasses?

Love,

May 25, Wednesday

Hi,

I forgot to enclose the pictures last night. Now I can send the one of Jack with his grandson at the same time. He looks so much like the typical proud grandfather. I know how he feels. You just wait. I would like to be there when your first grandchild is born.

I had a miserable work day. There were two long meetings, and in between I started the new project and ran into so many problems. I had to have Phu help me try to figure one of them out. After a couple of hours of going bonkers, I went to the Coordinator who originally had the project. She apologized and said she forgot to tell me that it was originated from Word Perfect 6.0a and not 5.1. This made a big difference once it was converted into my 5.1. Then while we were talking about it the Manager comes in and decides that she wants me to finish it in 6.0a. (I'm still trying to learn the 5.1 version.) I asked her, "Where are the reference books for 6.0a?" (There aren't any.) She tells me I'll figure it out "intuitively." (Right) The 5.1 program uses keystrokes and the 6.0a uses a mouse and icons. I left there kind of depressed, came home and ate a whole, but small, pizza all by myself.

Yes, I think I am going to love my new job, once I learn it. But, it may take me months to get to that point. Obviously today was not one of my better days. I phoned the new employee at the Anaheim office to set up the one on one training. I had wanted to set it up for Thursday as:

1) I don't know what I'll be hearing at the hospital on Friday morning and,

2) I have to finish packing my office Friday afternoon for a move over the week-end to our new offices on the same floor.

As it turned out the appointment was already made by someone else for one-thirty Friday. When I talked to her I found out that it's not the usual Quickstart training. She needs all these extra and very complicated things explained. (This is an exceptional training.) The Coordinator that I had observed doing the other one said that even he didn't know how to do all the things which she needed. I had to ask Phu, who is the expert. This should be interesting. I hope I know what I'm doing when I get there!

And, of course I haven't heard from Dr. Cheng. Waiting for the biopsy results is always in the back of my mind lately. My stitches drove me nuts all day, but I think it's because they are dissolving.

No, your job never sounds boring to me. It sounds like a clothing store "Cheers," and I often wish I had a job like that. I'm afraid I am boring you about my new job. But, I have to admit that the people I am now working with have their funny sides, and we have some lighter moments. It's a good working environment for a change.

I gotta go.

Bye. Love you,

May 26, Thursday

Hello again,

Well, I swore I wouldn't write another letter and that I would just call tomorrow night, but here I be.

This machine is acting weird and I don't know why. I also told myself that I wouldn't touch it tonight, but I am. I spend hours on the one at work, and then I come home and play with this one! Last night I didn't sleep good. I stayed up late playing PC Solitaire. I've got PC Blackjack down and I decided to try the other game. I've got to see if there is software for a Backgammon game somewhere.

Dr. Cheng never called. I wonder what that means?

Karen, my boss, came into my office just before I left tonight. Since I am scheduled to give two trainings tomorrow afternoon I thought I'd better let her know that at this point I'm not sure what shape I'll be in after going to the hospital in the morning. We also have to finish packing our offices tomorrow for the move. I told her about the biopsy. She said that she had the same type of biopsy done years ago, and that the hospital kept her overnight. She didn't find out the results right away either. She said her report came back negative, but she had prepared herself for the worst. I told her I was just telling her about it in case I got bad news and I couldn't handle it. I wanted her to know that I had the hand-outs organized for the training. I also have everything in my office just about all packed, except for the bare essentials and unhooking my computer equipment. She was very understanding and sympathetic. I'm glad now that I told her what was going on. She told me that if it is cancer, the surgeries these days are much improved. I stressed to her that I never win the lottery so there's no chance that I'm going to be told that I have cancer!

This afternoon I went to the Unisys Co. with our Systems Managers and Analysts for a demonstration of some new software that the company would like to sell us, and which we are in need of. It's a text retrieval program and it would be used for all the zillions of documents and manuals that our agency relies on in order to operate. If we get it, all the bookcases of manuals which everyone currently uses for research will be on their computers. The presentation was well done. Of course I was there for the experience only, but Sandi told me to not be intimidated, and to just jump right in with any input since I'm newly arrived from the districts. I didn't say a word, but I learned a lot.

The County is looking at different companies before deciding how to fill this need. I am really glad that I am in Systems right now as this is the direction we have been going for years. No matter where I go next in our agency I will have acquired invaluable knowledge. Of course I'm still a "baby" compared to the others, but I'll learn.

Enough. I didn't get much sleep last night and I have a big day tomorrow. Thank you for the notes and the cards. I will call you tomorrow night, or Saturday, with my **good** news.

Love,

May 27, Friday

Hi,

Well this should be a long one. I know you are going to return my call, but in the meantime I have to get it all out on paper. I talked to Jack and he was so sweet and kind. He told me that you, also, have to go in for a second mammogram, and that made me cry even harder. You never said a word. God I hope that you are okay. The both of us going through this together would be way too much. I can't wait to talk to you, but I didn't want Jack calling you at work to upset you there.

I couldn't sleep again last night. I forced myself to go to the appointment this morning. It was something I just did not want to do. Catherine walked into the examining room, and just came right out with it. She said that I do have breast cancer and another surgery is necessary as soon as possible. They want to operate the first week in June. I have the week-end to think over my options and decide what type of surgery I want. I am supposed to call her Tuesday, and then she will set up another half day of pre-op appointments.

The tumor was small at 1.3 centimeters. (They hope to find them under two centimeters.) I am so glad it was found now instead of later.

My options are to have either:

A LUMPECTOMY — where they will remove tissue from only the area where the lump was, and some lymph nodes from under my arm. But, this involves daily radiation for six weeks in the Los Angeles or

Hollywood area and I will be pretty tired after them. Also, she says I have to be approved by the radiologist as the radiation would be right over my heart.

Or to choose a MASTECTOMY — where they would remove my whole left breast and some lymph nodes from under my arm. I would eventually have to wear a prosthesis and in several months I can have my breast reconstructed.

They won't know about chemotherapy until after the surgery. Oh, she said that either surgery has the same chances for survival. One is not better than the other for determining future problems.

At this moment I don't know what to do. I go first in one direction, and then in the other, trying to make a decision.

Of course I started crying when she told me, and I have been crying on and off all day. I drove home, which involved three freeway changes. I swear I don't know how I did it without getting into an accident. I think Catherine should have told me to bring someone with me to the appointment.

When I got home I called my boss and told her that I wouldn't be in today, and that I would be needing time off in the future. I feel so bad. Here I am starting this new job, and already I'm going to be out a lot. Karen said not to worry about it though. I also warned her that I can't promise her what my emotional state is going to be like. She said that's okay, and that I can just sit at my desk and cry if I need to.

Then I called you and got Jack. (Poor Jack) Next I called my brother, Bud. He is so good to me. I kept crying. I told him that he is always offering to help me, and right now I need all the emotional support I can get. In the future I may need some financial help, too. I've always known he meant it when he said to just ask, but I didn't think I would ever need to do that. He offered to fly me to San Francisco and Sonoma this week-end, but I told him that I need to be home with myself, and my thoughts.

I also called the Program Assistant who took over my old job so that she could tell my former staff. They have been waiting for the results too.

And, I called Arthur at work. He is so cool about everything, but I could tell that he was shocked. We'll talk more tonight when he gets home. He did say that if I needed to talk, to call him at work anytime during the day.

I will have to tell the other kids soon. It's just too much right now. And I don't want to get Bridget upset, what with her being pregnant and all.

Then I start thinking stupid things like: this is the first year of my life that I treated myself to a whole bunch of new bathing suits all at once. Then it pops into my head "there goes my dancing." (It's a good thing I'm taking up computers). There is no way that I could go out there, and get thrown around the dance floor, wearing a make believe "boob." And, I think how glad I am that I didn't find a male dance partner/boyfriend with my newspaper ad! My brain is like on some kind of auto-pilot trip of it's own.

But, I feel better already just writing everything down.

I hope you don't mind, but I am going to keep doing it as therapy. I'll get this letter out now so that it'll go in today's mail.

Bye. Love you,

May 27, Friday, Journal Writing

Today I found out that I have breast cancer. There is no explanation why, and I have no guilt that I have done something wrong to cause it. One person said she believes that cancer, in general, is on the increase and that it is caused by pollution in the environment. Catherine at the HMO told me that there is an overall increase in breast cancer in women.

I tell everyone it's not from my smoking. I know smoking doesn't cause breast cancer. I eat a low fat diet. I am under weight and I'm not on estrogen. There is no known breast cancer in my family. And, I had my babies young. So, why do I have this?

I talked to Rita tonight and we cried together. On Wednesday morning she is calling her health clinic to get the results of a second mammogram recently ordered for her. The suspicious lump is in her left breast too.

When we were talking she joked and asked, "Who will I write to if you die?" We laughed and cried over that one. I said that at this point I am not even considering dying. I said my concern at the moment is to make a decision as to what type of surgery to have, and then I'll go from there. But, then when I got off the phone I walked around the apartment with a pad of paper deciding to make a will, and a list of who gets what. I have so little to leave anyone anyway. I want to make the decision as to where our little family heirlooms go. I want to know that my debts get paid, and that I decide who gets what, if anything is left.

Danielle called and she, as has been everyone who knows, was magnificent. She told me that she has plenty of vacation time, and if I need her help to call her. Bud has offered his help. And Rita, with her own breast cancer threat hanging over her head, said she can fly out here for one week to be with me if I need her. Even Dr. Cheng left a comforting message on my answering machine while I was with Catherine this morning.

I was in shock, and maybe I still am in shock. I've cried on and off all day. I know it's not the end of the world. I am a strong person. I will get through this. I may be in denial, but I don't believe this cancer will take over my body and my life. It may inconvenience me for awhile, but this too shall pass.

Later:

I think I'm okay, and under control, and then I start crying again. I was doing dishes and I just started bawling. I'm so thankful that I have a long three day week-end to work my way through this.

It's not like it's the end of the world, or that I am going to die or, anything drastic like that. It's just that things like this **"DON'T HAP-PEN TO ME."** It's an annoyance, and an inconvenience, and I can't even think beyond that. I am only feeling sorry for myself. I am telling myself over and over that this just is the way it is, and that I can handle it.

I want to talk to the radiologist oncologist to see if I am a good candidate for the radiation treatment. If I'm not, then I have no other option but to go with the mastectomy. If I am a good candidate for radiation then I will have to figure out some way to go to Los Angeles every day for the six weeks after the surgery. Danielle has offered to use her vacation time to drive me places if I need her. She is so incredibly generous.

It'll work out, and I will just keep telling myself this. By Tuesday I am going to be ready to go back to work and I will have my emotions under control.

May 28, Saturday

Hi L.S.,

I am so glad that I got to talk to you this morning. Just talking about all this is a big help. I feel so lucky to have such special, loving friends. I appreciate so much the support that I am getting. I feel better already!

When I got off the phone with you, my phone rang almost immediately. It was Rita calling from Massachusetts. She said, "Hi. I'm going to the store, — do you need anything?" Without missing a beat I said, "Could you pick me up some milk?"

I know how I pick my friends. Just hearing your story about little Kevin and his family, and how caring you are makes me love you more. Yes, I know you give off that tough "redneck" attitude at times, but let me enlighten you, none of us are fooled one bit.

Then Rita is attempting to help a sixty year old, illegal alien Mexican lady, who is being held in a form of slavery by some awful person in Massachusetts. It's a long story, but a very touching one, and one that makes me see the compassion in her once again. You are both this way. You are strong ladies, but your hearts are so big, and ever so soft.

Enough.

I got my long curly hair chopped off today. What the heck. It'll be easier to manage for awhile, and it was long and curly to fit the country western dance image. I can live with this for now. It will grow again.

I am in a much better state of mind than I was yesterday, and I expect tomorrow will be even better. Today I only got teary eyed maybe six times. Yesterday I went through an entire box of Kleenex.

Thank you again and again for being my friend, and always being there for me. I haven't called Art Z. He and I continue to be good friends. I really don't feel up to telling him about this though. His mother, Laura, and I remain pretty close. We meet every once in awhile for dinner. On Easter I met her for church and we went out for brunch after. I think I will tell her, and if she wants to relay the information to him, then that's fine. Also, his older sister, Joan, had breast cancer years ago. She spent a lot of time in treatment and today she is cured. I think talking with her will shed some more insight my way.

I got a funny video to watch tonight. It'll be a nice break from my thoughts and computers.

Love you both,

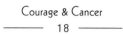

May 28, Saturday

To my "bosom" buddy:

If you could see me now. I got my hair cut real short. I thought it might be easier to take care of in the near future. It looks "old," but that's okay. It's different than anything I've ever had before because it still has some perm on top. And, of course, it's a tri-tone color with brown, gray and golden brown.

I went to the beach for about an hour. It was hot, but not unbearable. There were a lot of families at my little beach. Do you remember the one I showed you where I married Rob? It's close by my apartment. There is always parking available. It is almost a private beach and so perfect for my short, sunbathing stints. *And* I wore one of my new bathing suits. It was my skimpiest two piece. I might as well get some use out of it now.

What else did I do? Oh, I got the form to add Arthur as a joint owner to my bank accounts. This is something I should have done a long time ago. Not that there's much in them, but my paychecks do go automatically into my checking account.

You know I feel so lucky that you have been my friend all these years. Thirty years is a long time. We really have more history than a lot of blood relatives do. I can't imagine my life without you in it. I tell Arthur all the time that I don't know what I would have done all these years without you. Who else can make me laugh while I'm crying? Enough mush. I know you aren't into that.

Well, I'm doing laundry, fixing a frozen pot pie for dinner and then I'm going to watch another funny video tonight. Last night's "Mrs. Doubtfire" was hilarious.

Bye for now. Tell Jack I love him too.

May 28, Saturday

It's me again. . .

I already wrote you one today. I was tempted to call, and then I remembered that you were going to New Hampshire. Plus, my phone bill is going to be screaming at me soon. I'd better cool it.

I have to write all this while I'm thinking about it. I called Laura to tell her what was going on. I also wanted to get Joan's phone number.

I called Joan, but she was on the other line with her mom. She said she would call me back. It was a very nice gesture on her part as we wound up talking for over an hour. She was wonderful about explaining to me what she went through with her treatments, and the choices she made. But, now I am even more unsure as to what choice I want to make. As she said to me, it is my decision to make and one I will have to live with for the rest of my life. She said that after she chose, and had the lumpectomy, there was a period when she questioned whether she had made the right decision. At the time most women were choosing the mastectomy. Also, she said her breast is permanently burnt and hardened from the radiation treatment. She also has lung tissue damage from the radiation.

Joan did not have the lymph nodes removed and they gave her chemotherapy based on the lumpectomy. (Oh, her biopsy was her lumpectomy.) She was getting radiation and chemotherapy at the same time. She had the radiation for six weeks and the chemotherapy for months. She continued to work, but she says she was beyond exhausted. She realizes now that she should not have worked in and around the treatments. The treatments not only wear you out, but they break down your immune system. She took mega doses of vitamins, and when she could she would come out to California to go to a clinic in Mexico for one of the controversial cancer treatments. She also ate extremely healthy foods.

So I'm back to the question of whether (if the radiologist says I'm a good candidate or not) to go ahead and have my breast removed and get a prosthesis. Or, do I choose to keep my breast and endure six weeks of radiation that will leave me exhausted, out of work and probably without a pay check? And, I could possibly wind up with a deformed left breast anyway. This is too much. I never realized how much this breast meant to me before. Do I want to continue to dance? Yes. Do I want to have to deal with an expensive prosthesis? No. Do I want to drive to Los Angeles every day for six weeks, and go through all Joan went through to keep a breast that I may wind up disliking anyway? No.

God I hope you are going to be okay. Why should the two of us have to go through this? Please let you be alright.

I know it doesn't sound like it, but my emotional state is much better today. I'm no longer crying. I just get weepy every once in awhile when I'm not expecting it. And, occasionally I feel angry, but then that passes too.

What I hear is that emotionally I will be going through ups and downs and, that this is normal.

Joan has the same Science of Mind beliefs as me. We discussed how much the church's philosophy can help me to deal with this. She said I sound positive and that is the key in the recovery to all this. I know she is right.

All in all I am really glad I talked to her. I am also trying to get a lady from work's home phone number. It is unlisted, but I would like to talk to her this week-end if it's possible. She went through this a few years ago. All I remember hearing about what was that she had a rough experience, and she was off work for quite some time. For awhile there her staff didn't know if she was going to live. She is back at work now and doing fine. I would definitely like to talk to her about what she went through.

The more I hear, the more I have to weigh before I make a decision that I can be satisfied with.

And, that's all "she" wrote.

Bye. Love you,

P.S. I lied. I just remembered one other thing. I called and left a message for a Social Worker from our church who holds a cancer support group one Saturday each month.

May 29, Sunday

My therapy . . . Here it is the "witching hour" again and I can't sleep. I was going to write you a long one tomorrow, but since I'm wide awake, for about the fifth night in a row, I might as well "talk." I sure hope you don't mind all this. I think I will just ramble from one subject to the next. (Poor you being on the receiving end of all this.) But, I thank you with all my heart. How you have put up with my kookiness all these years I'll never know.

I have had my ups and downs. I mean I am so sensitive to everything and everybody, and lord knows, or at least you know, that I am normally very sensitive anyway.

I almost didn't go to church this morning, but then I decided that right now I really need to hear the messages there. I looked like **poop**. I mean my hair cut is not all that great, and then I threw on very casual clothes. I'm walking through the patio area and who do I see but that guy, Larry, that I met through his personal ad just before all this happened. He was so hot to meet me remember? Then after one phone call, following our date, I never heard another word from him. So, he's all dressed up and looking really sharp. I felt like hiding, but instead I went over and talked to him. He asked me how I was. I told him not so good and explained why.

I said "Whatever happened to you?" (It just came out. You know me.) It wasn't that I felt rejected, but I was curious. Larry said he was going to call me the other day. (Right) Come to find out he was meeting another blind date for the service. They were going to meet in front of the book store where we were standing. So I said "Oops" and made my good-byes. A few minutes later he and this younger, gorgeous lady (all dressed up) came into the sanctuary. They made a nice looking couple, but of course I compared myself to her, and felt **UGLY** and **OLD** and thought "no wonder he didn't ask me out again." (This is just me being down on myself once more.) I really didn't think I cared, but obviously I must have cared a tiny bit to think these bad thoughts about myself for a little while.

Arthur helped me to re-arrange my bedroom. Actually he did all the work. I didn't like the computer workstation where it was, plus I needed the computer near my phone jack to hook up the modem. I got the modem set up, but I haven't tried it out yet. He also attached the drawer to the computer table. I refused to do it the day I put the table together.

I decided to finally type up all the questions I have for the doctor, the radiologist and the prosthesis store. Every time I thought of something these past few days I'd write them down on various scraps of paper. I have quite a list going at this point.

I want to postpone the surgery for one week so that I can get more information from multiple sources before I make a decision. I have a call in to the American Cancer Society. They have a program where a volunteer who has had breast cancer will come out to the house to talk to me. I also left a message at a local hospital that has twice a month support group meetings. I found out that the next cancer group meeting at my church is this coming Saturday, and I'd like to go to that before the surgery.

It's late. I'm tired. Thanks for listening to all this jabber once again. Bye. Love you,

May 30, Monday, Journal Writing

I am ready to go back to work tomorrow. I have not cried much all day. I am ready to deal with the next step in this new experience. I have my questions for everyone written down. I'm more accepting of the way things are. **I can handle this!**

My questions for the doctors are:

To first, ask them to make an appointment with the radiologist oncologist, and then:

1. Was an estrogen receptor test done when the lump was biopsied? If so, what was the result? Will I be able to have estrogen replacement if needed in the future?

2. What is the HMO's referral process in order for me to get a second opinion prior to making a decision regarding the surgery?

3. Can I have copies of all the reports since the 1992 mammogram?

4. Is it necessary to remove the lymph nodes? Is there any other way to determine if the cancer has spread?

5. How severe is my cancer? What is the name of it?

6. Will I need the drainage apparatus for both types of surgery? If so, how long will I have to use it?

7. What other options are available to me other than radiation therapy if I choose a lumpectomy?

8. How limited will I be with my left arm once the lymph nodes are removed? (Example: Will I be able to drive myself to and from Los Angeles or Hollywood every day?)

9. If I have a mastectomy how soon after the surgery will I be able to get fitted for, and then start wearing, a prosthesis?

10. How soon after a mastectomy will I be able to start driving?

11. How soon after a mastectomy can I return to work, and without

going in looking like one breast is missing?

12. After a mastectomy, and wearing a prosthesis, will I be able to West Coast Swing dance again?

My questions for the Prosthesis store are:

1. What is the price range of, and what are the, different styles?

2 How comfortable are they to wear?

4. How soon after the surgery can I be fitted for one?

5. How soon after the fitting will I receive it, and be able to wear it for full days?

Questions for the Radiologist:

1. How much damage to my lungs can I expect? (And please take into consideration the fact that I currently smoke half a pack of cigarettes a day.)

2. How much damage will occur to my heart muscles?

3. How will the radiation affect my immune system?

4. How much damage can I expect to occur to the breast itself? (Example: burn marks, hardening of my breast and nipple)

5. Where exactly will I go in the Los Angeles — Hollywood area? And what time of the day will the appointments be? How long will I be in therapy?

6. Will I be able to drive myself to and from the treatments?

7. Will I be able to go to work each day either before or after the therapy?

8. The brochure I received from the State Of California mentioned that this therapy incurs additional expenses. What are they?

9. The brochure also mentioned that there are other side effects. What are they?

May 30, Monday

Dear Bud and Lynn,

Thank you so much for putting up with me on Friday. Thank you for just being there every time I need you. I am so grateful that I can pick up the phone and call you when it seems like I don't know what I'm doing. You must be turning into surrogate parents or something. Arthur says "Well, he's your big brother." (Simple enough.)

My emotional state is greatly improved. I am glad I've had the long three day week-end to get used to all this. Now I can even laugh about it at times. I find I only get weepy eyed a few times a day, versus the all day cry out on Friday. I actually look forward to going back to work tomorrow to get my mind busy on other things, and get a sense of normalcy back with a daily routine.

I feel very fortunate actually. I realize how lucky I am with the support system which is out there for me. Friends from everywhere have said, "Just call and let me know and I'll be there." We are not talking down the street either. My friends on the East Coast have said they'll hop a plane if I say the word. This type of love and nurturing feels so good.

I had a long talk Saturday night with Art Z's sister. She had breast cancer years ago and she is my age. She gave me a lot of insight into this disease. Also, hearing from a female who has been there, or I should say " here," was very real. She of course could tell me the things which are not found in medical books.

Yes, Lynn I continue to read and re-read what information I can. I finally, after many hours of absorbing and thinking, have come up with a plan, and my questions, but still no decision as yet. I want to tap on all the resources which I can prior to that. I want to postpone the surgery for one week while I get more information. I do not think one week's wait will make that much difference, and I do not want to be pressured into making a decision too hastily. I would like to know that the decision I make was made with as much information as I could obtain.

When I call the HMO tomorrow I will ask for a referral to the radiologist oncologist. And I have my list of questions ready for him.

My week-end hasn't been all that bad. I've been to the beach. Also, I had Nick over and took him for a much needed haircut. He loves getting his haircut. They are always amazed that he is so good while they are cutting. Of course they don't understand that this is a treat from his perspective. Then we went to the shoe store. This has become part of the ritual. He gets a haircut and new shoes at the same time.

Do not worry about me. I am going to be fine. This is just another one of life's challenges and I like a good challenge.

Love you both,

May 31, Tuesday

Hi,

This letter is not going to have fancy fonts or anything. It's going to be your basic, plain, old typing. I know. I'm calling you in the morning, but I had to at least attempt a letter. There has been so much information coming in. And believe me *you* are in my thoughts with all this input. I hope you won't need all this information that I am gathering.

First I have to say that people's kindnesses and sharing is so wonderful that, this in itself is overwhelming at moments. This "event" has restored my feelings about the goodness in the world. See there is a positive side to all this.

I went to work today and did the whole nine hours without crying once. When I got home there was a card and a check for $1,000 from my brother, and I started crying again. I will put the money in the bank and hope I won't need it.

At work it was chaotic because we moved offices over the week-end. But, through it all people were so kind to me. My new work room-mate, Bruce, hooked up my computer and gave me his personal beeper number in case I cannot do the trainings tomorrow. I can beep him tonight so he'll "dress up" tomorrow, instead of wearing casual clothes to finish the move. Another Coordinator's wife is a Social Worker who works with oncology patients. He gave me her name and their home number. I talked with her tonight for a long time. She gave me more information and insight into all this.

I called Catherine and she asked if I had made a decision. I told her that I hadn't and I had a lot of questions for her. Then I also asked her for a referral to the radiologist. She said, "Oh, you must be leaning towards the lumpectomy." I said that at this point I had not decided one way or the other, but that I had questions for him also. I have an appointment with Catherine and the surgeon tomorrow.

I also tried to contact the prosthesis store when I got home from work, but they were already closed. I hate to call them from work. Maybe I can do it when Bruce is out of our office.

I also talked with a lady from the American Cancer Society. She had a mastectomy years ago. She said that she had large breasts, and she chose to have the remaining healthy breast made smaller when she had her reconstructive surgery. She has never regretted her decision to have the mastectomy. She is going to have a lady who had a lumpectomy call me so that I can talk to her too.

Oh, my co-worker's wife, Crystal, the Social Worker, told me that radiation isn't fun and has a lot of side effects. She said that in some cases the breast becomes "wedge" shaped from the lumpectomy and on top of that, a hardening of the breast can occur. She said that the women she has counseled, who have had a mastectomy and recon-structive surgery, have not been displeased.

Everyone has been so supportive and helpful. Hopefully by next week-end I will have made a decision regarding the surgery. Beyond that I can't even think at this point.

I have my modem hooked up and I "talked" with people from all over the United States yesterday through the "America Online" pro-gram. I get one month's free service. Today my boss asked if I had a modem. I said yes, it was set up and working. She said that she is going to see if I can telecommute while I am convalescing. This is a long shot, but if it's approved it'll be great. That'll be less time that I'm off payroll.

Well, I am thinking about you constantly. I hope your news is good news in the morning. Let's just let one of us do this, okay?

Love you,

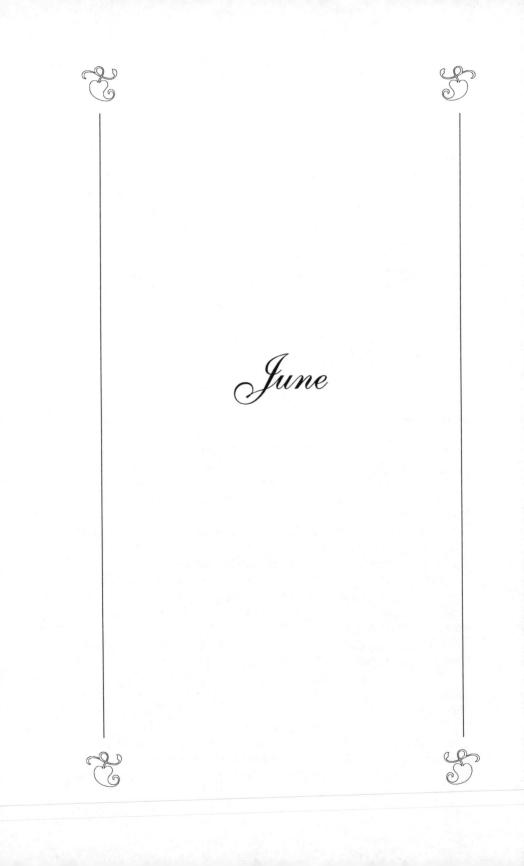

June

June 2, Thursday

Rita,

I have thought about you off and on all day. As people talked to me about what's going on with me, I shared with them what is happening with you. I hope that's okay. This is just so weird. I love you and I can't believe that we are both going through such an ordeal.

I went to work on very little sleep. But, I have to emphasize again how wonderful everyone has been. A co-worker told me that he had a relationship with a lady about five years ago. She had a mastectomy before he met her. Today she is totally healthy and cancer free. They are still friends and he asked if I wanted to speak with her. I said "yes." Then he told me her name. I know her and I've always admired her, but I never knew about the cancer. I hope she calls me.

Then one of my prior Manager's, John, was in Administration this morning for a meeting. He dropped by my office to say hello. We hugged, and I told him about the breast cancer. I immediately started babbling that I can't get over how good everyone has been to me about all this. Then, John made me feel so special. He kissed my cheek and said, "Marilyn you are not just well liked by a lot of people, but you are very much *loved*." I almost started crying again.

I wore a new dress to boost my self-confidence for the two training sessions. I think I did a good job on them. Since I had extra time between the trainings I went to a bookstore and got two more computer books and two about cancer.

I arrived an hour early at the hospital after the trainings. I was glad as it gave me time to devour the section on breast cancer in one of the books. Then, I added even more questions to my list.

I met the doctor who did the biopsy. (I was slightly out of it that day.) He and Catherine answered my questions, and she gave me a copy of the pathologist's report. Knowing more about my condition makes me feel somewhat in control.

I have an appointment with the radiologist oncologist tomorrow afternoon, and I have my list of questions for him too.

Today I talked with the owner of a prosthesis store. She gave me some information over the phone, and she will mail me some of her brochures.

I am not sharing this with anyone else as yet but, I believe I have made a decision as to what treatment I am going to choose. Catherine wants me to call her Friday morning to let her know what the radiologist oncologist says. I told her that, after my meeting with him, I would like the week-end to think things over, and that I will give her my decision by Monday morning. It looks like the surgery will be one week later. My mind is almost made up, but I want to allow a little more time.

In the meantime tell me about Linda's sister and her experiences. **PLEASE**. I want to have as many facts, from as many different sources as I can. I feel like I am cramming for an exam which was sprung on me, and it's a critical one that I need to get a perfect score on.

The good news from work is that I finished my second project and routed it today for comments. I am learning this job in spite of everything else going on around me.

Tomorrow I hope to get out to my old office and do a training for the new clerk. She is the one I interviewed, and hired. She started working there after I left. My only concern is that I will see my old staff and start crying.

I'm thinking of you constantly.

Bye. Love you,

June 2, Thursday, Journal Writing

After much reading, talking, questioning, listening and thinking I have made my decision. I will call the doctor tomorrow and tell her to schedule me for a mastectomy.

My decision is based on numerous issues. There were no "pros" to weigh. It's been a matter of which "cons" I could live with the most. Now I have the week-end to work on my acceptance of this decision.

I have surprised myself (sort of) with how well I am handling this. My boss said that she felt I was being very centered and balanced. Mostly I am. But, I feel in control, or I should say more in control, now that I have done my research.

When I called Rita tonight I worked on reassuring her that I do feel positive about my future prognosis. I have learned that my cancer type is a "stage one," and that is good. The doctors aren't able to feel my lymph nodes which, is another good sign. In my heart I do not believe that they will find that the cancer has spread. I believe that by removing my breast I will end this disease in my body.

I understand that I will have some discomfort, and some temporary incapacity, and also some "black" times in the near future. I will need time to grieve for a breast that I have lost, and did not appreciate, until all this occurred. And, I know that I will get past this.

There have been positives to all this. People have been so loving, caring, and understanding. I have a whole new perspective on us as human beings.

I am just so in awe of the love I am receiving from so many. It is the kindnesses shown to me which now make me weep. What with all that has happened, and what will be happening, I feel very fortunate to know that I am not going through this alone.

June 4, Saturday, 1:30AM

Rita,

This is not one of my up periods. I cannot sleep. I needed to talk to you. Finally I got out of bed and decided to write another letter. I've already written one tonight, which I tore up and deleted from my disk. I say to myself, "Don't write her all this." Then I say, "If I don't, I won't be honest." I've told you everything as it has happened, or that I have thought, up to this point so I might as well continue with it. I wish you were here with me. I don't like this one bit, and please understand that this gloomy period will pass. By tomorrow I will be okay again. Tonight I just feel so dammed depressed.

I'm in one of my crying moods, and this time it is all just for "me." (I hate feeling this way!) Hopefully when I go to the cancer group today, if I ever get any sleep, I will be supported and lifted up, and will feel more positive about things again.

Please do not become alarmed when you receive this. (If I mail it.) By the time you get it I anticipate that I will be okay again. I don't expect this will last long. (I sure hope not.)

One of the books I bought is, "Breast Cancer The Complete Guide" by Yashar Hirshaut, MD and Peter Pressman, MD. Finally I have a reference book that is answering all my questions. It is well written, easy to read and tells about breast cancer the way it really is. I don't think they left anything out.

This morning I left a message for Catherine to schedule me for a mastectomy.

Of course I later thought that maybe I am giving up my breast for nothing, and that I'm not trying hard enough to keep it. After reading this book I realize that I have made the best decision for me and my type of cancer. Even though I do not like either of my options the mastectomy is the one I must choose.

I also do not feel as optimistic regarding the lymph nodes, or about chemotherapy either. I was missing pieces regarding explanations of my biopsy report. This book, in layman's terms, helped me to translate the pathologist's comments. Joan was right when she told me to get copies of reports and read them, because there's stuff in them that the doctor's don't explain. We have to do our own research. Previously when I saw the description "in situ" I thought I had it made. Well, there is another term in the biopsy report called "infiltrating ductal carcinoma." This book explains what that means. Now I feel that I am being more realistic when I say that there is a good chance the cancer has spread to my lymph nodes. The tumor which was removed was 50% in situ and 50% infiltrating, and it extended to the margins. At this point I will be surprised if it hasn't gotten to the nodes, especially because of the location where it was found. Now I understand why the radiologist oncologist said that he felt I would be having chemotherapy. I now believe that this is a strong possibility. My bubble has been burst some.

This book also explains the size of the tumor, versus the size of the breast, versus the location, versus whether to have a lumpectomy or a mastectomy. I realize now why Catherine told me that my breast would be disfigured if I had a lumpectomy. Since my tumor was so deep inside me, even though it was small, and because of the size of my breast there would be an obvious part of me missing. Also, now that I suspect I will have to have chemotherapy, no matter whether I go with a lumpectomy or a mastectomy, I know that I personally could not handle surgery, radiation, driving to Hollywood every day and having chemotherapy administered all at the same time. My better option is to forget the lumpectomy, with the radiation, and have the mastectomy.

So now I'm lying in bed thinking how I'm going to have a disabled left arm, a missing breast and no hair. See why I'm crying and feeling sorry for myself? I mean you'd think I could see past this and be happy because my prognosis, I truly believe for curing this disease, is good. It's just all the stuff I have to go through to get to that point that is depressing me. I believe that the mastectomy and the chemotherapy will rid me of all the cancer. I am *not* going to die and that is the goal. But, the thoughts of all this, and then wondering where my rent money is going to come from, leaves me feeling a little bit down to put it mildly.

This is just one of those dark times I've been warned about. I know it'll pass and I hope they don't come too often. I have also bought some positive affirmation type books for people with cancer. I guess it's time for me to get those out and start reading them.

And, I need sleep desperately!

Please continue to put up with me. I don't know what I'd do at this point without you being there.

Love you lots,

June 4, Saturday

Dear Joan,

I just got off the phone with your mom. I wanted to write you a short note to thank you for last week's long phone conversation. It was a big help. You gave me good advice, and insight, at a time when I was not thinking too clearly.

Since Saturday I've been doing my homework. I've gotten about a half dozen books.

I've met with the surgeon, and the radiologist oncologist. I've talked with a lot of women who have had breast cancer, and one oncology Social Worker who does support group sessions for women. Everyone has been so helpful. I've also contacted the prosthesis store and asked my questions there. And, as you advised, I got a copy of the biopsy report.

Weighing everything that I could, in this short period of time, as of this moment, I have chosen to have the mastectomy. It will be the modified radical with axillary lymph node dissection. As I was telling your mom, I think I am dreading the lymph nodes removal more than the mastectomy. **And,** the Physician's Assistant has assured me that I have the right to change my mind about which surgery I want right up until I am taken into the operating room.

The one good thing which has come from this is my renewed appreciation for how wonderful people are. I feel quite loved and that, you know, is a really nice feeling.

Rita is going in for an ultrasound on Wednesday. She will see her doctor for a possible needle biopsy. As yet she is still in the period of not knowing what is going on with her left breast. I do not envy her the anxious waiting period.

I hope all is okay with your job and Joan, thank you again.

Bye. Love you,

a much brighter day

June 4, Saturday

Dear Rita,

I hope last night's letter didn't upset you too much. I'm sorry. I debated whether to even mail it or not. I guess I should just go more with the flow of all this. I finally got about six hours of much needed sleep. I woke myself up scratching at the last of the scab on my biopsy scar. I wondered if it was itchy, or if sub-consciously I was just trying to remove all of it!

Laura called. I told her my decision and I got Joan's address. I wrote to Joan to thank her for all of her advice and help last week. Oh, Laura said that Joan did not lose her hair while having chemotherapy. That is really nice to hear at this point.

I'm now showered and dressed in a bright shorts and t-shirt outfit to go to the church support group. I am looking forward to it. I think it will raise my spirits. This letter probably won't be finished until I get back from the group.

I keep thinking that I have to write to Elaine, but I'm dreading it. I have been a horrible friend to her this past year. I never write or keep in touch, and then to write her a letter telling her all this.

This will be continued.

and the beat goes on. . . .

Later:

What an incredible day after all. It has been a good one considering what I put myself, and you, through last night.

I was at the church for three hours this afternoon. It was a humbling, yet beautiful experience. The group members told their stories. Compared to them I am in great shape, and I have very little to complain about. One older lady is on her fourth cancer. She's had skin, lung, colon and now liver cancer. She is a feisty little thing and she refuses to let the cancer win. Like me, she had not slept much last night. She said that she was going home after the group, putting on her pj's and curling up with a sexy book. I loved that idea! It's time for me to stop reading about cancer and PC's and go back to "escape" books.

Three women in the group have had breast cancer surgeries. I cried when it was my time to share. I couldn't talk much. On break the three women came to me with hugs, words of encouragement and love. One of them unbuttoned her blouse, pushed aside her bra, and gave me a good look at her "reconstructed" breast. There was a scar around it, but I can live with a breast like hers!

The facilitator was dynamic, but I had a problem with some of what she said to me and the group. At break she told me how she had a malignant lump removed during a biopsy. She was told that she would need to have her lymph nodes removed and have radiation treatment. She went up to Hollywood, as she has the same HMO as me, and got a second opinion from a female radiologist there. She was told that she did not have to have the additional surgery and radiation treatment, and she would survive just fine without them. She gave me the radiologists name. I thought I might call her for a second opinion until later, during the meeting, when the facilitator told us she has had "four" biopsies, and her mother died from breast cancer.

Okay, I believe in the power of positive thinking. I believe that I have some control over my body through my thoughts but, I shudder at the thought of playing Russian roulette with breast cancer. This lady most likely has a much more tuned mind than me since this is what she does for a living. She teaches workshops in metaphysical thinking. I too believe in metaphysics, but in my case I do not have enough self-confidence to believe that I can rid my body completely of all it's cancer cells. I do not want to take any chances in having cancer cells recurring, and then later thinking that I did not do everything I could to rid myself of this disease. I prefer to have medical assistance to go along with my positive thinking. (Enough said here.)

Ann came by after her second job. She only had two hours of sleep last night, and here I am complaining. I have only known her a short time, but I consider her a really good friend. You know how it is that with some people you just "click." She had a glass of wine and we talked about everything. She is leaving Wednesday for a business trip in the mid-west, but she said she would call me when she got back in town. She also asked if I had called Barbara with the news. I said, "No." (Barbara was in Texas when I found out.)

Just as Ann was leaving, Sandra, my landlady came by. She wanted to know if I would like to move into the two bedroom/two bath apartment next to me when my neighbors, Jerry and Gloria, move to the downstairs one. I told her I probably would have before all this. I told her my news. She was very encouraging. I really like Sandra and her husband. They are the best landlords I've ever had. She said that they would help me move, and for me to think about it over night.

I talked it over with Arthur and decided that I have way too much going on right now to even consider changing apartments. It's not much more a month. The extra bathroom, larger kitchen, dishwasher, and having a spotless apartment again would be nice, but right now my life is kind of busy and expensive. I think I will tell her "no." Maybe it'll become vacant again once all this has passed.

Then I called Barbara. She was distressed when I first told her my news, but she is such a positive person, with such a loving way to her. She immediately let the negative thoughts go, and was very reassuring that this is going to come out fine. You can see why we all adore her. Then she told me that she just found out that our favorite cocktail waitress at the Cowboy has a reconstructed breast. She wears the most outrageous sexy, tight clothes and obviously none of us could tell.

All's well again. I hope my last letter did not get you too upset.

Bye. Love you,

June 4, Saturday

Dear Elaine:

I just wrote a letter to Rita. I told her that I needed to write you, but I was feeling guilty because I have not been a very good correspondent this past year. Please forgive me. Maybe now that I have a computer it'll be easier for me to stay on top of my letter writing. I got the computer about three weeks ago and I love it. Remember when I was back there a couple of years ago, I was saying then that I needed to get a PC? It took my starting a new job in our Systems Division to finally do it.

Well, there is a lot of news here as usual, and especially because I have been negligent in writing regularly.

Did you know I broke off the engagement? Actually it was six months ago today. It is a long story as to why but, it was for the best. I did date some, but no one that I was really interested in, or vice versa. It's just as well that I didn't meet anyone special.

I recently found out that I have breast cancer. This has changed my life around considerably. I have spent the last week researching the subject, and talking to women who have survived this disease. I feel like an expert at this point. It is a sad thing that so many of us have to go through this not very pleasant experience.

Anyway I will be having surgery the week of June 13th. I anticipate that all will go well and I will have a full recovery. I have been receiving tremendous support and love from family, friends, co-workers and strangers. I think I needed this wake up call in order to be more appreciative of all that life offers us. So, there has been a positive side to what could be considered a negative situation.

In case Eric hasn't written, he and Bridget are expecting a baby in November. (Will this make you a grand-god-mother?) Needless to say they are overjoyed, and we all are so happy for them. They are the cutest, nicest couple and ever so much in love. It is a pleasure to be in the midst of their love for each other.

Even though this letter brings some distressing news please know that we all are doing fine. There are no complaints as of the moment.

When you have time, and I know you are a busy lady, please write, and know that even though I don't write often, you are still in my thoughts.

Bye. Love you,

June 6, Monday

Hi,

I got your note and pictures today. Little Michael is so cute. I just want to reach into this picture, pull him out and hold him. I am going to return them with this letter, along with a little money to assist Maria. I hope it is successful. You have a lot of guts and, of course we know much, much heart. Let me know how it goes.

My new online "computer" friend from Alabama answered my note. I sent him e-mail Sunday morning telling him how much I enjoyed our "date" Saturday night. He responded Sunday night and said that we have to do it again. I e-mailed him and suggested we do it next week-end. (We'll see if I hear from him again) It was fun and interesting. He sounds like a nice man, but I know there are a lot of people out there on the network to beware of.

I went to church, and the beach Sunday, came home, had dinner and then one of my former staff came by with her husband. I had ordered that little gift for you before I left my old job. Chau had to get it from her son. I hope you receive it in good condition and that you like it. Her son is so talented. The pieces on the tape were his original compositions and they are performed by him. (They also brought some fancy chocolates, but I'm trying to cut down on sugar and chocolate, so I put them out for the kids to enjoy.)

All of the kids came over tonight. After they had been here awhile I told them that I wanted to talk to them about what was going on with me. I started to cry, but I was able to get myself under control. While I was calming myself Eric reached across Bridget and patted me on my leg to give me comfort. (He is such a sweet son.)

I explained everything that I know so far to them, as best I could, and they didn't have any questions. Bridget wanted to come visit me at the hospital, but I told her that I wouldn't be there long enough. I think that it was awkward for them. They really don't know how to handle this. But, I do feel better knowing that they all came and that I was able to tell them.

It was a good evening. Eric played Blackjack on the PC. Nicky was a doll as usual. He kept raiding the refrigerator. He ate so much, and such a variety, that I thought he was going to be sick. (No wonder he is getting so big so fast.)

Today at work my new co-workers, and boss, took me out to lunch to "welcome" me. I told them all about my private room experience on the computer Saturday night, and how I learned that "computer sex" exists out there in cyberspace. They were all laughing over my latest computer escapade. I want to write to my aunt and uncle yet.

Bye. Love you,

June 6, Monday

Dear Aunt Dot and Uncle George:

I got your nice letter. Thank you so much. I have been meaning to write you, but it has been hectic here. Hectic, but nice because I know that I am loved and cared about. There have been non-stop phone calls and guests. Although I feel like I am getting behind in other areas, I know that those things can wait. Now is the time for me to be with the people I love and who love me.

Please excuse me if this is written like a telegram. It's late and I have to get to bed soon.

My surgery will be some time next week. Actually I will find out the exact day and time tomorrow. I will only be there for twenty-four hours, or less. I doubt I will know much that is going while I am there.

One of my former staff, Danielle, has volunteered to take me, and also bring me home. She is a sweetheart and I consider her more than a former employee. She is a really good friend.

My new job was not another promotion. They don't happen quite that fast. I have to be at this level a little longer before I will qualify to go higher. It was a lateral transfer so that I could gain more experience. Since computers are the thing to know I felt it would help me tremendously in the future.

I am so glad that you are both doing well. We are all fine too. I am 90% cheerful, and then I allow myself the luxury of some down times too, and I have heard that that's normal.

Love you both.

June 7, Tuesday

When friends are united in the heart, it matters not, they're miles apart . . .

The above was sent to me for Christmas, from my very best friend. It's imprinted on a magnet which is on my refrigerator. Recognize it? (Nice, huh?)

Actually when I talked to you on Sunday you said that you were always thinking about me. Well, I can honestly say that you are in every room of my apartment. In the kitchen I have magnets on my refrigerator, and a monkey bank on the window sill. In the living room there are two love struck dinosaurs in my hutch. In the bathroom there's a vase from Venezuela, and in my bedroom your picture, and a picture of the Old Grist Mill in wintertime. See, you are here, there and everywhere!

I just called and left you a message about my brother calling you, and the date of the surgery. He called last night after I had written you. He and Lynn are in Montreal for a few days of rest and relaxation after his reunion in Vermont. From there they are going to Boston to spend time with my niece, Erica. While with Erica they are going on to Connecticut. I asked him if he would have time to meet you. (After thirty years it's time my best friend and my big brother met.) He said he honestly didn't know if they would have time to see you, based on the schedule that Erica has planned. But, he would definitely make a point of calling you while they are there.

Afterwards I thought about it, and decided I'd better call you and let you know. I didn't want you to get alarmed when you got a call from my brother "out of the blue." He really is the best brother anyone could have and you, the best friend, so I would like you two to meet somehow, even if by a phone call.

Also, late last night one of the ladies who was a referral from a cancer support group called. She is only thirty-six and had a mastectomy three years ago.

Her story is quite sad. It was so depressing that I could not fall asleep afterwards. She was very nice, and very honest. She gave me more insight on a deeper level about the way this disease can affect our lives.

Because you've heard everything else so far I'll try to tell you her story as briefly as I can. (She and I talked a long time.)

She is single, has never been married and is a work out and health food person. She was adopted and never knew her real parents, so she does not know if there is a history of breast cancer in her real family. She had been in a long term relationship with a man who died when she was thirty-two. Naturally it devastated her. She had also been with the same company for ten years in a professional position. After he died she got another job. About six months later she met another man. They started dating and began a relationship. Four months later she was diagnosed with breast cancer. She said that she is a private person and could not talk openly about it to anyone. Fortunately her new boyfriend was very supportive. (They are still together, but are now having problems over issues unrelated to the cancer.) She said she went into shock when she was diagnosed.

Her tumor was small. As it turned out there was no cancer in her lymph nodes. But, she did have to have six chemotherapy treatments.

Her new employer wound up demoting her because of all the time she missed from work as a result of the mastectomy. She was too worn down to fight it. (She was off work for six weeks after the surgery.) Then when she started the chemo she missed work as she was so sick from the treatments. Her employer started "documenting" her time off, and her punctuality, so they could "fire" her. Meanwhile the chemotherapy was ruining her immune system. She said she had diarrhea, lots of vomiting, and continuous yeast infections. She kept catching colds and the flu. She didn't lose her hair, but it thinned out.

She chose the saline breast implant because there was so much controversy in the news about silicone at the time. The reconstruction was done at the same time as her mastectomy. She has had to go back twice to have it re-done because, although it is safer than the other, it keeps leaking.

Finally she got so upset at the way her employer was treating her that she took them to the Labor Board. It was only recently resolved in her favor.

So, now she is thirty-six, never been married and in a job where they are really mad at her for winning the lawsuit against them. She hates to go in there every day, but she can't change jobs. She needs the health insurance, and since she now has a pre-existing condition it is difficult to get on another health plan. She and her boyfriend are having problems. She says that she can't even imagine getting into a relationship with someone else because she is so self-conscious of her reconstructed breast that keeps deflating and leaking.

Poor thing. And, she has no clue as to why this has happened to her. She says the only thing that she can think of is that the stress from her prior boyfriend's death may have caused her very healthy body to get this disease.

She worries about all women based on the statistics. She said that if this were a male disease, at these proportions, our government would be doing much more research into how to prevent it.

Do you see why I couldn't sleep last night?

Then this man who works down the hall from me invited me into his office today and expressed his concern over my health. Newton is a very sweet man. He said his wife had breast cancer three years ago and she is healthy today. He was being so kind to me.

A short while later a clerical supervisor that I've known for years called me about line dancing. Jacqui and her staff have a video that they watch at lunch time, and they are learning the dances. She knew I danced and wanted to know where they could go to dance outside of their practice sessions. I told her about some of the clubs in Orange

County. At the end of the conversation Jacqui invited me to go with them. I said that I wouldn't be dancing for awhile, and she asked why. I explained. As it turned out she had a lumpectomy seven years ago. She said it was a very tiny lump and her lymph nodes were negative. She had no chemo and she is fine today.

It is an epidemic Rita. It is extremely upsetting to think that so many women are experiencing this, and we don't know why.

The girl I talked to last night said that she is in counseling today and it's probably because she couldn't talk about it when it happened. She said she has bad and good days still. Sometimes she feels okay. At other times she looks in the mirror and gets very upset. She said that this will be the norm for the rest of our lives. All her friends and family say how great she looks, how healthy and lucky she is. She wants to tell them that they just don't know that she isn't always all those things.

This is another depressing letter, but I am not depressed now, honest. Last night I definitely was. Actually, today was a good day considering I did not have much sleep. I am glad I am in this new job instead of the one I was in before this happened. This office is so calm. The people are so nice. I get hooked into the computer, and get focused on what I am learning and doing. I forget about what is going on in my life outside of work. I think getting this job was a blessing.

I am finishing the projects assigned to me. (Of course I am still getting the easy ones.)

And, this is all I'm writing for tonight.

Bye. Love you,

June 8, Wednesday

Hi,

This is the new WordPerfect 6.0a which we are testing at work for possible use by all the district PC users. It's got a lot of neat features. I am trying them out. So, you may get some weird things in future letters. (More so than usual.)

My surgery will be Wednesday morning, June 15th. I have to be at the hospital before eight. Arthur is going to drop me off on his way to work. Danielle will pick me up the next morning. I am somewhat prepared, and getting more prepared each day. I will try to call you the night before. I want to hear what happened at your doctor's appointment that day.

I'm tired and it's getting late.

Bye. Love you,

June 9, Thursday

Hi,

Since I spent all day working on this new program at work I thought I'd have some fun with it tonight while I wrote you, although there is not much to write about. I learned how to make newspaper columns. Don't be surprised if you get Marilyn's version of the "Moody Blues." (Remember the newsletter that Rob used to send out?)

Your pictures are terrific. I especially like the one of your diningroom with the lilacs. Those are my favorite flowers for "scent." My favorites, for their simple beauty, are white daisies.

Well, how do you like this imprinted **cowboy**? I thought it would be a change from all the different style fonts I've been writing to you in. It is just amazing what can be done with one program as powerful as this one. It has all kinds of ClipArt and TextArt in it. I tested the whole workbook today and I only came across a few minor problems. Of course I can't retain all that I tested, but at least I have an idea now as to what's in it.

Guess that's it for tonight. All's well.

Bye. Love you,

P.S. Good luck on Saturday. I hope everything goes okay with "Maria's escape."

June 10, Friday

Dear Rita,

Here's a bird for you.

I got your card. Thank you. I am thinking of you all the time too and wondering how your plans are going for tomorrow with getting Maria out of that house. I hope it goes smoothly. She is so lucky to have met you.

This bird is weird. As I space down he flaps his wings across the page. It's interesting to watch. It's like he is in flight.

I am loving my job more. As you can tell I am making progress daily in this program. I'm also learning more about our e-mail system, but I want to know it all *now*. We get too many phone calls for me not to be doing my share. Also I hate telling people I'll have to get the information and call them back. (But, it will come in time.)

Enough for tonight. Once I am through this I'll hardly write at all, and then you'll miss these letters.

Bye. Love you,

June 11, Saturday

Hello,

I thought about what you said regarding Jack worrying about me being alone. Tell him I'm not. You have been here with me every step of the way.

I am at the point now where I just want to get this over with, and get on with my life. It's taking up too much of my time and thoughts, and there is so much more to life than this breast cancer issue.

Did I tell you that I'm taking vitamins? I started over a week ago. I'm taking a large multi vitamin, a vitamin C and a calcium tablet every day. I'm trying to make sure that I am extra healthy before the surgery, and for the recovery. Even though I eat tons of food I've lost weight. I'm down to 106 pounds as of this morning. It seems like all I do is stuff my face. The weight will come back on, and probably extra once I quit smoking next week.

Friday nights must be a curse lately. Last night I didn't go to sleep until four in the morning. At least this time I didn't cry. I just played computer Solitaire all night!

I haven't heard from my computer friend since Sunday so guess I don't have a "date" for tonight. Arthur was teasing me and said it's because I wouldn't "put out" with computer sex in our "private room." I think I'll go rent a movie and eat caramel popcorn. I'll forget about computers, men and breast cancer for awhile.

And, I guess I can stop thinking about your escapades with Maria for another week. I'll probably be out of it while you are helping her. Afterwards you can entertain me with the story of how you got her out of that lady's house.

Did you know that Nicky will be three years old next Saturday? I was just thinking of the date for Maria's escape and it is the same as Nick's birthday.

We just talked last night and there really isn't any news, but since I skipped a day of letter writing, and you noticed, this one is to make up for it.

Bye. Love you,

June 12, Sunday

Hi,

I wasn't going to write again for awhile, but I had to. Read the enclosed. This morning I went on America On Line (AOL) again for a little while before going to church. I "chatted" with some people in one of the large rooms. I began talking with a man from Northern California. He lives near the Sacramento area. We were talking about wineries in Sonoma and Napa. He sent me an "Instant Message." As it turns out he is a metaphysician too. He reads my church's daily affirmations. I told him about the breast cancer, and the soon to be surgery, and he was so wonderful about it. People are great. Anyway I had to get to church so I told him I'd like to talk more with him sometime and could he e-mail me when he was going to be online again.

When I got home from church this was in my messages. I printed you a copy to read. I got goose bumps from it and I almost cried. What a beautiful person.

I saw Paul at church and told him I liked his new beard. (You know I am a lover of beards.) Then he asked me why I cut my hair. I explained and he seemed pretty shocked. (I just kind of spring it on everyone.) We talked about it and then I told him I had to get into the sanctuary, and I knew that he needed to get to his Sunday school class.

This is it for tonight.

Bye. Love you,

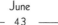

*J*une 13, Monday

Hi,

I'm feeling like there is so much I want to write tonight so bear with me. I suspect that this is going to be one of my rambling letters. I just feel antsy, like I am going to come right out of my skin. Won't you be glad when these letters have ceased?

I got the box of clothes tonight. I already tried them on. I like them a lot. They fit perfect, and yes I *am* too going to iron them anyway, but not tonight. I plan on calling you tomorrow night. And, Rita, I have to return this check. I still have a paycheck coming in. I can pay the phone bill. I really appreciate this, but I *can't* accept it. You have a big phone bill coming in too. You just mailed me a box of new clothes, and you are mainly the financial support behind Maria's escape. Are you trying to support the world? I promise that if I get to a point where I need money I will say "Send money **NOW**." Okay? What am I going to do with you?

I know you care. I know all this must be driving you nuts, and must be frustrating the hell out of you. I read last night that cancer is considered the "lonely" disease. I have my moments of feeling that way. But, Rita, I swear I don't know what I would do without you. You have been here with me. I don't know how to put it any better. I just can't tell you how much it has meant to me to have you to talk to, and write all this stuff to. I feel at times like I am being a big baby about this. You are the only one I can be whiny with. Do you understand?

At work I go, and I do. And, I have to admit that some days lately I do very little. At home I'm going through the motions, but I'm sort of zombie like. People call and I get all "up." But, after the calls, it's back to zombie time again. It's hard to explain. I just want to get this, and the next year, over with.

They say that if there's no recurrence in five years then the cancer is "cured." I now understand why the women I've talked to have mentioned their "anniversary" dates. Each one is a celebration. When I get to the fifth I'm going to celebrate big time. Want to join me? Also, June 15th will be the day that I finally quit smoking so I will have lots to celebrate on that day each year.

I've installed the recent version of Lotus 123 for Windows onto my PC. It's the next program I have to learn for work. I might as well learn it while I'm home recuperating. It's going to be difficult for me as it is a spreadsheet application. (I'm more of a word processor person, or haven't you noticed?) Actually, I am feeling pretty comfortable with this 6.0a and it has only been a week since I installed it. I've spent a lot of time at work going in and out of the different functions. I would say I have an intermediate knowledge at this point. To get to advanced will just take a little more experimenting on my part.

Tomorrow I work until two o'clock. My pre-op is at two-thirty. I have more questions for Catherine. Such as: If they send me home Thursday morning, and I still have the drainage tubes in me, am I really going to be able to drain and measure them myself with one hand? I'm worried about this.

I guess I am scared somewhat, but I know that usually for me, the anxiety before something happens, is usually worse than the actual event, with the exception of public speaking of course. I have prepared myself as much as I can for this experience. I have my moments, like now, when I feel overwhelmed by all of it but, on the whole, I am able to remain calm. I think having the new computer, and my new job to learn, has really been a plus in keeping my mind off of the medical problem.

Rita, thank you so very much. I hope the doctor has good news when you see him tomorrow.

Bye. Love you,

June 14, Tuesday, Journal Writing

Since I am calling Rita in ten minutes I obviously can't write her. Tonight is journal writing night. It's a place for me to talk. I need this therapy.

My emotions are going haywire today and I am worn out from them. It's almost nine o'clock in the evening and I should be fighting to stay awake. Instead I am doing, and then doing more. Eventually I will crash.

Being at work today was very difficult for me. I could not concentrate on any one thing. I probably should not have gone in at all. My boss and co-workers were wonderful though.

Karen mentioned that she was concerned about my not my having clothes to wear. (Clothes that I could get in and out of with my soon to be disabled left arm, and hanging bottles and tubes.) I told her how Rita had sent me a box of laundered, but un-ironed, big shirts.

I slipped out of work five minutes early. I really didn't want to have to talk with anyone before I left because I thought I might start crying.

At the hospital Catherine and I further discussed the surgery. I asked her about my left arm movement. She says I should be fine. The arm will be sore, and it will take awhile to get the movement back, but I can use it to do minor things right away.

My estrogen receptor test came back "positive," which is a good piece of news. Now I'll be able to take an estrogen suppressor drug. This will stop the estrogen which the cancer cells have been feeding on.

After doing all the pre-op requirements I stopped on the way home and got my hair cut again. It's really short now, but it will be much easier to take care of after the surgery.

Everyone has called tonight. (This is a slight exaggeration.)

Rita did not have her lump aspirated today. She now has to go back for another ultrasound and have it done at that time. And, Maria is finally out of that wicked person's house. Poor Rita has been dealing with her own suspicious lumps, my cancer problems, and Maria. She must be emotionally worn down.

I just want to get this over with and move on to the next phase. I want all the cancer surgeries and treatments done, and then I can get my life back in order again.

My moods swing from high to low, and I'm starting to feel like a manic depressive. But, other women have gone through this, survived and have gotten on with their lives. I will do the same.

June 16, Thursday, Journal Writing

I'm home. I'm in a bad mood. I wish the hospital had let me stay one more day. It is hard for me to believe that they could insist on sending me home in less than twenty-four hours after this type of surgery. Normally I would want to get out of the hospital as soon as possible. This time I wanted, and felt that I needed, to have someone with me for another day. Last night the drainage came apart. The nurse had to strip me and the bed, and then redo the tubes. What if that happens tonight? Then they said that I have to go back to the hospital tomorrow morning to have my dressing changed. Again I asked why not just keep me one more night? Catherine said the hospital couldn't keep me because it wasn't "cost effective."

Danielle came to see me at the hospital last night. I was pretty out of it. She brought flowers, cards and a gift from the people at my old office. After she left the hospital she was involved in a two car accident. I feel so bad. She and the other driver are okay, but still I feel badly about it, like some how maybe it was my fault. I know this is stupid thinking again.

She got up early this morning and fixed a rice, green bean and beef casserole for my dinner, and then came to the hospital to get me. When she got there I was in a foul mood. She is also going to take me back to the hospital tomorrow. Poor Danielle.

I haven't called Rita yet. That will be next. Danielle called her last night though. I really am okay. I'm not in as much pain as I had expected, and I'm not as depressed as I had expected to be. Maybe the anger I'm feeling at the HMO right now is my way of temporarily dealing with the surgery and the loss of my breast.

Even though I have some left arm movement, I can't type with my left hand. This one entry has taken me forever.

June 17, Friday, Journal Writing

Each day will be better. I am able to use my left hand more for typing.

Right now I am waiting for Joyce. I look forward to seeing her for two reasons. First, I miss our "gossipy" phone calls since I changed jobs, and second because she is bringing dinner and I'm so hungry.

Last night was an up and down night. Finally at about four I decided I'd had enough. I took over the bathroom and carefully washed my hair and body. It took me an hour, but it felt so good. I was so tired afterwards that I took a pain pill and went back to bed.

Danielle is such a sweetheart. Here she has a zillion things of her own to be doing, and with a banged up car, but she is still willingly and joyfully taking me back out to the hospital. She is the right person to be around when I'm feeling down or helpless. She knows how to make me start feeling good again.

My tubes were leaking like they were in the hospital. I was frustrated and mad that Catherine expected me to be changing the dressing at the site where the tubes enter my back.

When the nurse came into the examining room she immediately rushed back out to get Catherine to help her with the mess. Fluids were pouring out of me onto the exam table. And, when Catherine came in I let her know that I was still pretty upset with her for not allowing me to stay one more night in the hospital. She started giving me an explanation that I did not have a medical need to stay another night.

I became aggressive (for me anyway) and said that yesterday morning she indicated that it was a monetary reason. She denied this until I quoted her "cost effective" terminology. Then she said it wasn't herself that made these decisions. I asked her who did because I wanted to write a complaint letter.

The long and short of it is that I feel like I won a small victory. Catherine made a referral for a visiting nurse to come out to my apartment each day to do the dressing changes. This is what I had suggested on Tuesday during the pre-op, and what I asked for before being discharged from the hospital.

Actually I feel it has worked in my favor as the visiting nurse will be coming every day until Wednesday. That's actually more than I had originally requested.

One of the books I am reading says that cancer is not the time to be quiet and to act like a "Mr. Nice Guy." It says that we need to speak up and say what's on our mind, or else no one will hear us. I like Catherine. I didn't mean to upset her, but I was so angry, and I did not like the way I was being treated.

Flowers, plants, cards, calls, notes. It's so wonderful to receive each and every one. I thought I'd want to be alone right after the surgery, but I am loving all the attention, and care that people are showering on me. It does make me feel loved and it will help me to recover more quickly.

My underarm is throbbing from all this typing, but I can do it and that's the wonder.

June 18, Saturday, Journal Writing

I am doing remarkably well. People continue to be so kind to me. The power of positive thought works. There are so many people sending me love, good wishes and prayers that I think all these thoughts are what are speeding up my recovery.

Yesterday Joyce came and brought me dinner and flowers from her office staff. It was so great to have her here. She lost her husband a few months ago. He unexpectedly died from heart failure. They are younger than me and I've known them both for almost twenty years. Women are so strong. I admire our inner strengths that keep us going when times are tough.

Joyce was fun company, and the food she brought was delicious.

Last night Rita called. I think I am surprising both of us with how well I'm doing. I truly expected to be depressed at this point, but it's not happening. I have some pain, but the pills take care of that. I am keeping busy, yet getting lots of rest too.

This morning I got up early and washed my hair and did a sponge bath again. It took forever, but it was worth every minute. I'm also eating regular meals. I even stripped my bed and did two loads of laundry. I feel like life must be getting back to it's familiar routine when I'm taking out trash, and washing clothes and dishes again.

This morning I called Nick to wish him a Happy Birthday. Instead, he said "Happy Birthday Grandma." That's fine. I'll take whatever kind of good wishes I can get.

As soon as the visiting nurse goes I plan to take a well deserved nap. Laura should be coming to visit this afternoon and I want to be energetic again.

June 19, Sunday, Journal Writing

Rita called twice yesterday to see how I was doing, and then I called her once in the evening. She mentioned that now that I've had the surgery I am no longer writing to her. I explained that I felt bad sending her all the bizarre letters, and I'm trying to keep my weirdness in a journal. I don't want to keep her in distress. I will still write, but I want to try to get back to normal with her. I feel I've had her go through hell with me for this past month, and enough is enough.

I continue to feel wonderful. I am amazed at how rapidly I am recovering. The movement from my arm is returning. I think once the tubes are out it'll be even better.

I am not horrified by my stapled chest. It's okay. I would prefer my breast being there, but that's not the way it is. My right breast now looks big and kind of lost all by itself. But, looking at it does not get me crying, or repulsed or anything like that.

I just completed a book "Now That I Have Cancer I am Whole." It is spiritual, truthful, funny, and sad. It has been very beneficial for me. Knowing how another has experienced his cancer, and dealt with it, helps. Once again I am reminded that I am not alone. I find this too when I talk with other women with breast cancer.

June 19, Sunday

Hi,

This is two handed, so here goes. You missed these letters, huh? Okay, just so we keep in practice here's another. Between you and Arthur it'll be a miracle if my staples remain in place. He keeps me laughing too.

Here's a story I know you can appreciate. (In all it's gory details) I have not had a bowel movement since before the surgery, and I am eating and drinking lots. Yesterday the nurse told me to get an over the counter laxative. When she came today and I still hadn't gone to the bathroom, I promised her I would have Arthur get some at the store tonight.

I gave Arthur a small shopping list and at the bottom I put "ex-lax (sorry)." He takes the list, and the money, and goes into his room. All of a sudden I hear him say "No Way! You're sorry? What about me?"

He plots and he plans how he is going to get a laxative out of the store without being seen with it. He was even joking about stealing it. We decided he'd be more embarrassed if he got arrested, and in court the judge told everyone what they caught him stealing!

Finally he goes to a new store, instead of the one he usually shops at. He comes home just as pleased as can be and says, "I figured it out." He hands me a pretty package that says "Correctol, the 'gentle' laxative for *women*." He said, "I knew the cashier wouldn't think they were for myself." I thought I'd wreck my stitches. My son and you, his Godmother are definitely two of the same kind.

I'm off now to splurge on a root beer float. Sound good? I'll fix you one too.

Love you,

June 20, Monday, Journal Writing

I am up early, and just *doing*. It feels so good that I just want to do more and more. I've got laundry going. I've had another shampoo and "sink" bath. Now, to just get these tubes out of me, the staples removed, get a real shower and start driving myself again. At the rate I am going I will be back to my old routines in no time, and then back to work.

I plan to take a morning walk while people are still sleeping, or at work, and then do some ironing.

When the nurse called this morning it sounded like a man. I wish it was a female again, but that's okay.

Life is good, and considering what I have recently gone through, and will be going through in the near future, I am happy and content overall. There are some things I would like to change, but if they are not within my power, or control, I am instead learning to accept them the way they are.

Later:

The nurse was a man. I don't know if he's gay or not, but it was still a little awkward for me to expose my stapled chest to a man. Maybe it wasn't that bad. I'm just so sensitive and modest.

He said I look great and everything is healing nicely. I am *ready* to get these uncomfortable tubes out of me, and of course I want the staples gone too.

June 20, Monday

Hello,

This will be a short one. I *had* to write because I got "the" card from you today. It is hilarious. I was sitting on the couch, and I couldn't stop laughing. It hurt, but it was a nice kind of hurt! I don't know where you are finding such perfect cards. Do you hunt forever? This was definitely "*us*."

Okay, that's the extent of today's letter. See, I am running out of things to write. Actually it was either write you about receiving the card or call. So here I am.

You want more? Hmm Okay, I went for a little walk around my neighborhood this morning. I went up and down the streets, and the birds were singing and the weather was perfect. Tomorrow I'll go even further.

I got the biggest, most beautiful plant today from the Systems Division. They enclosed a funny card signed by all the staff. The plant had a huge balloon on it. The florist knocked at the door. When I answered the door he just handed it to me. I almost fell down it was so heavy. I thought my staples were going to pop for sure. Fortunately the end table is right by the door. I put it down pretty quick, but it gave me an instant of fright.

Barbara called to confirm Wednesday. She is going to take off work at one o'clock so that she can drive me to my appointment. I am really glad that she is going with me. I think I will need her support that day. She has been through this before with another friend of hers.

Ann called last night. She went dancing and saw Don. She said he was sort of with his girlfriend, but not really. Anyway she said she told him about me and he almost fell off his bar stool. He had no idea that my biopsy came back malignant.

This is plenty considering I had nothing to write about. When do you go to have the ultrasound done again? I will probably call soon to find out what's going on.

Bye. Love you,

June 21, Tuesday

Hello,

My visiting nurse just left. She was a sweet older lady. I've had three different nurses. When I told her that I have a doctor's appointment tomorrow to get the staples out, and hopefully the tubes, she said she didn't think they would remove the tubes just yet. There is still a lot of fluid draining out. I'm bummed. The tubes are what are uncomfortable at this point. They go through my back, and then into my chest and my underarm areas. I think I would have more left arm movement if they weren't there. (But, whatever.)

I cannot wait to be able to drive and do things. I'm getting so bored here. I'm reading lots, playing games on the PC, and eating continuously. I gained one pound as of this morning.

I want a real shower and shampoo. I want to be able to shave my armpit. I want to be able to sleep on my stomach. (I want. I want. I want.)

I ended my free month on AOL. I'm now on Prodigy which I don't like as much, but I also get one free month. I contacted Rob through it. Actually I had wanted to send Jon some e-mail, but I could not locate him in the directory. I found Rob with no problem. He is so surprised that I'm hooked up to a computer. We are messaging each other and he gave me Jon's online address so that I could send him a note too.

Hey, I've gone one whole week without a cigarette. Actually it will be one week tomorrow morning. But, this is close enough for me to be bragging about it.

Bye. Love you,

June 22, Wednesday, Journal Writing

This WordPerfect 6.0a program seems to be working slow, or maybe it's me and I'm impatient lately.

I want to get today's doctor's appointment over with. I hope they take out the tubes and tell me that I can take a real shower. Maybe then I can get a comfortable nights's sleep, and wear clothes that aren't intended for hiding tubes.

Of course the one thing that I'm hesitant to admitting to is my fear of hearing the results of the lymph nodes. I want to hear that they found no cancer cells in them, but I don't want to get my hopes up too high.

In the mail yesterday I got the copy of my favorite picture of Rita and I, which was taken when she and Jack were out here on vacation four years ago. I had ordered an enlargement made. It's now framed and on my computer table. I can look at her hugging me as I type these crazy letters. This is mushy, but I swear I don't know what I would have done without her all these years, especially through this crisis. And we still don't know for sure that her lump is a cyst. Friday, finally, she will have the needle aspiration done. The doctors tell her not to worry, but I want to hear that she is okay!

Considering all that has happened in the past month, or past six weeks, I really can't complain about my life. I am happy. It sounds bizarre I'm sure, but I am.

Later:

Where to begin? All the **good** news! I had my appointment with the surgeon today. Seventeen lymph nodes were removed, and all were negative. This is such a relief. I started crying when Dr. Gruber told me. I had dreaded hearing the results, but I got good news all around. The tubes were removed. And, it was very **painful**! Nothing had prepared me, or warned me about their removal hurting so much. But, they are out. If there is any swelling I have to go back to have the fluid drained. If there's no swelling then I don't see Dr. Gruber again for six months. The staples were also removed and they didn't hurt a bit after having those tubes yanked out of me! She said I can shower in two days, which was more good news. And, I can start driving. I will probably be back to work by the 11th of July. She suggested that I wait until I meet with the oncologist, and have a couple of the chemotherapy treatments before I return to work.

On Monday I call the oncologist for an appointment. I hope it'll be next week. In the meantime Dr. Gruber is making a referral to the Los Angeles clinic for my reconstruction appointment with a plastic surgeon. Things are progressing. Soon this will be behind me.

Now, I am into celebrating. I have some country western music blaring in the background. I could not bear to listen to it before. Now I *know* that I will be dancing soon.

In the mail I got more cards and good wishes from friends and co-workers. I feel very fortunate to be receiving such great support.

I called and left messages for Bud, Rita, Karen, Danielle and Arthur. I wanted to tell everyone all this good news right away. Karen called back first. She was happy for me and my good news. And, she had her own good news. She will be gone from Systems before I return as she got a promotion. I told her that I am happy for her and expressed how glad I am that she was there while this was happening to me.

Rita called. We were both so excited and happy about this news. I am looking at the picture of us, the one with her arms wrapped around me, and I can feel her love.

I am ready to move to the next step in this experience and to get on with **my life**.

June 23, Thursday

Hi,

This is going to be a quick one. I have laundry going. I'm all "bird-bathed," as Danielle, calls it and I have country music blaring. The weather is beautiful. I have on such a **cute, bright,** outfit. Originally I bought this blouse for dancing. It's a Liz Clairborne with red, purple, blue, gold plaid and metallic gold thread, which ties at the waist. I never got to wear it. I'm wearing it with purple shorts, and gold socks. *I* am ready to go somewhere today, and anywhere will do. I plan on cleaning the apartment, but first I want to get in my car and drive. It'll probably be to the dry cleaners and the car wash, but just getting out on my own sounds fantastic.

Yesterday an incredibly beautiful, huge bouquet mix of all kinds of spring and summer pastel flowers was delivered from Arthur and Darleen in New Hampshire. I put it in the dining room. It is below my watercolor print of the same type of bouquet.

My other bouquets are slowly dying. At first I was getting all upset. I think the thought of anything dying these days can set me off. I wouldn't even consider killing a bug right now. Of course this is going to change when my pesky ants come back any day now.

I want to dance. There is a *fantastic* swing song on the radio. Before I thought the lack of a breast would stop me. Now I can't wait to get my left arm movement back and then I know I can do it. The missing breast part doesn't even bother me right now. I want arm capability!

Love you,

June 23, Thursday

Hi,

Boy it didn't take me long to get back to the plain old style of writing, huh? I got tired of playing around with the fancy stuff in this word processing program. As long as I know it's in there, and where to find it when I need it, then I'm okay. By the way, whatever happened to the computer/typewriter that you and Jack got? I know you said it needed a new ribbon. Is that why you don't use it anymore? I can't imagine handwriting a letter now. I mean maybe a short note, but a long letter? No way.

I got two cards from you today with the "rubber" check which is "bouncing" between Massachusetts and California. Thank you. I'll keep it and mail it into the Credit Union. These pictures came too. They are wonderful. How can you stand it? I'd be wanting to enlarge, and frame all of them. And, little Michael is *so* cute. I think he's got Jack's smile. What do you think?

Also, I got a "computer" type home-made card from Paul which was very sweet of him. Today was productive, yet pleasant. I did a few errands. I went to the church bookstore and got some greeting cards, and rented some Louise Hay, "motivational" tapes. I cleaned the apartment, and I actually enjoyed doing it. Then I got my ironing done. I've also had numerous phone calls. My ex-boss, Shannon, called to see how I was, and to tell me that she had just finished my annual evaluation. She said it was "glowing" as usual which was nice of her, and she is going to mail it to me.

John, the boss I had before her called. He just got back from a two weeks vacation in Tennessee at FAN FAIR. John said that I should be getting lots of mail from his staff in the next few days as he posted my address on their lunchroom bulletin board. That's cool. These are the people I worked with when I was in Quality Control. He and I talked quite awhile, but then I had to go because the volunteer from "Reach To Recovery" was knocking on my door.

The volunteer brought me a padded "thing" to put in my bra until I get a prosthesis. She said they really don't work too good because there is no weight in that side of the bra, and since I'm numb from the surgery I won't realize it, but the bra will creep up around my neck which could be pretty embarrassing. (I think I'll go to the prosthesis store next week and check out what they have instead.)

She was very helpful and she kept commenting on how "up" and adjusted I am to all this. And, I really am Rita. I mean how else could I be?

This lady had her first mastectomy fourteen years ago. It was her left breast and there was no cancer in the lymph nodes. After two years, and three biopsies (benign lumps as they turned out) of her right breast, she told the surgeon to remove the right breast too. She did not want to spend the rest of her life going through the anxiety of having lumps biopsied. At that point she had not had any reconstruction surgery. She had always been very small breasted. When she had the right breast removed she had them save her skin and nipple and put in a silicone implant. On the left side she had her own abdominal tissue moved up into her breast area. She went in two months later to have an areola and a nipple added to the left breast. The left nipple eventually scabbed and fell off. But, her husband doesn't mind the missing nipple, so she decided to leave her one breast without it.

She showed me both breasts. She is probably about ten years or so older than me. Her breasts looked great to me. She wears a 36b, which is my size, and her breasts are pretty firm and young looking. (I can live with that.) Actually I was glad that she came and talked to me, and showed me her breasts. I have been thinking of having the abdominal tissue breast reconstruction surgery done. I hope my HMO sees it that way. I know it's painful, and it will involve a big scar on my abdomen, but it would be "my" tissue. If I gain or lose weight it would go up and down with me. We'll see. I have plenty of time to decide yet.

The volunteer also said that she did not have chemotherapy after the lymph nodes were found to be negative. I have thought about this since yesterday. I dread the chemo, but I have gone this far with attempts to protect myself by having the mastectomy and quitting smoking. Why would I not choose to have as much done to me as possible, to be sure that there is no cancer left?

Oh, she and her husband are dancers too. They swing dance almost every week-end. She said she was out dancing three weeks after her mastectomy, but she did have physical therapy for her arm. I keep thinking that I wish there was some way I could have this also. Two of the other lady's I have talked with had physical therapy. My arm is doing okay, but I cannot complete all the exercises. I have lots of shooting pains from under my arm to my elbow. It feels like things are ripping inside my arm when I try to continue the exercises. The volunteer said to keep doing them, and to push myself a little further and harder each day. Maybe I am expecting too much for the first week after surgery. She said that if I had a Jacuzzi it would be a big help in getting the movement back in a gentle way.

Here I was going to stop writing to you about cancer stuff all the time, but I got carried away.

Change of subject:

My roommate at work called me today. Bruce said that they are planning a luncheon for Karen on Monday if I want to meet them at the restaurant. I told him I should be able to make it. They are also having a potluck for her in the building for everyone to attend on Wednesday.

I am eating like crazy. My weight is still 107 pounds.. The way I'm eating it should be going up real soon.

Tomorrow is shower in the morning day!

And, that's all she's writing for this one.

Bye. Love you,

June 24, Friday

Hi,

Yesterday one of my next door neighbors moved their "midnight plant" closer to my patio. She said that in the Philippines this plant only blooms occasionally in the evenings and the person who sees it blooming can make a wish. She wanted me to watch it last night. I did, and it had bloomed. I made my wish, — for left arm movement!

I am bathed, and "cute," and ready to go out to do some light grocery shopping. I had THE luxury shower this morning. I feel so c-l-e-a-n now. I have on denim shorts, a white t-shirt and a plaid denim vest over it. (The top button is unbuttoned to give it a little puckering out in front) I figure if I go braless and wear clothes that normally made me look small breasted, that it'll be difficult to tell that one is missing.

Also, I did arm exercises like crazy last night. Today I've promised myself to not baby my left arm. I am going to use it as I normally would, other than carrying heavy things with it of course. I want a very, close to normal arm by next week. We'll see.

Today I am going in search of an electric razor so that eventually, when the swelling goes down, I can shave under my arm. (It is *so* hairy under there.) And, some sun block too, which I have never used before. (I'm not supposed to get any sunburn on this arm for the rest of my life.)

I'm out of here to shop.
Thanks for listening again.
Bye. Love you,

June 24, Friday, Journal Writing
I can't call Rita yet. It's too early. I've been thinking about her all day. I know she is going to be fine, but I want to hear these words spoken to me. I almost wish I had told her to call me as soon as she left the doctor's office, because now I'm saying to myself, "Well, she would have called if everything was okay." Lately my mind jumps to wrong conclusions so quickly. I'm trying to think positive most of the time, but I can't help but worry about this. I know she is okay—I just want to hear it!

I replied to a person who had put a note on the Prodigy medical bulletin board regarding chemo questions. I had read her note and all the replies she got. I posted a message to her stating that I had read them for my own benefit, and that they had helped me with my fears of chemotherapy. A lady from San Diego saw my response and messaged me that she just finished her chemotherapy for Breast Cancer and wished me luck. I immediately sent her some e-mail with questions regarding her own chemo experiences.

I went to the prosthesis store in Seal Beach. The owner was so helpful. She showed me several types of prosthesis. We discussed prices and comfort. She suggested that I call the surgeon to find out when I can be fitted. She thought it was too soon for me to do it today. While I was there I was talking to her about my arm. She also suggested that I ask the doctor to refer me to physical therapy.

I bought an electric tooth brush with a WaterPik. I am having problems flossing my teeth. I don't want to incur dental problems too. I also bought an electric shaver. I'm afraid to use a regular razor on my left armpit for fear I'll cut myself. The only thing is that when I got the electric razor home, and read the brochure, it doesn't say anything about using it for shaving underarms. It just mentions legs. I'll have to experiment on my right underarm tonight. All this is just way too much.

I am watching the clock. I'll wait a little while longer before I call Rita.

Later:
Rita called. She said that her doctor has assured her that the lumps

are only cysts. They tried to do needle aspirations, but nothing came out because the lumps are so small. She is sore from the needles, but feels there is nothing to worry about. I guess I am just being extra paranoid lately. I need to stop worrying so much about cancer.

She and I could even talk about other things for a change.

June 25, Saturday, Journal Writing

I must have been driving Rita crazy all this time. Now I feel selfish. I am making myself a promise that from here on I will not write her all this weird stuff. The anxieties which I feel I need to write about are going in this journal, and that is that.

I started reading "The Race is Run" last night by Nancy Brinker. She is the lady who founded the "RACE FOR THE CURE," in memory of her sister who died from breast cancer. I am half way through the book and it is very sad, but also quite informative. Nancy herself had breast cancer. What a difference between her treatment and "cure," and her sister's failing to receive correct treatment when she was diagnosed.

My arm is improving, but I am impatient. I want it the way it was before the surgery **right now**. I do the exercises and then wonder if I'm doing them often enough, or maybe too much, or if I'm doing them right. (I could make myself crazy with worry over all this. I've got to stop.)

I have continued my online Prodigy contact with the lady from San Diego. She said she will help me with hints and tips on how to deal with my chemo.

June 25, Saturday

My questions for the oncologist are:
1. What chemo drugs are being recommended and why?
2. How many months will I need these treatments?
3. How frequent are the treatments?
4. How will they be administered?
5. How long will each treatment take?
6. Should someone accompany me for the treatments?
7. What are the possible side effects?
8. How should I prepare ahead of time for the side effects?
9. Is there anything I can do to lessen or relieve the side effects?
10. Will I be able to work?

11. What type of hormone therapy will I have and how will it be administered?

12. How often will it be administered?

13. How long will I be on this hormone therapy?

14. What are the side effects?

June 27, Monday Journal Writing

I improve more and more each day. Although I get discouraged with my left arm. I am obviously making progress. I can't believe it has been less than two weeks since the surgery and I feel this good. Even though I am anxious to get back to work I'm now starting to enjoy the time off. I've never had this much continuous time off work before. I feel so relaxed and stress free.

Yesterday I went to church. I sat with a man from the cancer group. He didn't remember me, but as soon as I saw him I felt as if my dilemma about my arm being raised during the "Peace Song" was resolved. He doesn't have cancer, but he has a type of chemical allergy which makes him very ill. He said his only defense right now is to move out of Southern California, and also to use holistic approaches. I feel so bad for him. It's not as if he can have a surgery, or take medication, to ease the symptoms to rid him of his infliction.

In the evening Marvette, the secretary from work came by. We went to Marie Callendar's for dinner. It was a very pleasant evening, and I enjoyed myself. She told me her story regarding back surgery two years ago. Marvette was working in our agency for only three months, and she had never had back problems when one day her back just went out. She was taken to the hospital by ambulance. The terrifying part was that ten days after her surgery the hospital told her she had to leave or they would charge her, and not her insurance, for staying there. She was completely bedridden, living alone in Laguna Beach and had no one to drive her home. Marvette has no parents, no siblings, no children and the one close girlfriend she has doesn't drive. She finally called her boss and he came and got her.

She had a visiting nurse, but that was only three times a week. She had no bath for ten days. The only way she could get herself out of bed, to go to the bathroom, was to take a pain pill first. Her story was sad, and so scary. What do people do who don't have someone to help them at times like that? And, here I've been complaining about my minor problems.

June 27, Monday

Hi,

I'm really trying not to write as often, but now I have lots of reasons to write, and I won't be writing as much soon.

First, I got the package and everything fits. I was worried when I saw that the shorts were a size six, but they fit too. And I like this cowboy boot t-shirt!

Now, ready? I met my unit and my boss for lunch today. It was Karen's good-bye luncheon. They all said how wonderful I looked, and I agreed with them. I told everyone I would be coming to the potluck on Wednesday since I don't see the oncologist until Friday. After I left them I went to the antique area of Orange County known as "the Circle" and browsed through the shops. I bought a Max Parrish reference book. (Do you like his art? I've always been intrigued by it). Anyway, I started thinking how dumb it was for me to be using up precious vacation time when I'm going to need it in the future.

I called Dr. Gruber and she agreed to let me go back to work half days for a week, and then full time thereafter. She is going to write a note for me to pick up tomorrow. Afterwards I called my boss. Then I called the County Doctor's office to make an appointment for tomorrow afternoon so that I can get a release to return to work.

Tomorrow I'll have a million things to do, but it feels good to know I'll be going back to work, and not be using up all my vacation time. I told my boss I might just as well be sitting at work doing the Lotus 123R4 practices on the computer there, and get paid for it, instead of sitting at home forcing myself to do it.

Thank you for the "friendship" book. I'll put it on my nightstand and read little bits each night. It'll be a good way to end each day.

Rita, I love life and all sides of it. I cannot tell you how my outlook has expanded.

Bye. Love you,

June 28, Tuesday

Hi,

This really will be the last letter for awhile. I just got home from the Employee Health Office. I met with the nurse, Jeannie, who is a breast cancer expert. We talked about breast cancer, and her experiences, and the things I have read, or discovered in talking with other women. And, we talked about you.

Now, don't get upset with me for this. I promise I won't keep bringing it up, but I love you, so I have to tell you what I feel and think. Even though you told me on Friday that the doctor assured you that the lumps you have are cysts. I'm still concerned. I have not stopped thinking about it, but I did not want to bring it up with you again and get you all aggravated with me, and thinking I am terribly paranoid.

Today I told the nurse all this. She encouraged me to try to convince you to have someone, either from the HMO, or out of your own pocket, do a biopsy. Jeannie said she and her physician have the theory that any lump is malignant until a biopsy proves otherwise. The fact that *no* fluid came out when he did the aspiration leaves me feeling quite leery. People keep asking me about you and I tell them that we found out Friday that the lumps are cysts. But, we didn't really. Do you honestly feel certain yourself that they are cysts?

Jeannie told me this story:

Her younger sister had a lump near her nipple. She had her doctor check it out. He told her not to worry because it looked like a cyst to him. Jeannie told her to have it biopsied, but she didn't. The next year she went in and the doctor did a needle aspiration. Nothing came out, but again he told her not to worry and that it was probably a cyst. Jeannie got upset and begged her to have a biopsy. Her younger sister got mad at her and said things like, just because she was a nurse in the breast cancer field, she did not know more than the doctor, and that she was being an alarmist and to leave her alone.

The "cyst" kept growing. The next year she called Jeannie and asked her where she could go to have it biopsied. It was almost five centimeters by then and it was cancerous. She had a radical mastectomy and chemotherapy. This was, I think she said, a year ago. Today she is fine, but she should have had it removed and treated sooner.

Then, this past year Jeannie found a lump in her own breast. It was cancer and she had a lumpectomy. She is doing okay also.

Rita, please consider getting it biopsied. I promise I won't keep bringing it up. I asked Jeannie how I could convince you to get a biopsy. She said to just ask you to do it no matter if you got upset with me or not. So I am.

Okay. I'll drop it.

It seems like I had more to write, but this is enough. Aren't you glad I'm going back to work?

Love you,

P.S. When I walked into Tamsin and Nick's apartment today, he said to me "Grandma, did you have your boob cut off?" I couldn't help but laugh because it was said so innocently. I wonder where he heard that?

June 29, Wednesday, Journal Writing

I am getting ready to go back to work in two hours. I have my make up on and I feel very good about myself. I am well rested. My arm is behaving. I am doing much more strenuous arm exercises which involve my left chest. My hair only looks so-so, but I'm waiting to hear what the oncologist says on Friday regarding chemotherapy, and the future status of my hair. If it looks like it's going to fall out then I'll just leave it as it is. If I'm not going to be losing my hair then I might go ahead and have it colored again.

Even though my dress selection is limited right now I have picked out a very feminine dress which I can wear with a vest.

Since this cancer scare everything is new again. I don't feel I have much anger or hostility towards anything or anyone. This is a very freeing feeling. There have been many positives to this crisis. One big plus is my having quit smoking. Occasionally I think about cigarettes, especially after eating, but I can't imagine that I would ever go back to them.

I'm faithfully taking extra vitamins and calcium, something else I could never seem to get into the habit of previously. I'm trying to be more conservative and cautious with money and my accrued vacation time. I know that I have future responsibilities coming up where I will need both. Still, I am not depriving myself of anything that I want.

Although I am not up to a love life as yet, I am, as always, hopeful that that day will come again.

Once more I feel as if my life is on track, and in balance. I am grateful for all this.

Later in the evening:

I loved being back at work today. I picked a "fun" day to do it, and it was productive too. I feel lucky to have this new job with such wonderful co-workers. I got lots of compliments from everyone and that made me feel good. Sometimes I felt embarrassed with the descriptive praises of "brave," "inspirational," and "strong," which were being showered on me, but then I decided that maybe I am these things.

One kind person said to me, "You are still the same person inside." I replied, "No, I'm a better person inside. I now appreciate things that I used to take for granted."

Bridget came by in the evening with her ultrasound pictures of the baby. You can see it's whole body and little face. It looks healthy, sweet and beautiful to me. Bridget and Eric are such an exceptional couple. They inspire me with their love for each other.

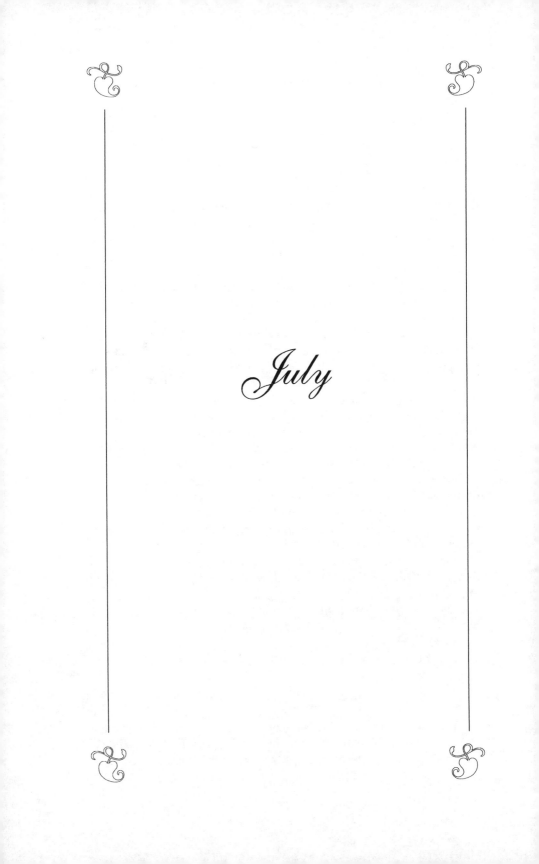

July

Hi,

I am ever so tempted to call you and tell you the great news, but I'm chicken to call you in case today was the day you got my last letter!

I went to see the oncologist today and **NO CHEMOTHERAPY**. He decided that based on my age, the negative lymph nodes, the positive estrogen/progesterone receptor, the fact that the tumor was found early, and that I had the mastectomy he is not recommending chemotherapy. I had been in the examination room for about ten or fifteen minutes before Dr. Nielsen told me. Rita, when he told me this I almost jumped off the table I was so excited. I had prepared myself for the chemo based on what the radiologist and the surgeon had said, and also on what I had read. I even had a wig picked out. I was *dreading* it!

I will be taking Tamoxifen twice a day for at least the next five years, and it is going to put me into an "instant menopause." He said to expect hot flashes. He even wrote me a prescription to alleviate them. The Tamoxofin is going to suppress the estrogen in my body.

I had some swelling under my arm. It has been extremely sensitive. Dr. Nielsen said it needed draining and he tried to call my surgeon, Dr. Gruber, so that I could go right from his office to hers. But, her office was closed. Instead I went to the Urgent Care Clinic. The Physician there used a local anesthetic and he aspirated seven cc's of fluid. It feels much, much better. He said that it will probably continue filling up with fluid until the "flap" adheres to my chest wall.

When I got home I called my hairdresser and scheduled an appointment to have my hair colored tomorrow. This is in celebration of the fact that **I am going to have hair!**

Now if I could just rehabilitate my arm, and get my chest to heal so that I could get fitted for a "make believe boob," I'd be out there dancing again!

Did I tell you that Arthur is moving out pretty soon? He and his best friend's brother are getting a place together.

Please don't be upset with me.

Bye. Love you,

Rita, honest my intention is to not write so often, and I'm trying to give you a break by taking it out on my Prodigy pen pals. Amazingly I am meeting lots of interesting people through this computer service.

But, today I got this surprise package from you. I love it so much! Arthur and I flipped out. You are extremely talented. Well, I walked from room to room, and wall to wall, and finally hung the photograph in the first hallway as you leave my livingroom. It is hung so that you can see it immediately upon entering the livingroom. And just in case someone misses it that way, it'll get them as they are walking towards the back of the apartment. It is really beautiful. I had forgotten that you were making me something, and when the mailman handed me the package I couldn't imagine what it was.

I had thought about going out to look for a couple more vests today, but I was pretty tired. When the vests came in your package, I matched them with two cream colored long sleeved blouses, and a skirt and a pair of slacks. I think I have enough changes of nice clothes now to wear that will disguise my missing part until I can get into a bra again. I thank you, but please you have got to stop as I'm starting to feel guilty.

I tried to wear a bra with the padded "thing" that the cancer society gave me. Right! I wore it around the house for two hours and it had "escaped" the bra and was up around my neck, even though I had put "weights" in it. Also, my skin is tender under my arm from the swelling. It hurts there still.

This afternoon I sewed some weights, and the "thing," into a bra. I'll give it a try again on Monday. I am anxious to start looking whole again.

I got up at about five and started cleaning the apartment and doing tons of laundry. At nine I was at the Credit Union and a half hour later I was at my hairdresser. Fortunately, because of the holiday weekend, it was very slow. Regina did a terrific job of coloring my hair. I like it. She also trimmed it some more. She said that she thinks I look better with short hair, except for when I have really, really long hair. I told her that right now I am just ever so thankful to have any hair, and that I will never complain about "bad" hair days again.

I have been so into reading computer and cancer books lately, that I decided to treat myself to two novels for this holiday week-end. Maybe tonight I'll start one.

I've taken two of the Tamoxifen and so far I haven't had any hot flashes. Maybe I'll get lucky and I won't experience the side effects. I'm also trying harder with the arm exercises. I swear it is getting more painful to do them instead of easier though. I guess I am just impatient.

Oh, I've also met some Backgammon addicts. They are putting me in touch with places that carry software so I can install the game onto my computer. (See I'm not the only one in the world who is nutty about this game.) I found out that these people actually hold tournaments. Two guys who have met through the computer, and live in different states, are attempting to set up a competition between themselves through their modems.

Forgive my rambling on and on again.

Bye. Love you,

July 4, Monday

Dear Rita:

How was your Fourth? Mine has been quiet, but it's been a nice one so far. Bridget came by early with Nick and we took him to the Huntington Beach parade. We only stayed for half of it because he had to go to the bathroom. He refused to use the porta toilet, but he didn't wet his pants.

Then they stayed a couple of hours at my house munching, talking and playing. This little boy is just too cute. And, when we say that to him he'll say "I'm not too cute!"

I'm wearing my "boot" t-shirt, and I wore a bra under it to the parade this morning. I looked normal from the outside. I couldn't wear the bra all day though as my skin is still very tender. I'm going to call Dr. Gruber tomorrow to ask if I can go in this week to have it drained again.

Ann just called. I told her I may be up to going out for some "line dancing" by next Saturday night. If I line dance I'll be dancing solo. Then I won't have to worry about getting my arm yanked out of me.

Arthur and Reid think they've found a place downtown. If they decide on this place he'll be moving out in two weeks.

Oh, I gave Bridget the big green t-shirt you sent, and which I wore when I had the tubes in me. She needs maternity clothes and it fits her like one. Also it looks good on her because of her green eyes. I got the baby a cute outfit of blue pj's and a matching bib that says "I love my Daddy." She and Eric were thrilled over it. I also got her a baby's name book. They have a boy's name picked out, but not a girl's as yet.

I've been meeting so many interesting people through this computer service. I correspond with two ladies who have had mastectomies. One lives in Pennsylvania and had hers the week after me. Her arm is still pretty messed up too. She is preparing for her reconstruction and is going to have a saline implant. I talked to another lady who has a saline implant and she has had no problem with it. Also, some people have advised me that the abdominal tissue reconstruction is extremely painful, but in the end it's worth it.

I've been meeting men too. Unfortunately, they are younger than me. One is forty and one is thirty-eight. I'm trying to fix up a blind date for one of them with a co-worker of mine. Here's a letter from a guy in Los Angeles who is thirty. I just happened to print his. Usually I just read them, respond and then delete their letters.

It's been fun, interesting and entertaining of course. I don't know which service, if either, I'll use once my free month on Prodigy is up. I canceled America On Line when I went onto Prodigy.

Jon called me last night from Rob's. He and his girls are visiting Rob and his wife for the holiday.

I started this much earlier and have had some interruptions, and now I'm hungry again.

Bye. Love you,

July 8, Friday

Hi,

I got your card and letter when I got home from work tonight. It was a treat, and no we are not getting *too* mushy. I love mush and you know it! I wish I was joining you up in New Hampshire. But, guess what? I talked to my brother today and asked him if *we* could have the Sonoma townhouse next year, and the "we" includes Jack. He said "yes" and to let him know as far in advance as we can, so that he can keep it free for us. (The managers in his company use it too.)

Summer may be a little too warm. How about May of next year? Do you think you can save some money and vacation time for then, or maybe even early June? Actually I guess the spring is the prettiest. When I was there in April it was beautiful, but it was windy and cool at times. I need to save some vacation time and money too. I will probably drive up so that we will have a car for transportation and sightseeing. I could go up a few days early and visit with Bud and Lynn, and then meet you at the airport. It'll be fun, except I hardly ever drink wine anymore. But, there's still plenty of good food in that area too. Here I am talking about eating again.

Dr. Gruber told me that there is more fluid building up, but she doesn't want to keep putting needles in there to drain it because they can cause infections. I had read this in one of my reference books so I wasn't surprised. When I asked her how to shave under my arm she said, "Just do it." I said, "I can't." I showed her the "bulge" in my underarm. She seemed surprised that it was so big. It's something she calls a "cord" and it is what is bothering me so much when I try to stretch out my arm. This "cord" thing sticks out from my underarm to my elbow. Actually, not only does it hurt in that whole area, but it also hurts all the way down to the bottom of my ribs. It's weird. She said to give it another three weeks, and to put hot compresses on it at night.

What else have I been up to? Well, lots. I told you I have met quite a few people through Prodigy. Every night when I get home from work there is a bundle of e-mail waiting for me on the computer.

I've been asked out too! The ages range from twenty's to fifty's. Most of them are younger than me. My favorite is Blaine though. (I sent you one of his letters.) Since then we have written almost daily. I gave him my phone number and he called last night. We talked for over an hour. He sounds like such a sweetheart. It is too bad that he is young enough to be my son.

I am going off Prodigy this week-end as my free month is up. I want to think about which online service I want to use on a regular basis. It can get expensive and I need to cut back on my spending.

The women online have been so supportive. I met a forty year old in Maryland who just had her second mastectomy. She is a nurse on an oncology ward. My heart just breaks for her. She has written a book ("Welcome to the Club: The Realities of Breast Cancer") and it will be published soon. She started the book after her first mastectomy, and now has had to add another chapter regarding her second surgery. She is also a spokesperson for the American Cancer Society down in the South. These younger women who are being diagnosed with breast cancer just tear me up. They are all so brave.

The men I've met have been from all over the United States. There is one in St. Louis, Missouri who wants me to write him when I sign off Prodigy. He gave me his address. He's twenty-two and in college, majoring in criminal justice. I've been "counseling" him regarding his disappointments over women. Then there are the Backgammon addicts like me. I am getting my own Backgammon software this week-end.

I will miss all this, but I am getting too addicted to it and I think I need a break. They'll be there if I decide to return online a month or so from now. But, I tell you there are so many men on these services. It's the way to go to meet men these days. Forget the old newspaper ads.

I love my hair color, and I'm ready to let my hair grow out again. Maybe by the time you get here it'll be long, and I will have two boobs and be beautiful.

Somehow I'm losing weight. I told my brother that maybe it's a side effect of the Tamoxifen. According to what I've read though, and the women I've talked to, I'm supposed to be gaining weight. Arthur says that maybe I'm having a delayed reaction to the surgery. All I know is that I eat, but I just don't have the same appetite that I usually do.

(And you know I can always eat no matter what I'm feeling.) My weight is down to 105 pounds and I really don't want it to go any lower. I thought that if I ever quit smoking I would get fat. I also thought that once I went into menopause I would gain weight too. It's not happening. As a matter of fact I've been taking the Tamoxifen for one week now and it seems that I'm going to escape all those menopausal side effects after all.

Work is okay too. I get frustrated with myself because I don't have all the answers. It's going to take me longer to learn this job, to my satisfaction, than any job I've ever had. There is so much to learn, and computer technology changes daily.

Next week I will only be in my office for one day. On Tuesday I will observe my roommate giving AOS support, at Staff Development, for a new users class. One of the Staff Development Program Assistants does the training, but we provide the classroom support. On Thursday I'm "it" and I'll be providing the support by myself. On Wednesday I have an off site meeting, in a park, to help write our Mission Statement. And, Friday is our flex day. Next week should just fly by.

Well, this has been another long one.

Can you tell that all is great here?

Love you, and Jack too,

July 12, Tuesday

Rita,

Congratulations on passing your sailing test. I am amazed and impressed with how you have gotten into this sport. And, now your sister has too. You know that it won't be long before she's buying a boat!

Yes, I continue to do okay on the Tamoxifen. Two nights ago I might have had a side effect. I mean it didn't wake me up or anything. I woke up to go to the bathroom and I was soaked in sweat. That is not like me. But, I fell right back to sleep. I don't know if the problem I had with my appetite was from adjusting to the drug or not. I think I've got my appetite back and my weight seems to be stabilizing at 105 pounds. I definitely don't want it to go any lower. At this weight my bony butt is uncomfortable to sit on.

I am kind of worried about my arm. I exercise it, use it and every night I put a heating pad on it to loosen it up, but it's not getting better. I don't know if it's me wanting it to be normal too soon, or if it's my arm. I think the "cord" is too short for my arm, if that makes sense. When I try to stretch it out, it hurts like hell. I get it sort of loosened up, but then it goes right back to being too tight. I've exercised it, and stretched it so much that it actually hurts down at the bottom of my left rib cage. When I touch myself there it is sore and tender. It feels terribly bruised.

I wore a bra to work yesterday and today. I wore it with that thing that I sewed in it. Forget it. It comes way up high, and gets flattened from my seat belt. Tomorrow I'll do without it. Maybe on Thursday I'll try it again. I hope to get a prosthesis and some mastectomy bras when I'm flexing on Friday.

Arthur and Reid got the downtown apartment. It sounds like a nice place. It is theirs as of tomorrow, but they are not going to move all their belongings in until Saturday. Arthur is worse than me. He's spraying the place for bugs tonight. Then he and Reid will be cleaning and fixing things over there for the next three days. They have a little yard, which is good because Reid has a Doberman. I'm going to miss Arthur. I'll really miss his cleaning the bathroom every week!

He and I went to the store last night and I ordered a TV. It's 20" Sony Trinitron with stereo speakers. (Not that I have a stereo, but maybe someday.)

I know I have more to write, but it's time for me to quit.

Bye. Love you,

*J*uly 15, Friday

Dear Bud and Lynne:

This is my catch up on letter writing night and you are first since you both have been with me, and my check book all day. This was my Friday (flex day) off. It's also one month from the surgery and the day I have been anxiously waiting for.

I was at the Prosthesis store as soon as it opened. I had visited the store two or three weeks ago, and today I was ready to get fitted. The lady who owns the store was extremely helpful. She's been where I am. Just writing this gets me all teary eyed.

I was like a young kid getting her first bra, only much more excited. She asked me what size I wore, and I told her I had no idea as I have lost weight since the surgery. As it turned out I'm one cup smaller now. I tried on three prosthesis out of all the ones I had looked at when I was there previously.

I look so normal, and I feel so normal! It is wonderful. When I decided on this one I refused to take it off. She said "Are you going to wear it home?" and I said "You bet." I got one extra bra and got out of there at $400, and felt good about that. But, I think I would have paid three times that amount to feel this good about me. I can't wait to go to work Monday in one of my pretty dresses instead of a baggy jumper or vest. I look great!

I have my appetite back mostly. I did lose a few pounds, but I figure it won't take me long to gain them back. Also, the swelling and the fluid build up problem seems to be clearing up. Next is my arm. I am just impatient. When I asked the lady at the store how long it took her to get her arm back, to where it no longer hurt, she said it was about six months. I plan on meeting my doctor's estimate of six weeks.

Work is going smoothly. I am really proud of myself there too. I do not profess to know as much as my team members, but I'm learning. Yesterday was my first day as the support member to a new users training class. For eight hours I rescued the students who were having problems while the trainer was lecturing to them about the keystrokes for our e-mail system. I actually got them out of all kinds of weird computer places.

I have a few other letters to get to tonight that I have been negligent about. I wanted you to know again how much I appreciate everything, especially the fact that you are there.

Bye. Love you,

July 15, Friday

Dear Elaine:

Thank you for your note and the card. They are much appreciated.

Today is a big day for me. It has been one month since the mastectomy, and since I quit smoking, and also today I got my prosthesis. I love looking normal again. Of course when I get the reconstruction surgery I am going to feel even better.

I have made an incredible recovery, and I feel very fortunate.

Yes, I agree with you, this breast cancer disease has become an epidemic. It saddens me. What is especially upsetting for me is hearing about the number of younger women being diagnosed with it. Some have not been married yet, or had children, and my heart just aches for them.

I hope you are enjoying your summer off. I know you must work hard. I don't envy you your job. Being an elementary school principal is a big responsibility.

Originally I was planning to be in Boston one month from now. I was making arrangements to spend my birthday there with Rita and Jack. We were going to visit different places than when I was out there two years ago. Of course, it's all been suspended for now.

This has been a long day, but I had to write. I feel so bad that I don't write more often. Forgive me, but know that you are not being forgotten.

Bye. Love you,

July 15, Friday

Hi,

I wish you were with me today to share in my excitement. Notice the date? It's one month since the surgery.

Rita, it is too wonderful to describe. I am so proud of myself and I feel so normal. I look like me. I haven't taken the prosthesis off since I put it on in the store. I got two bras to go with it. They were expensive so I just got one white one and one in a flesh color. (I'll eventually get reimbursed for the prosthesis from my HMO though.)

I left the store in tears, because it felt so good. I keep getting tears in my eyes when I think about it. Can you imagine what I'm going to be like when I get the reconstruction surgery, if I'm like this over a prosthesis?

This has been one incredibly busy day. Well, actually it's been a busy week.

But, before I go any further. Have you heard any more from Maria? Did you send her the clothes and the money? Did she write to you again? Let me know the continuing story there.

Your week-end with Linda and Larry sounded like so much fun. I'm glad you have her there. Really, I know we tease about the situation of "best" friend, but I am glad she is your best "Massachusetts" friend. I hope you took some pictures of the week-end and the Mt. Washington Hotel. I'm jealous. I loved that place when we were there.

Your mother cannot be seventy years old. She looks like she is in her fifties. That's amazing. But, then again, of course she has to be about that age because of your (our) age, but I never thought about it because she looks so young.

Work is wonderful. I had a fun week, but I was tired every night. On Wednesday we did the offsite at the park to write the Mission Statement. I work with some really funny people. Mostly I work with men, and you know when they get together they are just like little boys. I had so much fun doing the off-site that I felt like I was at a summer day camp.

Bruce brought a croquette set, and I haven't played this game since I was about ten years old. We played a "rough" game on our lunch hour. They had me laughing so hard. Myself and one other female played with the men, and it was hilarious. The meeting itself was productive, and funny too. All in all it was a really good day, and I am glad that I was back at work so that I could enjoy it.

Yesterday I did the AOS support for Staff Development all by myself. It was an eight hour class. What I did was (from the back of the classroom) watch eight students and their monitors during the lecture. When they hit the wrong keys, or got themselves into a jam, it was my job to bail them out, and fast, so that they could get right back into the lesson and not miss anything. These were brand new users. It was very busy, but I enjoyed it. And, I actually got them out of all their problems. (That was the amazing part!) This class can be up to twelve students so fortunately for me it was a small group. When it was over the students thanked the trainer, and then me, for helping them. The trainer gave me a nice compliment. She said I did perfect, and you'd never have known it was my first time. Considering that I am new I felt really good about this.

The TV that I ordered, and paid cash for on Monday night, and that Arthur was supposed to pick up on Thursday night, turned out to not exist. When he got there they told him that there were none left, and it would take until at least next Tuesday to get me one from another store. (They are a big chain here in Southern California.) Arthur asked for my money back and they refused him. They said it would take about ten days for me to get a refund. When he got home and told me I was not too pleased.

I said, "No Arthur. I will have either a TV, or my money from them by 6:30", which was in a half hour. To make this short, I got the cash. I went to the store and very calmly, but firmly told them they would give me back my cash right then, and they did. I went to another store and got the same TV for a little bit more, but it was still a good price. I think the first store was advertising falsely.

Bye. Love you,

July 18, Monday

Hi,

I got these pictures today so I thought I would send them to you. They were taken on May 12th, my last day at the old job, and the day I found that out I was going into the hospital to for the biopsy. Do I look stressed, or what? This is my previous boss, Shannon and the other picture is the Medical Social Worker, Linda. She and I became friends while I was working there. Her office was next to mine.

Thank you for your offer of the heating pad. My arm still hurts to stretch it, but I am using it for everything, including three hours of non-stop dancing yesterday afternoon. The first dozen dances hurt, and after that either my arm was all stretched out, or my endorphins had kicked in and I was just too happy to feel any pain. When I got up this morning I felt it, but I don't care as much now that I know that I can dance again!

And guess who was there, and I danced with him? Rob was there with his wife, Sherry. He asked me to do a West Coast Swing dance with him and it was fun.

Allen was there. He had just gotten back on Saturday from his Alaskan cruise and was leaving today for New York. It was good to see him and dance with him too. Actually the whole evening was wonderful.

I had started the day by meeting Ann at a dance/brunch in Long Beach. It was okay. I danced about half a dozen dances. But, they felt so good that I decided to go to the Cowboy in the afternoon, and I'm glad I did.

The men that I normally dance with asked me where I had been. I told them what has been going on. They were wonderful about it. Some said really kind things to me. One didn't. It was male humor again which I couldn't appreciate. When I said "mastectomy" he started laughing and said, "You had a vasectomy?" Yuck.

I might even go to a dance graduation party Wednesday night after work. Do you believe this? I am just thrilled that I am dancing again.

My dance clothing is sort of limited. I kept trying on things for both dances, and most of my summer dance clothes are v-neck, or too low cut for any "ducking" type moves. I tried some on, and bent over in front of my full length mirror. "Nope." You could see down in there, and there was a big gap between my bra and my skin!

Arthur got moved. It is quiet and extremely peaceful here. It's nice living alone again. The bathroom is all mine. The phone is quiet. (I like that.) I'm not saying that Arthur was any problem to live with though. Actually, he was the ideal roommate.

This got longer than I anticipated, and it's time for me to get in the shower.

Bye. Love you,

July 22, Friday

Hi,

Would you believe it is before eight in the morning and here I am at the PC? Today is my short day. I go in at nine so I thought I'd sleep in, but wrong. I was up at five. I've gotten lots done: laundry, changing bed linen, washing dishes, and other mundane chores.

Tonight I'm going to a party after work. It should be interesting. Remember my friend, Rick, who got promoted to the same position, as me, at Systems right after I transferred here? This is his promotion party which is being held by some of the old timers from our West District office.

I also went to a party Wednesday night. It was my friend Ann's dance graduation party. There were a lot of people there. I saw and danced with that guy, Larry, whom I met through his personal ad. (Remember the ad that read like mine?) He's the one I also ran into at church when I had just found out about the breast cancer. I'd forgotten to tell you that he also called me a few weeks ago to see how I was doing. There's something "hokey" about him. I mean he is out there meeting all these women and saying he wants a relationship. He acts really interested and then "poof" he's gone.

I asked him about the lady that I saw him with at church. He met her through his ad also. She was young and good looking. But, he said he never called her again after that morning. (That's what happened to me too.) Anyway, he was at the party as they had a meeting for a dance cruise that he'll be going on in September. Allen is going on it too.

I asked him to dance. Surprisingly, he was a good dancer. While we were dancing he asked me which arm was messed up because it wasn't obvious to him. I said , "If you don't know, I'm not telling you." Then he laughed and said, "Well, if I knew which one I could be more gentle with it." (Right. I know what he was trying to figure out.)

Saturday I am going to babysit Nick over night.

I'll take Nick to church with me, and then take him home afterwards. So, I've got my "hot" date with a cute, and funny little man planned for this week-end!

Bye. Love you,

P.S.I got kind of upset Wednesday night. I have met three wonderful women through Prodigy. I had signed off for ten days because I am getting really addicted, and it is running up my phone bill. (It is a toll call to use this service, plus the charges for the "extra" features.) Anyway, I missed being online. I also missed hearing from my new friends so I signed up again. I sent a message to Sharon before I went to the dance. She responded and told me that Sue and she had been writing while I was off-line . She said that Sue was having another mastectomy. She just finished her chemo this summer. I was really sick over this news. I wrote Sue immediately, and I got the response this morning. She's okay. This is elective surgery since she is such a high risk for a recurrence. She has chosen to have her other breast removed, and then have both breasts reconstructed at the same time. Thank God. I thought they'd found another malignant lump. I'll tell you this bothered me a lot until I heard from her. My other pen pal, Lillie just had her second breast removed. It was not elective. I have put she and Sue in touch with each other. It's like we have this great friendship and support group going online. Strange, huh?

July 23, Saturday Journal Writing

It's time for me to call my own bluff. I've been saving copies of letters, and my journal writing, since this breast cancer experience started. I've said I'm going to write a book about it. When Rita was teasing me that I haven't been writing her letters as much anymore I said, "But, I'm writing you a book." My Prodigy pen pal Lillie has written a book. She pointed me in the direction of who to mail a manuscript to. Now it's time for me to start cleaning up all these miscellaneous letters and notes. This will obviously be a time consuming project in the near future. But, I've got the time, and the therapy of writing my story will be beneficial to me. Besides, I am bored with this Journal Writing.

Physically I feel wonderful. My arm is still feeling like the insides are shorter than the outsides, but I guess this is normal. I stretch it daily. I am dancing and that's a big plus. If I can dance, then my arm, and all of me, is *okay*.

Emotionally, mentally and spiritually I am in good shape. I am one lucky lady and I know it. I am lucky in so many areas of my life.

There is a country song that I can relate to lately that goes, "Life's a dance *you* learn as you go."

July 27, Wednesday

Hi,

I can't tell you how happy I was to get your long letter tonight. I've missed talking to you on the phone. I've felt like there hasn't been as much communicating between us lately. This long letter makes up for a phone call. The pictures are beautiful, and you sound wonderful. I am glad that Maria is writing to you. That is so neat the way things turned out for her.

Yes, my prosthesis is very comfortable. I think I lucked out again. It fits me perfectly and looks quite natural. Yesterday I even wore a summer sweater to work. My skin doesn't hurt at all. The only discomfort I have left is around my elbow area when I stretch my arm. I can feel that cord through my whole arm. It strains and sticks out, and the shortness ends at my elbow, and that hurts. Someday I guess it will be free of pain. Of course I will never get the feeling back in parts of my chest and underarm. When I shave my underarm now I do it looking in a mirror, and very carefully. (I cannot feel the razor there at all. I can't even feel deodorant when I put it on.)

Yes, my HMO will cover the reconstructive surgery. I'm looking forward to it with mixed emotions. Once again, of the types of implants, they all have so many "cons," and as I hear it the only "pro" is having a breast again.

Okay we'll aim for May as our vacation in Sonoma, Napa and San Francisco. We will have a lot of fun.

Did I write and tell you that I went dancing again Sunday afternoon for over two hours? I enjoyed myself immensely. I wore the silk vest you sent me over a silk blouse of the same color and my short black leather skirt. It was a different looking outfit, but I got compliments on how I looked so it must have been okay. I think some of the guys are trying to figure out which side of me is not real. I see them sneaking little peeks and it's kind of funny actually.

I called Danielle and told her you said to say "hi." Then she invited me to her house for dinner tomorrow night. This will be the first time I've been to her new house. She said it is almost ready for the open house party which she plans on having soon.

Oh, I also got a surprisingly pleasant piece of mail tonight. There was a card with a return address in New York. I could not figure out who it was from. It was a beautiful card from Allen. He wrote some really nice sentiments in it. I am very touched by what he wrote. I wish I could show it to you.

I'm writing "our" book. Remember I told you I would? Lillie my breast cancer sister in Maryland is giving me some direction as to how to contact Publishers. I got the "1994 Writer's Market" book this weekend. It lists who to contact. I thought I'd better get something together to send them so I work on it a little each night. It's probably boring with all my personal stories, which no one in their right mind would read except you. But, it's good therapy for me.

Last night was my first support meeting with the hospital cancer group. I thought it would be all breast cancer women. Wrong. It was a small and cozy group though. The Social Worker from the hospital facilitated, and also present were:

A girl in her twenty's, and engaged to be married. Not quite two years ago she went to her regular doctor for an annual pap smear. When she was there he was pushing on her while doing the pelvic exam. He asked her if it was "sensitive," and she said "yes," because you know it always is when they do that. Then he sent her for some x-rays. The next day she was in surgery having a huge tumor removed from her hip. She had to have part of her buttocks removed too. She didn't even suspect that she had anything wrong, and she was filled with cancer. She has had one set back this past year. They found more cancer and she had another surgery. Now she has to walk with a cane. She is so pretty, sweet and very upbeat and positive.

The other brand new member of the group is in her early thirties and she had cancer surgery last month. She is married and has two young children. She is also quite attractive, sweet and has a positive attitude. For two years she had a pain in her side that wouldn't go away. She kept seeing doctors for it and they indicated to her that she was a hypochondriac. Finally eight weeks ago one doctor decided to do some surgery to look at her gallbladder. (He did this when she and her husband became insistent that something was wrong.) When they removed her gallbladder they also removed some tissue surrounding it and sent it to the lab to be biopsied. She was not aware that this was being done. One week later she stopped at the doctor's on her way to work to have her staples removed. The pain had finally gone away once her gallbladder and the surrounding tissue was removed. She felt great, and thought that the appointment was just going to be a routine follow-up. The doctor told her that she had cancer and she had less than five years to live. She was so upset with this totally unexpected news that she crashed her truck in the hospital parking lot as she was leaving. As it turned out, when she went back in to the hospital for more cancer surgery, they discovered that the cancer was in her bile duct, and not where they thought it was when they gave her the five years prognosis. She plans on living a very long life.

The longest cancer survivor in the group is just so courageous. She is probably in her early forties, and you've got it. She is a also quite attractive and has a sweet personality. Ten years ago she was diagnosed with breast cancer. She had a lumpectomy with radiation. Her lymph nodes were negative and she had no chemotherapy. She was being monitored every six months by her doctors which is standard follow-up care. Shortly after, and I don't remember the time span, but maybe a year later, they found a recurrence in the same breast and some of her remaining lymph nodes. They did a mastectomy and put her on heavy duty chemotherapy. They thought they got it the second time. A few years went by. Then, at one of her follow-up visits they discovered that the breast cancer was in her liver. Again, she went through some very strong chemotherapy. She has been cancer free for a number of years now.

Is this scary stuff or what?

Our next meeting is the night of my birthday. When I mentioned this they were going to reschedule it, but I told them I really didn't have any other plans. I told them how my original plans to celebrate my birthday with you kind of got postponed until next year.

I told you about my online friends. There are four of us and I thought it was so unique to have a support group like this. We can just write each other when we feel like it, and respond when we feel like it. Usually there's a message from one or the other of them every night. It's excellent support. I was sharing all this with the support group last night. The Social Worker said she'd heard that some breast cancer women were forming online groups like ours. I guess we're not so original after all.

Quite a few of the men I have met online have given me their home phone numbers, but I haven't called anyone yet. I also have some addresses, and I gave my number to two of the men. One of them is Blaine and I guess I told you that he has called a couple of times now.

Some of the men sound interesting, but I don't think I'm quite ready for a relationship. The day will come, but between upcoming surgeries and my new job, my dance card is pretty full already.

This is a long letter and I hope it makes up for not writing daily anymore. (Joke)

Love you,

July 27, Monday

Dear Allen:

I cannot tell you how pleased I was when I got home and opened this beautiful, and very thoughtful, card from you. I couldn't imagine who was sending me something from New York. I hope I have read the address right and that this reaches you.

You are a good friend. I know we get frustrated with each other at times, but you are still my friend. I love you too.

Well, how is New York and your family? It must be wonderful for you to be with all of them again, and eating all your favorite foods. We'll just have to dance you lots when you get home and work all those calories off of you.

I have been dancing four times since the surgery, and have had a lot of fun each time. It's interesting how an experience like this can change your perspective and attitude. I appreciate everything so much more. The things I used to take for granted are very special to me now.

See you when you get back from vacation.
Bye. Love you,

July 30, Thursday

Rita,

Even though I wrote you only two days ago I feel like I need to write a long letter as a lot has happened since. And, you're right. All I talk about anymore is men, boobs and computers.

Well, let's see. How about if I write about men in this one? Rita, I met one of my online pen pals last night. He was truly darling. It was Blaine, the thirty year old from Los Angeles. He called me at eight and said he was going to be in Orange County later in the evening, and did I want to meet somewhere. I was in my pj's and watching a video, with a big bag of gourmet popcorn. But, he convinced me to get dressed and go out. (We've been going to meet before now, but it's never quite worked out.) As it is, he is on his way, this morning, to Las Vegas for a week of business meetings.

I got to the agreed upon club early. At about the time we were supposed to meet, and in the throng of many, I saw him. I mean I saw someone matching his description and then I thought, "Okay now picture him in an IBM business suit." As soon as I did that I knew it was him. He was so surprised when I walked up and touched his arm. He said, "How did you recognize me?"

We danced a lot, but I think I was wearing him out. He is a beginner Two Stepper and doesn't do West Coast Swing. He does have his own kind of swing that was great fun though. We talked as much as we could in a noisy place like that. After a couple of hours Blaine said he had to get back to his cousin's club. (That's why he was in Orange County. He was meeting relatives at another club where his cousin was singing.) He walked me out to my car, and he was a total gentleman. I'm glad I met him.

Thursday night I went to Danielle's for dinner. Her new house is big, spacious, and well taken care of. Danielle is in seventh heaven between her yards and her very own garage work bench. (I swear she reminds me of L.S. at times.) We talked about anything and everything, and ate way too much. She is a great cook. She fixed chicken, pasta, some kind of a cabbage salad and lemon mousse cake for dessert. Yum!

You would really like her. She is so interesting and smart. Danielle told me that she knows her fourteen year relationship would never have worked out if they had gotten married, or moved in together. She likes and values her independence, and doesn't want all the grief that comes from living with a man. She has her cake and gets to eat it too. I need to take lessons from her.

Today was "color my hair day." How often do you have to go to the hairdresser to have it done? I just had it done four weeks ago and already my white streak was declaring itself.

Dani called me. She's coming over tomorrow. I got her a little birthday cake and a purple hat. It's the kind that the little girls wear with the front flattened and a flower on it. For her birthday gifts I got her a Ken doll and some clothes for him. When I gave her a Barbie wedding dress a few months ago she was insistent that now her Barbie needed a husband.

My new neighbors next door are noisy. Thank goodness I spend a lot of time back here in the bedroom, and I don't have any adjoining walls or floors with them. I wonder how Jerry and Gloria, who used to live there, but moved downstairs, like having them living over them.

Jon is coming down again from Northern California in August. We are going to get together on the 10th, to visit and to celebrate my birthday by going out to dinner. I'm looking forward to it.

I know there must be tons more to tell you, but honestly I spend a lot of time lately typing letters to my Prodigy pen pals. I can't believe how many letters I write a day. I'm forcing myself to push these keys right now.

Love you,

August

Hello again.

Since we talked for an hour last night I don't think there's much more to write about, but I've got some new pictures to send you so I'll have to think up a few lines.

Here goes. In my mail tonight I got a post card from Atlantic City, New Jersey. It was from Allen. Again he sent a very sweet message. I am just amazed. I don't understand this, but that's all right. I've taken a new approach on some things and instead of trying to figure out everything that comes into my life I'm attempting to go with the flow.

I get to do my first solo IRMA support tomorrow which involves training a group of supervisors. The supervisors just got brand new PC's. On the average they are inexperienced with Windows and other types of software. IRMA is the access to our main frame programs, going through a PC instead of using a dumb terminal. Since this is totally new for me, I am kind of nervous about being the support person for this type of class. But, the only way I'm going to learn it is to do it. There are two classes, one in the morning and one in the afternoon. Wish me luck.

Love you lots,

August 3, Wednesday

Hi,

I'm sitting here crying my eyes out again and feeling the most depressed I've been since before the surgery. I am tempted to call you, but you'd be at work. I'd probably get Jack again, and then I'd get him upset and he'd call you at work.

I don't even know where to begin. Do I just come right out with it? Yes, and explain about it further on. I am going to need chemotherapy after all. I can't even type the word without gushing tears.

I am so upset right now I can't think, let alone try to write. I'll have to come back and forth to this letter. I can't stop crying. It's as bad as the day they told me I had the cancer.

I keep asking myself, "Why me?" Let me explain to you what happened today. Did I tell you I had an appointment with Dr. Cheng last Friday? I wanted to thank her for remembering to send me for my regular mammograms, and also to ask her for a referral for a cholesterol test. (I figured I'd had every other type of test done on me lately so I might as well get that one done too.) Since I had to fast for fourteen hours prior to the test I waited until today to go to the blood lab. I already had scheduled time off from work, because today was my appointment with Dr. Nielsen. I told my office that I'd be in at eleven o'clock after the appointment with him.

I fasted, and got to the lab before nine to do the blood test. Then I went to a pancake house and splurged on one huge breakfast. I had the high cholesterol, fatty works. (This is rare as I live on extremely healthy foods these days.) Then I went to Dr. Nielsen's for my ten o'clock appointment. I was all dressed up, and ready to hop on the freeway to go to work directly from his office. I was not expecting any big deal to come out of this "check-up" regarding the Tamoxifen.

He comes into the room and asks me how I'm doing with the fluid build up, the Tamoxifen and of course the use of my arm. I'm beaming, and I tell him that all are fine and I'm ready for the next step, so when do I get to see the plastic surgeon.

Dr. Nielsen says, "First let's talk about chemotherapy." I got confused, and I thought he must have mixed me up with someone else. I said, "But, I'm not on chemo." He says, "I know. That's what we need to talk about. After consulting with some of my colleagues I feel I made a mistake in not giving you the chemotherapy."

I was dumb struck. I was speechless. I started crying. I asked, "Why?" He said that he thinks now that because I am pre-menopausal, and young, that the Tamoxifen isn't enough. I guess he's worried about the estrogen in my body. (I think it's also because of that 50% infiltration in the biopsy report.)

We talked some, and I cried a lot. He was very comforting and apologetic, but I was, and still am, devastated. He said there will be no reconstruction until after I have completed the six months of chemotherapy. Here I go again bawling my eyes out.

My positive attitude has just gone flying out the window. I'm about as depressed as I was that night when I wrote you the horrible letter because I had figured out that my cancer was worse than I originally believed. It was the night I thought I would probably have to have the chemotherapy. Remember? I remember it well. It was a truly black night for me.

Dr. Nielsen took me over to the chemotherapy clinic to meet the nurses. They wanted to start the chemo this week, but I asked for it to begin next week instead. I want to celebrate my birthday "chemo free." I also asked for it to be done on Fridays so I would have the week-ends to recover, and also so that I can use some of my flex Fridays. **I don't want to do this!**

The nurses were very nice, but I was extremely emotional and couldn't stop crying. They didn't understand that this had just been sprung on me, and I was in shock over it.

I saw where it'll be administered and they told me the type of chemo, the side effects and what to do if there are emergencies from them. They gave me tons of reading material and scheduled me for Friday the 12th at ten o'clock for my first treatment.

The nurse said I may not lose my hair because it is so thick. She said it's usually the people with thin hair that lose all of it. My hair will thin out though, but she couldn't say by how much.

Dr. Nielsen suggested that I get a turban just in case it does fall out, and I feel the need to cover my head while I go out looking for a wig. I called the wig catalogue company in Massachusetts and ordered two turbans.

There are more side effects than I like to think about. Let's see if I can remember a few. I was not in good shape. I think I was having an attack of Attention Deficit Disorder. After I read through the material they gave me, and research through my cancer books I will know more. This is being written off the top of my head. The nurse said that I will probably have really bad diarrhea. I may start urinating blood. I may run a temperature. For a severe case of the "runs," or actually any of the above, I need to go to the emergency room. (Right. It's on the other side of the world from me.) She said I will have nausea, but they will give me a prescription to help with that. If the prescription doesn't work, and I can't stop vomiting, again I should go to the emergency room.

They will closely monitor my blood count to watch for any drastic reductions in the good blood cells. If necessary they will give me a transfusion to bring it back up to normal.

Rita, I hate this and I haven't even started yet. I'm angry. I'm depressed. I'm scared. I tell myself that by tonight, and then tomorrow, and as each day passes, I will be okay again. But, right now I am just plain miserable.

Another concern is that I will have sores in my mouth, and my gums will bleed. Between my immune system being stripped, and the unhealthy mouth, I am going to be very prone to catching any type of cold or flu from people who get near me. The nurse said I will have to be especially careful around little kids. This is not going to go over big this winter. Dani always has a runny nose.

Where was I? I left the chemo clinic and went to a pay phone. It was after eleven o'clock and I had to call work. I called the other team's supervisor. (My team is still without one.) I kept crying. Finally I was able to tell her that I wouldn't be in today after all. I felt pretty bad about this.

Then I had to drive back to the blood lab, which is in another city, to get my second blood test of the day. The chemo clinic needed a baseline cell count so that they will know what to compare it to once the chemo starts.

I hope I will be okay at work tomorrow. I told everyone in the world that I didn't need chemo, and now I don't even want to talk about this to anyone.

My phone bill is going to be outrageous from using Prodigy. I am going online one last time today to say good-bye, again, to my friends there. My breast cancer sisters have my address. I could use the support right now, but once again I am starting to worry about future finances.

I doubt you'll be getting letters about men much in the next eight months or so. I was beginning to feel like starting to date again, but now my week-ends, or a good portion of them anyway, are probably going to be spent in bed and hanging around the bathroom.

Actually, I won't be going every week. Hopefully I will have good weeks in between. I think Dr. Nielsen said that he is giving me a mild treatment, and I think he said it will be eight sessions over the next six months. That would be nice.

Oh, the nurse suggested I have someone accompany me for the first couple of treatments. We'll see.

I love you. Sorry about more bad news.

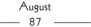

August 3, Wednesday

Rita,

Didn't I just mail you a letter? Well, here goes #2 for the day. I'm writing because I got a package from the mailman. There was a note in Spanish on it, which I think was telling me to not open it until my birthday. But, since I don't know Spanish and I needed a boost, I opened it anyway. I'm glad I did!

Yes, all the petites fit. I love them. You know how I always wash or dry clean new clothes before I wear them? I sewed a loose hem on the vest, and ironed the whole outfit to wear to work tomorrow. I need something to help me stay cheered up and daring, so I can make it through the day after this morning's blow. This outfit is wild compared to my normally ultra conservative work clothes. It will be especially outrageous when I wear the tan socks and a pair of flat shoes with it. I mean this is the County of Orange Social Services Agency Administration offices. Thank you!

Also, the book mark is special. Everything is perfect and lifted my spirits.

I've been doing my research so I can understand the current phase of this experience. I know this won't mean much to you, but I'll explain it briefly anyway. The chemo that I'll be having will be three drugs with the initials CMF. It's considered adjuvant chemotherapy treatment, and will be administered intravenously. The combination of the three drugs will hopefully stop and/or slow down the fast cell growth. I think I will be having it done every three weeks. On this schedule I should have time in between treatments to recover. Since CMF will be affecting all areas of my body that have fast growing cells, this includes the healthy fast growing cells which are in my mouth, bones, intestines, bladder and also hair follicles.

According to what I've read hair loss is only an occasional side effect from two of the three drugs. It is not a major side effect in any of the three. I am very pleased about this. Now I understand why the nurse is optimistic that I won't lose my hair, and if there is any loss it should only be some thinning out.

It's important that I eat lots so that I don't lose weight and that I eat foods high in protein, iron and potassium. And, I need to drink lots of fluids, especially water, which you know I love to drink anyway.

If I am lucky, which is what I plan on being, I should just need the week-end after each session to recover, and then I'll return to work on Monday mornings. I know I will be tired, but fortunately the job I have right now is the least stressful of any that I've had in years.

I got another post card from Allen. This one was from the Canada side of Niagara Falls. He sounds like he is really enjoying himself. He said he would be back on August 10th and he couldn't wait to dance with me again. Well, I doubt I'll be dancing that week-end. Allen is really shocking me with all this mail. I've known him for years. He has traveled all over the world, but he never sent me cards before.

Karen sent me a beautiful friendship birthday card also. I called her to thank her and told her what was going on. She said that she and Bob are dancing right after work Friday at "In Cahoots." She invited me to meet them there. I might just do that as I have to dance my little feet off while I still can.

I went online and wrote good bye notes to my Prodigy friends. I plan to continue corresponding with my breast cancer sisters. I gave the men my home number. (Of course I told everyone my news.) Then I contacted Prodigy and told them to disconnect me as of tomorrow. I'll miss it, but I don't think I should be spending money on that right now.

My brother is in Washington DC for the week. I talked to Lynn tonight instead. She feels badly that I have to go through this, but I explained to her that I do understand why it is necessary. I was really surprised when Dr. Nielsen told me last month that I didn't have to have chemo, based on my biopsy report and my understanding of the necessary treatments through the reading I had done. So, even though I do not want to go through this, I think that it is a good, extra precautionary step. If I refused this and had a recurrence in the future, I would never be able to forgive myself.

Tomorrow is back to work with chin up, and smile in place.

Love you,

P.S. I just called Danielle. She said that she will take me to the first session on the 12th. What would I do without the two of you to help get me through this?

August 4, Thursday

Rita,

You said to write so here I am. You're not getting enough letters, huh? Actually since we talked for so long last night about everything this will be short. But, I got your card and pictures. Your hammock looks quite inviting. And, I'm sighing over those flowers.

I finally took two sleeping pills last night in order to fall asleep. Between my shock from yesterday, and then being hung over from pills I felt like a zombie at work today. I had more problems with my work computer than I have had in the whole time I've been there. It was just an all around frustrating day.

As always the people in Systems were wonderful to me about this new development. (This must be getting old for them.) My Manager, Sandi, was so kind to me. She told me that they want me to get well, and they want to keep me in the Systems Division. She also said that one of the trainers, whose class I supported on Tuesday, called her and raved about me, and the way I had supported his class. She said he's a perfectionist and this is a big compliment from him. Sandi also said that the Manager over all of Systems expressed compliments to her about me and the new procedure I wrote, and how quickly I did it. I just couldn't thank her enough for all these good feeling type things she was sharing with me. I told her I'm still unsure of myself most days and the compliments help.

I wore my new birthday outfit today. It was quite a different me. You are the one who gets me to get out of my conservative clothes every once in awhile. That's good, and I thank you.

When I got home from work there was a message on my answering machine from my breast cancer sister, Sharon. She was crying, because of my message regarding the chemo. Sharon had just gotten my e-mail from yesterday and she thought I might be home again today. She goes back to work on Monday.

I called her tonight and we talked "Live" for the first time. It was as if we have known each other for years. She is forty, married and has a seven year old son. I think I've written you about her before. She is such a sweetie. Sharon had calmed down quite a bit since this morning when she had read my e-mail, called me and left her message. I plan to keep up a correspondence with her through postal mail.

Also, I was able to sign on as it takes a couple of days for them to process a cancellation request. There was a message from my "Boston Buddy." He had just gotten back from his business trip to Massachusetts. He said he would call me one night and we'd talk and get to know each other more than we have through our e-mail.

I have enjoyed the Prodigy program after all. When I first went on, it seemed old and boring compared to AOL. But, I met so many nice people through this service that it was worth it..

I had forgotten that I ordered CompuServe, which is another online service. I've already paid for it. When the software arrives I'll have to try it. I hope it is a local call.

I have to share a cute story which Bridget told me the last time she was here. She said that she called Eric at work one night and asked him to stop on the way home, and get her something "yummy" to eat. She was having a pregnancy craving and there wasn't anything that interested her at home.

Bridget said that Eric went to three different fast food places, and bought her, her most favorite foods from each. I think she said it was something like corn from one place, french fries from another and tacos from another. Can you imagine a husband doing that? I wish I had a husband that would be that good to me.

Bye. Love you,

August 6, Saturday

Hi,

Here's a short one. (At least I think it will be.) I have been getting all these terrific birthday cards from you. They brighten my days. Thank you.

Yesterday was a better day. I was actually able to function at work. This next phase will be okay too. I was just thrown temporarily.

Last night I met Karen and Bob at "In Cahoots." It's always fun to be with them. I was there for about five minutes, and was telling Karen that I had seen and danced with Paul on Sunday. I looked up and Paul was standing in front of me. He stayed at our table for about two hours. We talked and danced a lot. It was another fun evening for me.

Today I went to get my Tamoxifen prescription re-filled and the pharmacy clerk said that there is no charge for it. I had no idea. The last time the girl charged me. My prescriptions are minimal, but I'll be getting it refilled every month and this was a pleasant surprise. (I read somewhere that these little pills normally cost $1.50 each. That's $3.00 a day!)

I took Nick for his hair cut, because he told me that his hair was getting "too big." We also went on a spending spree at a Marshall's store. I let him pick out new shoes, clothes and a book. All the clothes were Power Rangers of course. He asked if he could come back to my house. While he played with the box of toys and puzzles I keep for them, I cooked spinach fettucini for lunch.

I also got Bridget more baby clothes and took Tamsin a box of fancy chocolates. I told both of them that I probably won't be doing anymore "splurges" like this for awhile.Since I had a one hour nap I hope to go out dancing again tonight. I want to get as much dancing in this weekend as I can. The rest of my week is booked pretty full in the evenings too. Monday I meet with a Practitioner from my church for a free counseling session. It's my birthday present from our church. We call it a "spiritual tune-up." I've had them the last few years and enjoyed each session immensely. Tuesday night is the Cancer Support Group at the hospital, and on Wednesday night I meet Jon for dinner. I'm worn out from thoughts of this coming week. I'm not used to having a night life during the week anymore.

Gotta go.

Bye. Love you,

August 7, Sunday

Hello there,

I didn't think I'd be writing again this soon, but I felt the need to talk so here I am. Actually, I've got to start getting ready to go dancing. I am going to wear my prettiest "frock" and get all decked out for my birthday dancing this afternoon.

My breast cancer sister from San Diego called, but I was taking a nap. She is the only one that I don't have a home number for, and she didn't leave it. She said that she would call again tonight. I hope it's after I get home from the Cowboy.

Even though I signed off of Prodigy I'm still able to continue logging on. I think they'll probably disconnect me as of tomorrow. I was glad I could get on today though. Rob sent me an online birthday card. Rita it was so neat. When it came on I just sat here going "WOW." Then when it started playing "Happy Birthday" I was laughing out loud. It was a "hippy bird" birthday card.

Last night I went to the club down the street. I got there early and sat at the bar. I started dancing and talking with a younger man from Los Angeles. We talked and danced for about two hours. He was shocked when he found out that I was a grandmother.

I charged up my VISA some more. This time I got birthday gifts for me. I bought: two pairs of shoes. One pair of Reeboks is to leave in my desk at work. (I walk twice a day on my fifteen minute breaks. I've been doing it in pumps, and I walk fast to get the exercise. These will be much more comfortable.) Also, I got some Avia aerobic/walking shoes for at home use. I got a Liz Clairborne purse in burgundy leather. I look forward to the day when I will have all new purses which do not have tobacco through out the bottoms and inside the pockets. I also got two work dresses. These dresses will be my "pick me up" clothes when I have meetings, or trainings on days that I'm not feeling too perky.

I have to start getting ready for my night on the town. I wish you were coming with me.

Bye. Love you,

August 9, Tuesday, Journal Writing

Today is my birthday. It has been an interesting year, what with a broken engagement, stalking type problems, a change in jobs, and now the breast cancer. I would never have made these predictions a year ago. A year ago I would have said that I would be married, and living happily ever after.

What are my predictions for the coming year? I have no clue. I foresee months of chemotherapy and then reconstruction surgeries.

Rita and I have talked about vacationing together in San Francisco and Sonoma next spring. I also talk constantly about getting past all these breast cancer challenges and then traveling to Knoxville, Tennessee to appear on TNN's Club Dance.

Professionally I think I will continue learning more about computers and will start taking on more difficult assignments.

In November there will be the birth of Eric and Bridget's baby. That is something which I am really looking forward to.

Men? Will there be any, or one, in my life in the coming year? At times I would definitely like someone to be here, but at other times I realize that that would be an additional stress which I can do without at this point in my life.

August 10, Wednesday

Hello,

I've been up since four-thirty and I didn't get to sleep until after eleven which is late for me. I hope I make it through the day, and that I make it to, and through this evening. Jon will be here at seven. I usually don't get home from work until after six, so I can see me rushing around to get showered and dressed. We are going to "The Olive Garden," which is one of my favorite Italian restaurants. I am looking forward to it, but I hope I have some energy left.

Last night my support group got canceled.

When I got home from work I called the twin from the Cowboy who had the mastectomy and chemotherapy last year. Did I tell you about her?

I have watched she and her sister dance for years. Then Pat dropped out of sight for awhile. She showed up twice this past year with really short hair. Normally she and her sister have long, curly, country style hair. She had also lost weight. I didn't really think much about it at the time.

A couple of weeks ago one of my dance partners told me that Pat had breast cancer also. This Sunday her twin sister, Betty, was sitting at the end of our table. I asked her about Pat and she gave me her phone number.

Pat was as wonderful as all the other women I have talked to. She is forty-three, quite beautiful, single, has no kids and loves to dance. One and a half years ago she discovered a lump. She said it was the size of a walnut and by the time they removed her lymph nodes three of them had cancer cells in them.

Breast cancer runs in her family. Her grandmother, mother, and younger sister have all had breast cancer. She said that Betty believes it's not a matter of "if," but "when" for her to be diagnosed also. This is too sad!

She had only four sessions of chemotherapy, but she had the stronger drug administered. Her hair fell out after the first session. Pat said that when I saw her with the short hair, it was her own hair just starting to grow back. She wore a wig when she was bald. Oh, and she had to have two or three transfusions because of her blood counts dropping so low. She said they gave her a blood test twice a week over the five months period.

Pat said that she tried to dance when her blood count wasn't low, but she'd get half way through a dance and her heart would be pounding so bad, that she would have to quit and sit down. She thinks that it's okay for me to go into crowds when my count hasn't dropped, but that on days when it's down I probably shouldn't leave the house. Pat was lucky and had an excellent disability plan so she hardly worked at all. Her employer told her to take all the time she needed and they held her job for her.

All in all she said it wasn't too bad an experience. Her HMO won't reconstruct her breast for five years as they are waiting to see if she has a recurrence in the other breast. I asked her if she thinks about having elective surgery to remove the other breast since she is such a high risk. She said "No way."

I'm not even as high risk as she is and I'd consider it. The mastectomy was nothing. It was the lymph nodes which were the most uncomfortable part, and now, of course, the chemo. I'm almost tempted to have my other breast removed and replace both of them if my HMO would do this. At least I wouldn't have to worry about ever going through this again.

I thought I was going to have a quiet night at home since the cancer group got canceled. I called one of the men from Prodigy just to talk. I got him on his car cellular phone. When Warren realized it was my birthday, and I was home alone, he decided to skip his chorus practice and he invited me out for a drink. (He sings harmony in a barber shop quartet and chorus.)

I met him an hour later at a restaurant at the end of my street. We talked for over an hour. Warren seemed very nice and he was also interesting. I wouldn't mind having him as a friend.

And, he got a birthday candle from the waitress, lit it in the parking lot while walking me to my car, and sang "Happy Birthday"!

When I got home my "Boston Buddy," from Prodigy had left a message on my answering machine. He travels constantly with his job. I called him back even though it was late, and then we talked for about a half hour. Finally I told him I had to get to bed.

He is an Aries. (I love Aries people.) He is forty-six and never been married. He actually likes living alone, which seems rare for a man. He's funny in a sarcastic kind of way and very outspoken. He said that he gets lots of mail from other women on Prodigy, but my notes were his favorite. He always looked forward to getting them when he got home from his travels. Anyway, the way we left it is that we are going to keep in touch by phone and be "Perfect Friends." This is our joke as he has a personal ad online which says he wants the "Perfect Lady." When I answered his ad, I told him I wasn't looking for a relationship, just a friendship. I told him I would be his "Perfect Friend." We also have an on-going joke about country western music versus opera. He hates country. I thought he was into opera, because at one point he said he wanted a woman who was comfortable in jeans at a baseball game and also, in an evening gown at the opera. Actually he listens to jazz and some classical, but I still tease him about operas. I have never met him in person, but I think he must be fun.

There's got to be more to write about, but I should start getting ready for work.

Bye. Love you,

P.S. I signed off Prodigy, and then the third online service which I had ordered, and already paid for, arrived two days ago. I'll have to try it out. I'll install it this week-end and make my way through their cyberspace community for at least a month.

August 12, Friday

Hello there,

I must be in worse shape than I thought I was because I can't even type. I remember when Sue wrote to me after a treatment. It was like she was drunk. I was going to start this letter by telling you that it wasn't so bad and that I'm fine, but if my typing is any indication, maybe I'm more wiped out than I thought I was. I am making errors in almost every word.

I am glad Danielle took me and stayed with me. She made it a not so negative experience. She kept me talking, and laughing, and was telling me all the gossip from the Work Program. She is so good. We were there for over two hours.

What was it like, and what did they do? I was settled into a big, comfy recliner chair. First, Betinia, my chemo nurse put in an IV with water and glucose (I think), and then added Zofran, an anti-nausea medicine. When that was done she put the Cytoxan into the IV. It made me a tiny bit nauseous and light headed. When that was empty she used the same vein for the other two drugs, Methrotrexate and 5-Fluorouracil which is known as "5-FU." These last two drugs were done with what's known as a "push." They went into me rather quickly, and were cold all through my arm.

I've been carrying a huge container of water around with me everywhere, drinking it and then running to the bathroom. It's really important that I flush out the Cytoxan.

I go back every third Friday, and I go to the blood lab on the Wednesday mornings before each treatment. Betinia said that there may be days when I just can't go to work, when my blood count drops really low. I am naturally worried about missing too much time from work.

Today in the mail I got some paperwork to fill out from an insurance company. I am going to apply for disability benefits through my union. It's expensive, but I thought I'd better do it. After completing the form I'm sort of guessing that they might turn me down because of the breast cancer.

I was going to lie down after Danielle dropped me off, but I had lunch instead. (And, yes, I can still eat which is good news.) Then I started thinking about all the errands I needed to do, so I went out. Tonight I plan on becoming a couch potato. It sounds good to me. I still have a few more errands to run, but I am out of energy. It could be the heat and not the chemo, but I decided to save the rest of the errands for tomorrow.

I truly have had a busy week. I can't remember when I wrote you last, but I think it was Wednesday.

Wednesday night Rob dropped Jon off. Rob didn't come up to my apartment with him. Jon and I visited for awhile and then we went to the restaurant. The food was delicious and, of course, Jon was, as always, good company. He is still cute, and he doesn't seem to age like the rest of us. I must have bored him with all my breast cancer talk, but I did manage to talk about other things too.

We came back to my apartment to talk some more. And, then I drove him to Rob's. It was weird to be back in my old neighborhood again.

Thursday night I met another man from Prodigy at the Airporter Inn Hotel across from the John Wayne Airport. He's fifty-one, and a pleasant man, but I was not romantically attracted to him. I stayed and talked for a couple of hours, and finally said that I had to get home so I could get some sleep for this morning.

When I got home there was a second message on my machine from Don. He'd left one earlier, but I didn't have time to return his call. I figured "What the heck," so I called him back and we talked for about an hour. He said he wanted to see how I was doing, but we mostly talked about his break-up with his girlfriend. Don says it is finally, really and truly over. Too bad it wasn't three months ago because I was really interested in him then. Now, I don't want to get involved. He knows that, as I've repeatedly made references to the fact that I just want a friendship and not a relationship.

I am having fun and I want to keep my life as normal as possible for the next six months. I'm not trying to be un-realistic, but I want to continue to have a quality life. I believe in order to do that it is up to me.

Someday I would love for you and Danielle to meet. She is such a treasure.

I know there must be more to write, but this is taking me forever because of typos.

I love you and I'm fine. Do not worry.

August 13, Saturday

Hello,

I had no intentions of writing you tonight, but I got all these pictures and I feel compulsive enough to want to return them right away. So, I guess we both can stand a short note. And by the way, I love the picture of you on the log over the stream. Your hair is beautiful, and you look like you have lost weight. This picture is one of my favorites of you.

You take the most unusual pictures. ("moss on rock") When are you going to start entering some of these in photo contests? (Or, even enlarging, framing and selling them? I bet some of those stores that you took me to in New Hampshire would be interested.) And, I wish I could be there hiking with you.

Christmas shopping already? Oh, yeah, I used to do that too. Now I have a hard time just keeping up with all the birthdays that keep popping up. I haven't even thought about Christmas yet. Maybe you can motivate me. Keep telling me what you're buying everyone.

Tamsin called tonight. She asked how I was feeling from the chemo. I could honestly tell her that the first treatment wasn't so bad. I had some weakness, feelings of being quite shaky, and a little nausea driving to the grocery store this morning, but all in all I feel pretty good. I feel so good that I'm considering going dancing tomorrow.

This afternoon I went to the support group at church. It was an excellent meeting. I enjoyed it even more than I did when I went in June. I felt very uplifted. We all made declarations before we left as to how we were going to celebrate life. I said , "By being, enjoying and *dancing.*"

I called L.S. today. I've been trying to reach her for weeks, and her answering machine was not working. She said that she and Nancy had just gotten back from a vacation with friends in Myrtle Beach, North Carolina. I am so happy for her that she moved back there to her roots and friends. She sounds much more content with life. L.S. says that she is working for a painting contractor. They are painting a school and she is putting in a lot of hours. I think this is probably good for her. This is physical work and it is giving her a break from all the emotional energy she was using with the AIDS patients.

Oh, one last thing. My landlady stopped me this morning and asked me about my new neighbors. I laughed and said, "You mean the neighbors from Hell?" Sandra said that everyone in the neighborhood has been coming to her, and her husband complaining about them. She said she has warned them if they don't stop all the noise, the swearing, the fighting, and all the other inconsiderate behavior going on that they will have to move out. Sandra said she'd rather the apartment was left empty than have people like them living in it.

I told her that one night I came home late from dancing and they were having a fight. He was at the foot of the stairs. She was standing in front of my door, and he was throwing things at her. It was kind of scary. They not only yell at each other, but at their two little kids too. It's hasn't been quite as nice here lately as it had been for the past two years.

Well, I thought this was going to be short, but as you can see it's growing rapidly.

Tamsin called again and we started talking about writing, and poetry and other interests that we have in common. She wrote me a poem for my birthday because she said that she couldn't find a card which she liked. She read it to me over the phone and I was very touched by it.

Guess this is enough for a short note.

Bye. Love you,

August 15, Monday

Sharon,

I am so glad you wrote. I have missed you and my other "breast cancer sisters" immensely. Sue keeps calling when I'm not home and she leaves messages, but no phone number where I can reach her. I have Lillie's address. I have thought about writing her. I didn't know what happened to her when she wasn't answering our e-mail. What did happen? Is she okay? I'm glad you are in touch with her again. I will write her one of these days.

I've thought about you lots, and your return to work. I don't envy you the transition. It was probably easier for me because I wasn't out of work that long.

Today was my first full day after the chemo on Friday. I am exhausted. I can't believe I am writing you now, that is how tired I am. But, I do feel better than I had hoped to. I even went to church yesterday, met a girlfriend for brunch, came home and napped for an hour, and then I went dancing. I was in a pretty weakened state and somewhat shaky on the dance floor, but I asked the men to be gentle with me and bless them, they were. I didn't stay as long as I usually do because I had a long drive home and I was afraid of over doing it.

When I got home there was a message on my machine from Rita. I called her, but I wasn't my usual energetic self with her. I think I was pretty out of it. There was also a call from the Prodigy gentleman, Warren, whom I had met on my birthday. He was calling to see how I was doing and I thought that was sweet of him. I returned his call, got his answering service and left a message thanking him. And, then I went to bed. It was about eight o'clock.

Bev, the lady at work who went through all this three years ago asked me how I was doing. When I told her "Okay" and that it wasn't so bad she said, "Cheer up. It gets worse." I cracked up. (I guess you had to be there.) She knows, that I know, that she is right.

Don't feel badly about your tears. This is an extremely emotional time for us. Let them flow. I know my own emotions have been quite erratic these past three months. It's healthy to feel them, and express them, instead of keeping them bottled up inside us.

How is your support group going? I didn't think I would need mine for much longer, but now with the chemo I think it's a good idea for me to continue with them. I have felt somewhat depressed lately. (It's off and on.) It'll be good to have somewhere to go where I can talk about it when I need to.

My girlfriend, Danielle, who took me for the chemo treatment, just called. I picked up the phone and said "Hello." She yelled, "I hear you went dancing last night!" I started laughing. She is so good. I don't know what I would do without her. She is fifty years old, Vietnamese, never been married and is the funniest, wisest, spunkiest little lady you'd ever want to meet. I am ever so thankful that she has come into my life.

Here is a picture that someone took last Christmas at my old job. I'm the one in red dress, and Danielle is the little lady beside me. The other is my favorite picture of Rita and I taken four years ago when she came out here for my birthday. Her fiance took it when we were in San Diego. I have a larger one framed and it's sitting on my workstation. I look at it as I write her all these letters. She is beautiful, isn't she?

Thank you for writing. I really have missed you too. Hello to the other "breast cancer sisters."

Love you,

August 17, Wednesday

Hi,

I feel like I have to be writing you, but I honestly don't feel like doing it. My butt is wicked sore and I'm using my down bed pillow to sit on. I've gone to the bathroom so many times today that my hemorrhoids are turned inside out. Maybe I exaggerate, but they are bleeding which isn't fun. It started this morning, but I went to work and made it through the whole day. Now I am just worn out. When I finish this I'm going to crawl into bed with a good book.

It's been kind of screwy here, or probably it's me. My moods lately seem to just bounce around. Yuck.

Did I already tell you that Elaine called the other night? I was so pleased to hear from her. We have known each other since we were maybe twelve or fourteen. (I'm not sure.) No matter how I have neglected her over the years she has always been there for me. Anyway, she is going to give you a call. I told her to go to your store and get some "back to school" clothes. I also suggested that the four of you get together. I think John and Jack would hit it off. Then I told her to take pictures and send them to me so I could feel like I was there with all of you.

At work I volunteered to do the testing of the Text Retrieval software that was demonstrated in May. (I think I wrote you about that meeting.) One other Coordinator and I will be doing the testing.

Today the Unisys company, and the company that owns the software, did a demonstration in our building for some of the managers and the Deputy Director of Financial Assistance. They were impressed. I'm looking forward to testing it. The company loaded it onto my PC yesterday, but I don't have the password yet to get into it in order to "play." I did spend most of the afternoon reading the handbook which the company left with me. I already have a list of questions for them just from my reading.

I'm also doing a lot more classroom support. I will do one of each type of training Friday and Monday. Let's hope I don't have to keep going to the bathroom on those days. The trainer just came out with the September schedule. I volunteered to take four of the ten training dates. I'm trying to plan the support days in and around my chemo.

Lately I have so many meetings, trainings, and other assignments that some of them over lap on my calendar. Today I had two meetings at the same time.

My current office roommate, Bruce, will be my new boss as of Friday. The Manager announced his promotion today. He has only been in Systems a short time compared to the other members of the team, but he is a whiz at this stuff. He also has thirteen years of supervisory experience.

The bathroom is calling again. (This has got to stop.)

Sorry. This is probably all typos, but I am really tired.

Bye. Love you,

August 19, Friday

Dear Sue:

I cannot tell you how good your timing was on this card and note. I miss you and Sharon and all the e-mailing we did online. Unfortunately I was just over doing it and I had to get out of Prodigy. I got a wonderful long letter from Sharon. That is terrific that you got to talk on the phone. Isn't she a sweet lady? I hope to call her next week when I have my flex Friday off. Have you heard from Lillie?

Thank you so much for your concern. Actually I am doing okay except for my hemorrhoids which are not taking kindly to the way my stomach has been the last three days. This morning was awful. I filled the toilet with blood and it scared me. The past three work days have been uncomfortable for me.

Honestly it's not that bad. I am not getting the Adriamycin like you had. That is the nasty stuff, and the one that made your hair fall out. Every morning I get up, wash my hair, and as I'm brushing it I say "Thank you."

Yes, the doctor prescribed the Zofran, and something which is in a suppository form. Luckily I have not had to use either yet. So far I haven't thrown up.

I hear that I haven't experienced anything yet though, and that as it builds up in me the side effects get worse. All I can do is take it day by day. I do know that I want to do all the things that I usually would, as I can. I want my life to be as normal as I can make it. I hope to dance again this Sunday afternoon. But, we'll see on that one though.

Now, what is happening with you and the second mastectomy and the reconstruction? I want to hear more. Sharon will be having her reconstruction soon too. I'm envious. Originally, before the chemo, I thought I'd have mine by Christmas. Now I realize that it probably won't be until next spring. I totally understand your decision to choose to have the other breast removed. Sue, I am not as high risk as you, but I swear if the HMO gives me the option I may choose to do the same thing. I'd much rather they removed a healthy breast now, as prevention, and reconstructed two matching breasts at the same time. I'm with you all the way on this!

I picked up an application today for "The Race For The Cure." Have you read the book about Susan G. Komen? Her sister, who was also diagnosed with breast cancer, started the foundation in Susan's memory. The book was quite sad. I sent my copy to my best friend. I plan to do the one mile fun walk in September. The reason I didn't sign up for the actual five mile race is that I have a scheduled chemo treatment the Friday before, and I don't even know if I'll be able to show up for the event, let alone walk the mile. I wanted to contribute though and be part of this excellent fund raiser. It is going to be held in Newport Beach.

Are you getting yourself geared up for "back to school"? I don't know how you worked (teaching kindergarten children, right?) while having chemo. Did you catch colds from the kids? Didn't they wear you out?

Say "Hi" to Sharon and Lillie. I really do miss having the constant contact with all of you.

Bye. Love you,

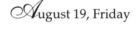 August 19, Friday

Hello there,

I just finished writing a long letter to Sue, so you are getting off the hook for one of the lengthy notes this time. There isn't much left in me to write another long one.

This has not been a really good week for me. My hemorrhoids totally rebelled this morning and burst open filling the toilet with blood. It scared me. I know how much you hate hearing about this kind of thing.

Things are really picking up in work. I am still enjoying it, but I have lots more to do all of a sudden. Today was another classroom support day. That is always intense, but fun. Monday is the same. It's challenging to switch back and forth between the two programs and to stay on top of bailing out the students. It sure keeps me hopping.

No real news, which means good news I guess.

Bye. Love you,

August 21, Sunday

Happy Sunday-funday.

Whatever you and Jack are doing I hope it's fun. I always like hearing about your hiking and boating. The weed pulling doesn't sound enjoyable, but your reward comes after the work is done.

I tried to take a nap as I would like to go dancing later, but my neighbors decided to have one of their dramas for all of us. Why do people find it necessary to yell and swear at each other? I feel so bad for their little kids. And, of course, my landlords are on vacation in Maine this week. I wonder how much longer they are going to be living here.

This morning I decided to call the HMO emergency number. It's been four or five days with my rectal bleeding. They told me to come right in to the Urgent Care Clinic. The nurse practitioner was a young guy. The exam made me start bleeding again, but he gave me a prescription for twice a day hemorrhoid suppositories. I asked him if it is possible for me to heal while I'm having chemotherapy. He said "Yes." I hope he's right.

Also, he wanted me to make an appointment for a colonoscopy to see if I had Colon Cancer. I flipped out just hearing about another type of cancer. I told him that I know I do not have Colon Cancer. The bleeding is from my hemorrhoids and that's a side effect, from a side effect of the chemotherapy.

I was feeling somewhat down after the exam, but I forced myself to go to church. As usual I am glad that I went. The assistant minister, Michelle, whom I adore, did the sermon. It was very good timing. She talked about "Why Wait?" I felt like I was picked way up and brought back down to a place I was supposed to be. It was truly inspirational.

Speaking of inspiration. You have motivated me to start Christmas shopping. When I went to buy a vegetable steamer I browsed the toy department. I ended up buying some toys for Dani and Nick. Now let's hope I can refrain from giving them to them early.

I just finished reading a book which I had picked up last weekend. It is, "How to Reduce Your Risk of Breast Cancer." It really didn't tell me anything much different from the other books I've read. I know it's important to eat a lot of fruit and vegetables, five to nine portions a day. If you are interested I will send the book to you.

Should I go dancing tonight or not? (To be, or not to be.) I live all week for Sunday's dancing . Maybe I will go. If I can't do it then I will just visit with people and leave early. I won't even bother dressing up.

Usually I try to look my best but, I think this is going to be a jeans afternoon. Write me.

Bye. Love you,

Good Morning!

YES! I feel wonderful today. There is no bleeding finally. I'm practically dancing around this apartment. I had to write you because I feel so good after having felt so lousy for the past week. I am even looking forward to going into work.

What a difference this morning is from where I've recently been. Maybe I'm going to survive this chemo stuff after all. The suppositories seem to be working. Yesterday I was still scared and wondering if I should just call Dr. Nielsen and ask to see him. But, then I told myself that I would give it one more week, and I would see him on Friday for my scheduled appointment. If the bleeding hadn't stopped by then I was going to request that he discontinue the chemo until my new problem was resolved.

I feel so good today. I feel like I owe you, and the people I work, with apologies for the way I've been moping around and feeling sorry for myself. I truly do feel energetic and like everything's okay again. Maybe it's because I'm not weak from loss of blood. Who knows? This is all too new and strange for me to be trying to figure it out.

Yesterday I did another classroom support. It's intense, but fun too. The best part is that it is rewarding. The students who, in some cases are my peers, are so grateful for the help we give them. I went into Social Services to help people, and you know that the last few years I was not feeling like I was accomplishing this. Even though my new assignment involves computers, I am helping people, and they are people who appreciate my assistance.

When I went dancing Sunday afternoon I had a blast. Again, I had to force myself to go, but when I got there and danced I was glad that I went. Don was there and he says (again) that it is really and truly finished between he and his girlfriend. This man is starting to drive me nuts. He is losing so much weight that I'm afraid he is making himself sick over their affair. The scary part is that I still love dancing, joking and laughing with him. He is so much fun to be with. I analyzed this somewhat when I got home. I'm trying to figure out if I still have a little bit of a crush on him. Not to worry though. I am being on my best behavior.

I'm glad this is going to be my short week. Last week was a long one and just about did me in at work. I have lots to do, and today I will start testing the new product. That should make the day fly by.

In the evenings when I have the energy I work a little on the book. What am I going to do with it when it's done? Right now I am just polishing up chapter one. Most of the time I enjoy working on it although sometimes it can be monotonous.

I've got to wrap this up and finish getting ready for work. Thank you for listening again and again.

Bye. Love you,

August 24, Wednesday

Good Morning,

Before rushing off to work I thought I would write just a short note because today is another glorious day here. I guess we get the bad days so that when the good ones come we can really appreciate them. I feel so normal and healthy it's like last week never happened.

My brother called last night. It was perfect timing since I had had such a good day and was so "up." I always love hearing from him. When he asked me what I was doing and I told him I was working on the book he jokingly (I think) said that maybe he could help me self-publish it. (Gulp)

Also, he said that he can't wait to meet you. He is looking forward to your visit in May. (I hope it works out, but right now it seems like there are so many obstacles in between.) He wants to take you and Jack to a gourmet, and very famous, restaurant in Napa. He said it is so popular that you have to make reservations two months in advance. We talked about how you will love it there, and will enjoy photographing the scenic areas and tasting the delicious wine. He got me all excited about this vacation.

I told him that the best part of it will be seeing you, and spending time with you. Do you think this will really happen? I don't want to be disappointed again after not getting back to visit you this month. I don't want to get my hopes up again if it's not a strong possibility.

I've decided to just love my body and it's new weight. I think I am meant to be skinny and I am working on accepting it. Except, like now, when I'm sitting here and my bony butt is uncomfortable.

The vegetable steamer is one of the best investments I've made ever made. I cooked my dinner in it last night and it was so delicious and easy. When I was telling my brother about it he started laughing and said that that was one of his favorite meals too. It's addicting. Once you start eating them your body just craves more. My favorites are the carrots, broccoli, cauliflower, mushroom, squash, red potatoes and yams. It's not even seven in the morning, I've already had breakfast, and just writing about the vegetables makes me want some.

Love you,

AugustAugust 26, Friday

Hello,

The mailman just came and brought your letter and the pictures. I am so glad you wrote. It seemed like it'd been forever since I'd heard from you. You do sound busy. It's funny you wrote about spending the day cleaning house. I was beginning to think you never cleaned house anymore!

I put one of the moose pictures on my bulletin board. He's cute. (It's the one drinking water by himself.) You did get awfully close to them in order to get these shots. No wonder the kids were worried about you.

The other pictures are beautiful. It is so green there. The pictures of you are terrific. I swear you are getting better looking. What is your secret? Also, I like your canoe. (Fun.)

It is hot and muggy here also, and we're not used to it. I can't imagine what it must be like to get things all moldy. I'd freak out over that. We just feel sticky and that's bad enough.

Today was my Friday off and I had an appointment with Dr. Nielsen. He was pleased that I am handling the chemo so well. We discussed the bad week I had with the bleeding and he gave me another prescription. I know you hate hearing all these things, but what we think happened is that the anti-nausea drug in the IV made me constipated. When I strained to go to the bathroom that's when I ruptured the hemorrhoids. Then, I started going to the bathroom a few times a day from the chemo drugs, and each time I'd bleed. I just couldn't seem to heal until I got the suppositories. He wants me to take this new prescription the day before the chemo. It is a "stool softener." (Sorry to gross you out.) I told him that I think I'll be okay, and I'll wait until after the chemo to see if I get constipated. If I do, then I'll take the medicine.

Anyway he was pleased that I wasn't nauseous and also, that I haven't gotten any sores in my mouth. Let's hope the next six months are the same.

When I was driving home from the grocery store, with all my fruits and vegetables, I was thinking how nice it was to just shop and prepare foods that I like and not feel pressured to cook major dinners for a man. I don't think I'm cut out for the wife routine that most men still want.

When I got home I steamed up some fresh vegetables. Then I made a huge tossed salad with all kinds of yummies in it. I made a big bowl of fruit salad too. And, then I cut up other fresh vegetables for munching. The refrigerator is full and I can just pick and poke through it and munch as I want to. Don't get me wrong, I still eat my splurges when I want to. But, I have definitely cut back on chocolate and sweets. I eat an even lower fat diet than I used to. And, of course, I told you that I haven't had a glass of wine since the surgery. Not to say that I won't have one when I want it.

Sometimes I think part of all this change is that down deep I am blaming myself for the cancer. Like, maybe all the chocolate candy bars, or the glasses of wine with dinner caused this, so now I can't over do on them again. This will pass.

I really am ever so much better now. The past few days I have felt beyond good. Now I'm starting to dread next Friday, but I say to myself that once I go on Friday I will have completed 25% of the chemo!

August 28, Sunday

Good Morning,

How are you today? I got your letter and pictures yesterday. The ad for Jordan Marsh almost gave me heart failure when I first opened. I wasn't expecting to hear a train. Then, I started laughing. Yes, I'll save it for the next time I see Nicky. He'll love it. That is quite clever advertising.

The picture of you and Jack is cute. You both look so happy and "sexy." I can see the elephant's forehead, and the beginning of the trunk, on the front of the rock in the other picture. You captured it nicely. I wish I was doing some of this hiking with you. I think I could handle it. If I can dance, then I can hike. Where was the waterfall? It is a very unique one with the rock formations on it's sides.

Please thank Clara for me. Rita, I have so many people praying for me that this is going to be a piece of cake. One night this week I got a card from someone I know from dancing. She and her husband, of forty-six years, are friends of Karen and Bob's. They are the cutest couple. I was very touched when I got their card and note. They are very religious people and she enclosed a religious type card, and said they were praying for me daily. When I least expect it lately I'll get a card from someone who just found out, and the sentiments are always so encouraging and beautiful.

So, when is Jack's party? Maybe the trip to Mexico can replace a surprise party. Which one do you think he would prefer?

Arthur came by last night to get his mail and the last of his things from the garage. (Eric is now using my garage for storage since their new place doesn't have one.) He looked terrific and said that everything in his life is going great. He brought me a "joint." I said it wasn't necessary and that I didn't need it. He told me to just put it away in case there is a day I need it. (Cute)

I've been Christmas shopping. (It's all your fault for reminding me that this is something I should be working on.) I used my VISA naturally. (Ouch.) One of my favorite discount stores was having a sale on down comforters. Last year when I got mine Bridget and Arthur both commented on how they'd like to have one. I got one for each of the kids. Also, they were having a sale on 14kt gold earrings with a variety of gemstones. I got Bridget an amethyst pair for her "purple passion." They are tear drop studs. I also bought some more toys for the kids and one bath toy for the new baby. It's a Mickey Mouse toy. Bridget said that eventually they are going to do the baby's room in Mickey or Minnie depending on the baby's sex. I'm getting there. It's a good thing I have the extra closet to put all this stuff.

My ants are back. I'm bummed. Last night I found a couple of "scouts" and the same thing this morning. I hate them. I have to put cereal, cookies, crackers and other open snack foods in the refrigerator. If I don't, they just swarm into the boxes and cover the food.

Today's my church's annual "Hoedown Sunday." It's always fun. People dress country. After the service there is food and country western entertainment and dancing. Today there's supposed to be some cloggers and square dancers.

Last night I stayed up late finishing the first chapter of our book. I'm mailing it out with a query letter to a publisher. I'll enclose a copy of the letter. I'm not expecting anyone to be really interested, or impressed by this effort, but I am going to continue working on it. I always like a sense of completion on things.

I have to get ready for church.

Bye. Love you,

P.S. Yesterday while I was ironing there was an interview on TV with a cancer specialist here in Orange County. The media is really pushing the information right now on breast cancer because of the upcoming "Race for the Cure." She said that 1700 women in Orange County will be diagnosed with breast cancer this year. The really frightening part is that 400 women in Orange County will die in 1994 as a result of this disease.

P.P.S. Tamsin just called and asked if she and Nick could come over to have lunch with me and also do laundry. I told her I'd pick them up after church. While she's doing laundry I'll take Nick to the Hoedown if it's still going on.

August 28, Sunday

Rita,

Bet you didn't think I'd be writing to you again today. I didn't think so either, but I got home from dancing a little while ago and I needed to talk, so here I am.

How do you spell "**ca ca**"? I looked it up in the dictionary and I couldn't find it. Anyway — **Poop**, and all those other words.

I danced for over three hours. I was having so much fun that I didn't want to leave. Don was there and that's why I'm cussing. (And, it's me I'm cussing out, not him.)

I'm at a loss for words. I'm sitting here staring at the screen with a blank mind.

What am I going to do? Am I hopeless? I am still attracted to him. I try not to be, but when I'm with him, dancing and laughing and having fun, I feel so comfortable.

Sometimes I think that I'd be nuts to get involved with him, but then other times I don't know why I think that.

When I finally decided that it was time for me to leave he said he'd walk me to my car. Isn't this how it started before? We small talked for a little while standing by my car. He told me how much fun he had dancing with me. Then we hugged, and it was great. We just kind of held onto each other and I said, "You still give 'good hug'." He laughed and said, "So do you."

I said, "Don, I don't want to get another crush on you. I worked hard at getting over the last one." He said he understood and he would try to just be my "good buddy." He told me that if I needed someone to talk to, or anything, to call him. I'd like to. I'd like to say "Come over and just hold me. No sex. Just hold me." But, I won't. I don't need any heartache right now.

Oh, I was teasing him and said, "I ought to fix you up with my best friend. You and she have so much in common between sailing, scuba diving, cats, Spanish language studies and photography." I told him I was teasing because you are engaged and that actually he and your fiance also have a lot in common.

I told Don, and my other friends, that I didn't know if I would be there next Sunday because of the chemo on Friday. Everyone told me to try to come even if I couldn't dance. Also, I explained to Don that the last time I danced, right after the chemo, I had poor coordination and was worried that I might fall down when doing the spins.

So, what do I do? If he and his ex-girlfriend get back together again then my problem is solved. Enough of this.

After I wrote you this morning I called Tamsin back and suggested that I pick them up before church. She did her laundry and showered while Nicky and I went to church. He and I stayed after for the entertainment at the hoedown. When we got home I fixed all of us a delicious, healthy, vegetarian dinner.

All in all the day was a good one. I always enjoy Nicky. He says the cutest things. He loved the train card from Jordan Marsh. He played with it constantly. When I gave it to him he started reading it and said, "Happy Birthday almost four years old." Bridget and I cracked up. When he didn't finish a banana I suggested he wrap it up and take it home. He says, "I'll save it for 'to-later'." (His version of tomorrow and later I guess.) He also told me that he didn't like green vegetables, the "little tree ones." But, actually when I cooked the broccoli, and gave him some ranch dressing for dipping them in, he ate every bit.

I'm out of stamps, so who knows when this will get mailed?

Bye. Love you,

P.S. Forgive the errors. I'm really tired. I danced a lot. Maybe I was trying to get it all in tonight in case I couldn't go next Sunday.

August 29, Monday

Dear Sharon — My little breast cancer sister,

I am so glad that your long letter came today. I am also missing all those great, daily messages from you and Sue, and yes, Lillie's occasional responses. It is so tempting to go back on Prodigy, but I have to behave myself financially right now. The letters from you are welcomed. Thank you.

This picture of you and your son is really cute. He looks like you. I think it is a nice picture. Why don't you like it of you? Oh, why am I asking that question? I'm the same way. I dislike most pictures of me.

I call you "little sister" because you look so little in the picture. Besides I am the elder here!

No, I never did hear from Lillie, but I sent her a card with a short note in it. Also, I've never talked to Sue. She finally sent me a note, with a card, and her address so I was able to write her. I think she gave up trying to reach me by telephone. Yes, I want to hear all the details of her surgery and reconstruction. She is the pioneer for us. Do you know yet when you will be having yours done?

You did do some shopping, and it sounds like you had fun at it.

And, so what? We both know that life is too short and we have to enjoy ourselves and take our pleasures where we can.

Speaking of "pleasures," do you want to hear about my love life? The one that isn't, but has possibilities? Actually, I should write to Rita about this tonight, but she will kill me if I tell her that Don called and I talked with him for about an hour tonight. Here goes.

A year ago when I had broken off my engagement, for about six weeks, I went dancing one night and met this cute "prospector." (This is his country western dancing dress style.) We danced and I was very attracted to him, but I was still seeing my boyfriend at the time, even though I had given him back the engagement ring. Well, as you know I wound up taking the ring back after the six weeks of not wearing it. Then I completely broke off the engagement in December. But, I never forgot the prospector. When I started dancing again in December I would see him every Sunday, but he was in a relationship. He met someone right after I met him in July. They made a cute couple, and looked like they were happy together.

In April he showed up on a few Sundays without her. We danced often and got to sharing more about ourselves. (We also laugh a lot together.) He appeared to be attracted to me too, except for his pining over the ex-girlfriend.

I was at that time running a very specific ad in the paper looking for a dance partner, with the possibility of it maybe becoming more than a dance partnership. One night when I was talking to Don I told him about my ad. He asked me what was in it. He actually met all my specifics. We joked about it, and he gave me his business card and suggested that I call him. He has a photography studio and he also has a regular night job. I thought about it. Before I left that night I gave him my business card and told him to call me, because I was too chicken to call him. He wound up walking me out to my car and gave me the greatest bear hug. He is about 5'8" and is a close Santa Claus look alike.

The next day I called him after all and said, "You give good hug." We both cracked up. He started calling me and we met to go dancing one night, but then he went back with his ex-girlfriend. A few weeks later they broke up again. He called and we danced again. And, then he went back with his ex-girlfriend. At that point I had a terrific crush on him, but I did not want to get involved with the "never ending relationship" he had with her. Also, it was right about then that I was going in for my biopsy.

He called me the night I got home from the biopsy to ask how I was. They had been broken up, but that night he told me that they were back together again. Dizzy yet?

I didn't dance for about two months. When I started dancing after the mastectomy he was there, and without her. They'd been seeing each other off and on though until about a week ago. Sunday I saw him at the Cowboy and he said, "It really is over this time." (I've heard this before.) We had a lot of fun dancing and laughing.

All day today I couldn't stop thinking about him. I said to myself that this was nuts and that he'd be going back with her again so "**STOP**." I was convincing myself that I could be cool about this and not go all ga-ga over him again. After dinner he called and I just melted. I rambled on about stupid things, sort of like I do in these letters.

Finally I just said, "Don, I like you." He said, "I like you too." I also told him that I expect he will go back with his girlfriend and I really don't want to get another crush on him. He seems to understand, but it was nice. (Sigh)

Rita told me to forget him since he can't make up his mind. We'll see. I'll let you know if anything comes out of all this.

Oh, he is very empathetic about the breast cancer. One of his ex-girlfriends had breast cancer while they were dating. She had a lumpectomy, and radiation, but didn't follow through on the chemo-therapy. They remain close friends and she comes to dance on Sundays when she is in California.

I've gotten carried away again. Sorry about that. But, it'll make up for two weeks worth of e-mail, okay?

Miss you too. Don't work too hard.

Bye. Love you,

August 31, Wednesday

Hi Lillie!

I got your card tonight and I had a double laugh on it, because I bought the same "drifting shoulder pads effect" card and sent it to my best friend in Boston. (And, I thought I had a sick sense of humor. Glad to see I'm in good company.)

You are one busy lady. I picture you as one whirling ball of energy. It doesn't sound like anything could get you down for long.

That's wonderful news about your lymph nodes and I'm glad that you won't need chemo. Sharon isn't having chemo either. So far I'm tolerating the chemo. I get my second treatment in two days. We'll see what I have to say after that.

I have much to do tonight so must go, but I had to write a little to let you know how glad I am to hear from you again. Stay in touch.

Bye. Love you,

September

Good Morning,

It is a good one here anyway. I've been up since four-thirty. It's not yet six-thirty, and I've got my laundry going, and all other "chores" for the day done. Am I a little bit anxious, or what? My chemo is at ten-thirty and I just want to get it over with and come home. The last treatment Danielle and I both had shorts on, and it was freezing in the clinic. Even though it looks like today is going to be a hot one, I've got long pants and a long sleeved, thick shirt on. I've also already started filling up on water so there's plenty in me to start flushing that nasty stuff out.

I can't remember if I wrote and told you that I got a really cute invitation to a birthday party for Karen next week-end at In Cahoots. She'll be thirty-seven. I called Don and asked him if he was still single. He was confused because he had just called me the night before and we had talked for about an hour. He finally got it and said he was. I asked him if he wanted to go to the party with me. He said he is doing a wedding shoot that night and sometimes they run really late, but he'll let me know how it looks before then. I called Karen to RSVP and guess what? The party was sort of a surprise. Bob sent out the invitations. He didn't write on them to keep it a secret. (Oops) She said that she had suspicions of it though. Her sister and Bob are doing all of the planning.

Last night I decided to color my hair myself with temporary hair color. My hair does seem to be thinning out a little, and I don't want to take any chances of losing any more of it than I have to. I'm afraid that the semi-permanent color that Regina puts on it might be a little too harsh right now.

Maybe my new neighbors are moving. Last night they were having a raging fight outside my bathroom window while I was coloring my hair. Finally I shut the window and went into the kitchen. They were both threatening to call the police on each other. I know everyone in the neighborhood will be happy if they move. It's been a daily brawl with them here.

I'm doing okay at work. More people have discovered that I exist and call me with computer problems. Most of them I can actually answer. About one call a day I still have to go to a co-worker to get help. Also, I finished testing the new software and wrote up the report on my results. I spent about fifteen hours working on this project. This is the fourth text retrieval program which our agency has tested. Since I was not there when the others were tested I have nothing to compare this one to. To tell the truth I am not that impressed with this one. But, I just do the test and give them my report. I don't make the ultimate decision as to whether we buy it or not.

Oh, one last thing. Newton came by my office. His wife is the one who had the mastectomy about three years ago. She had negative nodes and no chemotherapy. Her lump was also small. Anyway, he said that his wife has been having some problems with her lower ribs. They are very sore and tender. This week the HMO that she belongs to did a bone scan to see if perhaps her breast cancer has recurred. They will get the results today. I got a very sick feeling when he told me. I told him how sore my own ribs got when I was exercising my arm. I asked him if the soreness was on the same side as her surgery. He said it was, and he said that she had started a new aerobic exercise program recently. I suggested that she ask her doctor if maybe the soreness is being caused by stretching out that "cord." Possibly it wasn't completely stretched out after the surgery three years ago, and now all her exercising is doing it. I hope it is something as simple as this.

My own cord is finally stretched out, except for a small area near my left wrist. I can actually see the cord through my skin on my arm and wrist areas when I stretch it and look in the mirror. It makes my skin look scarred. None of the other women I have talked to have mentioned anything like this. Maybe on me it is obvious because my arms are so skinny.

I've been communicating with some women through my new online program. I met them in a Health Forum for Breast Cancer. One of them lives in Boston.

Enclosed is the letter we got last week with our paychecks. It's from one of our Board of Supervisors encouraging employees to take part in the "Race for the Cure." I think it is wonderful that they are doing this.

I'll close now so I can get this out in today's mail

Thank you for continuously hanging in here with me.

Bye. Love you,

September 2, Friday

Hello again,

There's one letter already sitting out at my mailbox for you. Guess this is a two letter day.

I'm pretty depressed again, but I know it'll pass. When I got to the chemo clinic Betinia said she tried to call me to save me the trip, but I'd already left. Wednesday's blood test shows that I am very low in my white blood count. They can't do a treatment when I'm this low.

She rescheduled me for next Friday and said for me to come home and get lots of rest. This was one of those weeks where I shouldn't have been working. Oh well. Betinia reviewed the list of do's and don'ts with me. For the next few days I stay away from crowds, people with infections (especially small children), fresh fruit and vegetables and animals. I'm sort of under quarantine. This disease is controlling my life and I really resent it. Betinia stressed to me that I am *not* to go dancing at all this week-end. I am so bummed out.

She said that I will have a new count done next Wednesday. If it is up on that day then they will administer the second treatment next Friday. If that treatment causes my blood count to remain low, after three weeks, then my schedule will be changed to every four weeks. I asked her if this meant I will be getting chemo for longer than the originally stated six months, but she didn't really answer me. (Does that mean "yes"?)

On the way home I stopped and bought a steak which I only eat maybe once a year. This was my lunch with some cooked vegetables. They even recommend that you eat liver when the blood count is down. Yuck!

I also got a couple of books and went to the video store for my reserved tape, "Schindler's List." It hadn't been returned yet so I got two lighthearted movies instead. It is just as well. They are going to reserve the other one for me for tomorrow night.

So, this is my long four day week-end. I get to read, watch movies, work on our book, pig out and write letters to you! I hope you don't mind sharing the week-end with me like this.

I really am upset about it. I'm not liking any of this chemo business. I'll be okay though as I bounce back fast from all these little set backs.

Bye. Love you,

P.S. I talked to Sharon. She gave me her 800 number so that I can call her when I'm home on Fridays. It is so wonderful to be able to talk to her. She knows exactly what I'm feeling about all this cancer junk. For example I was telling her about the statistics here in Orange County. I was quoting that letter from the Board of Supervisors. When I got to the part about "400 women dying this year," she jumped right in and said, "And, you said to yourself — and I'm not one of them, right?" I just said, "You got it."

She is doing okay now that she is back to work, except that she still hasn't gotten her strength back from the surgery. She asked me how I really felt. (This was before I was devastated one more time from the clinic's news.) I told her I honestly felt great and that I get so involved and busy doing whatever, that I forget I'm supposed to be recovering.

Rita, you don't think I'm doing too much do you? (That thought just hit me.)

$\mathcal{S}$eptember 3, Saturday

Rita,

I hate these letters lately. Don't you? I hadn't planned on writing again for awhile, but I tried to call you, and you weren't home, so here goes another gloomy one.

Your long, long letter arrived on the perfect day. I just devoured every bit of it. It makes me feel like you are here. I guess that's why I called. I couldn't get enough. Sorry about the message. I couldn't help it. I just started crying and now I can't stop.

This is nuts. I didn't use to cry so much. Ever since the middle of May it seems like that's what I do the best, and the most of lately.

This is not one of my better week-ends. I feel pretty lonely and depressed. I'm keeping myself busy and entertained, but I feel like there is a big world going on out there without me. First I miss most of the summer, and then I have four days off for Labor Day and I'm confined to my apartment.

The thing is that four months ago, before I knew about breast cancer, I was healthy. I didn't feel sick. I wasn't depressed. I was going my merry little way having fun, and my biggest challenge was in my attempts to meet a man that I was compatible with.

Now I'm sick, and I'm miserable. Just when I think the worst is behind me I get another set back that throws me for a loop. I wind up feeling sorry for myself, and that depresses me even more.

The highlight of my day was to return two videos and get two more. And, I cooked a chicken dinner just for me. I am trying to eat extra this week-end.

I talked to Don last night. I had called him and left a message on his answering machine at the studio yesterday. He told me last Sunday to call him whenever I wanted to talk. The problem was that I couldn't reach him when I needed to talk. Then when he called I was over the surprise that they gave me at the clinic.

Sometimes I think he is interested in me. Other times I don't know what to think. I know I am attracted to him, but I guess this is just the wrong time in my life to even consider starting a new relationship.

I am excited for you and the October trip to Mexico. Have you told Jack that you are taking him, or is this a surprise? It should be a beautiful vacation. You and he do have some nice memories from your travels.

When is Jack's birthday party? I wish I could be there for it.

I think you are the one who should be writing the book. Your love scenes and fantasies would make a number one seller.

I wish my hair looked good too, but I won't complain because I am still thankful to have any.

See, just writing to you makes me feel a whole lot better.

Thank you again for listening.

Bye. Love you,

September 4, Sunday

Hello again,

Thank you for yesterday. I felt much better after you called. Honest. Earlier, after I left you that message, I just put my head down on my bed and cried. I felt like I had sunk to the lowest form of despair. You cheered me up and let me know, once again, that I am not alone.

What do other women do, who are single, and living alone and don't have a "you," a Danielle, or cancer sisters to get them through these times? It must be awful. I am going to give that some thought. Maybe when I get through this myself I can find a way to be there for some other person who is in need of companionship and support. Actually, sometimes I think that, that is why I am trying to write a book. If there is some person out there, who has no one, maybe reading our story will make her feel like she has a friend who is going through it with her. (Does this make any sense at all?)

I had said that I would just go with the flow of this, and stop trying to fight it. This is the perfect week-end for me to act on my words. Usually the Universe knows better than I do what I need, and when I am in need of it. I want to be up, and out, and doing things like other people, but maybe my body needs this quiet time.

When I was at the clinic on Friday I asked Betinia if all the blood I lost that week could have contributed to this problem. She said "No," but that doesn't make sense to me. It seems logical that if I lost blood, and my blood count is low, there should be some correlation. But, what do I know? I've never done this before. We'll see what happens with my blood count after the next treatment.

My big excursion of the day will be to go to the video store, then to a mailbox to send you *two* letters and also to the market to pick up some milk and decaf. It should take all of twenty minutes. The rest of the day will be spent doing things around here, just like I did on Friday and Saturday. (Grrr.)

Bye. Love you,

P.S. My landlady stopped me again on Friday to ask me how I was doing and to talk about the neighbors. She said she worries about me living next door to them. I told her it has to be worse for Jerry and Gloria living below them. Sandra said that they are going to tell them they have to move out. Most of the people living around us are complaining. She feels badly that I am not well right now, and that these people are so loud and rude. I told her that I just shut my windows and work in the bedroom, and then I don't hear them, so for her not to evict them on my account. I'm not making a big issue out of it. (She is afraid that I am going to move out because of them.) I also told her that I feel bad for the two little kids. There is so much screaming and swearing by the adults, and the poor kids are crying continuously.

September 5, Monday

Happy Labor Day,

And, I hope you are doing something other than just working today. I know you said that your store was open and you had to go in. But, enjoy part of it in some way.

Once again your call last night was timely. I have been feeling pretty isolated, which is the idea I guess. Your call came at the time I would normally have been getting ready to go out dancing. It was tempting, but I don't want any further complications so I'll just hope that next Sunday I can make up for it.

I only got half way through "Schindler's List" last night, because there are two tapes, and the video store forgot to give me the second one. By the time I realized it, and called them, I was in pj's and not about to go out again. They said I can pick up the other tape today.

Last night I went onto CompuServe for a little while. I'm being very careful to not overdo it with this online service. I had two e-mail letters. One was from the lady in Boston, and the other one was from the lady in Philadelphia.

Anyway, the lady from Philadelphia finished her chemotherapy about ten months ago. She has had a heck of a time with this disease. She discovered the first lump herself about two years ago. It never did show up on any of the mammograms they took before, and after, she found the lump. She had a lumpectomy and was undergoing mild chemotherapy, like me, when the doctor found another lump in the same breast. She then had to have a mastectomy, and after that she was given the strong chemotherapy. Her hair fell out. She said that that was the worst of her losses.

Her letter was pretty sad, but spoken honestly and from her heart. She said it is so difficult to talk about breast cancer with someone who hasn't experienced it, because no one else can understand the loss and the fears. She isn't negative, but she says what her thoughts are, and they are pretty real. Listening to her has helped me to accept the fact that under my sometimes "Pollyanna" type act, I pretty much have the same fears.

What bothers me lately is that I am meeting and getting to know so many women who have gone through this. When I stop and give it some serious thought it is a very somber reality that one, or more of us, are going to die from this disease. And, of course I wonder who it will be. I get all choked up when I have these thoughts, and it's not just because it could be me.

I'm getting pretty heavy here. Maybe this is why I needed to stay alone this week-end. Possibly it was time for me to confront my underlying thoughts, feelings and fears.

I am not trying to tell you that I believe that I am going to die from breast cancer. I am still very optimistic. I know that my own prognosis is a lot better than some of the women I'm meeting. But, I know and accept the fact that it is possibility that I could die from this disease. I don't want to be known as a person in denial.

I hear the other women say that first they were involved in all the things needing to be taken care of with doctor's appointments, surgeries, and treatments. Then one day it hit them that, in their own words, which I hear over and over again, "I could die from this."

Well, my moment of acknowledging this fact seems to have come while I've been on this "forced retreat"and so, the past four days have not been a total loss. My next step with this inner reckoning is to decide just how I want to spend the rest of my life. I know that I don't want to waste one precious minute of it.

Whew. When I started this I never expected it to take this kind of a path.

Now that I've made it through the long week-end, and I feel that I have benefited from it with all my revelations, I don't regret the time spent alone after all. I actually feel like a big weight has been lifted from my shoulders.

I am looking forward to getting back to work tomorrow. I'm even looking forward to getting the next chemotherapy on Friday.

Love you much,

*S*eptember 6, Tuesday

Good Morning,

This is probably going to be my quickest letter on record since we just talked again last night , but I *knew* you would want to hear about my date with Don. It was wonderful. He was the perfect gentleman. (No he didn't have any "germs," and no I did not "lick" him anywhere! You are such a tease.)

I have another crush on him. (Who knows why?) The more time I spend around him, the more attracted to him I become. In my eyes he's cute, but knowing your taste you would definitely disagree with me. His interests are more like yours and Jacks, but I think he and I have very similar values, and our personalities seem to be a lot alike. Of course we have the country music and dancing interests in common. (Oh, and before we went to the show we played "Backgammon." He beat me!)

Then we went to the theater and saw "Corrina, Corrina." It was cute. Afterwards we came back here for about an hour and talked. (*Just talked*, Rita.) Then it was after ten o'clock and he said he should get going so I could get my sleep for work today.

The truth is that I can't tell how interested in me he is, but I'm okay with that right now, because even though I am attracted to him I still don't know that much about him.

I have to finish getting ready for work. Thank you for being with me over this long week-end. I enjoyed all your calls. Friday might have gotten off to a bad start, but the date with Don made it have a fun and happy ending.

Bye. Love you,

*S*eptember 7, Wednesday

Hello again,

Last night Laura called. She, also, was checking up on me. She felt bad when I told her about this past week-end. She said to call her anytime, and she will come over and keep me company. That made me feel really good.

Yesterday at work one of my team members, Juanita, told me the same thing. She said that if it happens again to call her, and she will bring a scrabble game and we'll lock ourselves in with it. When people are this kind to me I get a nice, soft gushy type feeling. I guess it's called love.

I'm off to the blood lab in an hour. Wish me luck.

Bye. Love you,

P.S. Oh, by the way, Don put down the toilet seat Sunday night. (Just for the record!)

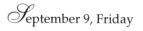

September 9, Friday

Hi,

I have two treatments down and six to go. **YES!** I am pretty wasted, but I have the evening to do "nothing" in. This time the appointment was in the afternoon so I got my errands completed before I went to the chemo clinic.

Betinia, the nurse, is so sweet. She explained the blood counts to me. She said that last week mine showed 2.6. This week I was 7.9. The count has to be at least a three in order for me to have the treatment. She also said that I would probably be able to go dancing Sunday, as long as I was careful and didn't over do it. She is amazed that I am able to dance though. Then, of course, she doesn't know me and my addiction to dancing.

I got the card which you wrote last Sunday. Thank you. I know I'm loved. It helps to keep me going. No I didn't eat two pieces of the chocolate pie. I didn't even have one. Maybe this week-end. But, when I grocery shopped this morning I got some chocolate-chocolate chip cookies. Do they count?

I got three copies of the Nancy Brinker book for each of my breast cancer sisters. I don't know if any of them have read it, but I know two of them have their reconstruction surgeries next month so maybe they can read it while they are recuperating.

In the mail I also got my paperwork to do the "Race For The Cure." I'm looking forward to participating in it.

Bye. Love you,

September 10, Saturday

Morning,

And, it really is that. I've been awake and miserable since two. It's now three. I was lying there thinking of one subject after another and finally decided to get out of the bed and write you. Actually, once again, I was saying how I couldn't write you all this, but I believe you are totally in this with me now, so here goes.

This treatment has hit me much harder than the last one. I know that people told me it would build up with each session, but at the moment I can not imagine it being stronger.

Last night I kept getting weaker and weaker. Finally it got to the point that when I was eating some watermelon I was having a hard time lifting the fork. I was in bed asleep by eight-thirty. I've been drinking water constantly. At two I woke up to go to the bathroom and I could barely get out of bed. My body felt like it was wearing cement. If I had felt like this last week I would have believed that my blood count was as low as they said it was.

Naturally, I was laying in bed thinking about the errands I should do today. I have my "list" sitting on the desk. Now, I'm contemplating calling Arthur and asking him to come get his mail, and then drop off a video for me. The thought of driving, or even walking there, is beyond my imagination right now. I will definitely have to miss Karen's party tonight. If I remember I will enclose her invitation so you can see it. It's a cute one. I'm glad I mailed her a card a couple of days ago. It was a precaution in case I couldn't make it to her party.

I would like to think that by tomorrow I will feel enough energy to at least go to church, and possibly dancing, but I am not going to push it. And, I am concerned over Monday. Monday and Tuesday I am scheduled to go to Staff Development from home, and spend both days, on my feet, doing the classroom support. If Monday morning comes and I don't think I can do it I have my boss' beeper number. I will beep him and he will send one of the other team members in my place.

Just like after the last treatment my face is "butt white," and I am pretty lightheaded and disoriented. When I was at the clinic I told Betinia that my hair has been falling out more so than usual. (Including my pubic hair!) She said this is normal, but my hair is so thick that I shouldn't worry. I told her that I was going to let my hair grow out again, but she suggested that I keep it short while I'm on chemo. I guess the thinning won't be as noticeable, and also if it does decide to completely depart my head it won't be quite as radical as it would be to have long strands falling out.

You are already wrapping Christmas presents? No, you aren't motivating me to do that yet. Wrapping gifts is usually a November chore for me. I am not a good wrapper so it has never been one of my favorite things to do. But, yesterday morning when I was out running errands I did pick up a couple of cute t-shirts for Nick. Also, I ordered some pink slip-on slippers for Dani. She always goes in my closet, and puts mine on and they are way too big for her. I found some for little girls in a L'Eggs catalogue. Now I'll have to find a bathrobe or nightgown to go with them. I also got more baby things for Eric and Bridget. (I've got to stop doing this!) And, I picked up some "pogs" for Nicky, and sunglasses for he and Dani. I can't resist.

I also have a wicked, bad head-ache and I'm not allowed aspirin. (Bitch, bitch, bitch.) See, once again I feel much better by just writing out what I'm feeling. You must be picking up half the load, and it relieves me. (But, poor you.)

I really do feel much better than when I started this.

Bye. Love you,

P.S. One more work story. We have team meetings every other week and the members take turns taking notes and writing up the Minutes. This was Bruce's first meeting as our boss, and my first meeting to be the note taker. He jumped around from subject to subject, and talked really fast, but I was able to keep up. I spent hours writing, and rewriting the minutes. I was so proud of it. Since it was my first time I wanted to do an exceptionally good job. I finished it Wednesday and I thought I put it on our team's shared drive. I also thought I copied it on my hard drive. I didn't make a paper copy, and I threw out my handwritten notes. Then, I e-mailed Bruce and the team members to please review it for corrections before I finalized it for the Managers.

Thursday I thought that I might as well make a paper copy. It wasn't there. I totally panicked and went to the team members and "nope." No one had a copy. They also said that they hadn't taken good notes because I was doing it, and Bruce was moving so quickly through the agenda.

I spent hours recreating, from this worn out memory of mine, what I could and wound up writing another three pages of Minutes. (The original version was five typed pages.) When I finished I made paper copies for the team and distributed it. Whew.

At five o'clock I was going through all my directories and drives, in an attempt to try to figure out what I had done. I found the original Meeting Notes in another directory. I cannot tell you how excited and thrilled I was.

Well, I had given everyone a good laugh. They understood my anxiety though as they have all done similar things in the past. This was my first "trauma" over losing a file though.

September 11, Sunday

Hello,

It is a glorious day here. What about in Massachusetts? The weather is breezy, but sunny and it is so clear out. It's one of those days where everything seems right in the world.

Yesterday I managed to get out and do the things that needed doing after all. I was pretty exhausted by the evening so I never made it to

Karen's birthday party. There will be another time for that I guess. To-day I'm still tired, but I'm much better. Mostly I ache. Remember after the first treatment I had a few days of sore glands? That's what I'm noticing most today. After I write you I am going to get a book and relax on the couch. I'm still hoping to make it to the Cowboy this after-noon. I want to go even if it's only for an hour, and even if I don't dance. It is Ann's birthday celebration.

I felt that this week-end I had to be making up for last week-end. I've been out getting my hair cut and yes, doing more Christmas shop-ping. (That's your fault.) Oh, I also sent you a small package. It has a little birthday gift in it for Jack. The other things are for you. (But, don't go wrecking your tooth on the lollipop!)

I keep meaning to tell you that Newton's wife is okay. The bone scan test came back negative.

We had a guest speaker at church today. She's very well known in the metaphysical community in California. I've heard her speak be-fore. Today's message was about "Acceptance" and I thought, as they always are, her lecture was timely for me.

I'm out of this one.

Bye. Love you,

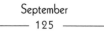

September 12, Monday

Hola yourself!

I'm not much in a letter writing mood, but since I got two very long letters today I am going to respond. Also, I know that the picture of Maria is very special for you so I want to return it right away. The whole story surrounding your meeting her, and your continuing friend-ship is beautiful. Will you go to Mexico with her some day?

If I ever see Don again I will give him your note. (Joke) I haven't heard from him since Thursday night and he wasn't at the Cowboy yesterday afternoon, so naturally I assume that he and his ex are back together. (Now, why would I even think that?) If they are that's not a problem for me. I just don't have much extra energy lately. Using what strength I do have, in the pursuit of any man, would be rather foolish.

Rita, I had to finally throw in the towel and leave work right after lunch. Today was what I thought was "support" day at Staff Develop-ment. I got to the classroom a half hour early as the Trainer prefers and the class was canceled. The secretary called all the students on Thurs-day, but forgot to call me. So, I drove to my office and got there at eight. It was a pretty slow day, but as it went on and on I just started sinking lower and lower in energy. At twelve thirty I put my head on my desk for about ten minutes. I started thinking that if I didn't leave soon, I wouldn't have enough strength to drive myself home. I had to use vacation time for this as I'm out of sick leave.

On the way home I made a quick stop at the pharmacy to get a fleet enema. (Double yuck!) Dr. Nielsen's stool softeners were not working. I hated to use this thing, but I knew that I didn't want to strain and wind up bleeding again. It was a situation of "the lesser of two evils."

After I performed this nasty little chore I totally crashed out. I was exhausted to the point of not wanting to move. Two hours later I felt much better and cooked a pasta dinner. And by the way as of this morning I weigh 104 pounds. I keep wondering why I'm losing more weight.

Yes, I did go dancing yesterday. I took a nap after I wrote you and then I went over to the Cowboy for about one and half hours. I was glad I went, but honestly it wore me out. I came off the dance floor at one point, and realized that my coordination was lousy and that, again in that situation, if I didn't leave **right then** I might not have the energy to drive myself home.

This letter got kind of long considering that I wasn't in the mood to write.

I'll let you know if Don calls tonight. He usually calls from his night job.

Bye. Love,

P.S. Pat, the twin who had the mastectomy, was at the Cowboy yesterday. I went over and gave her a hug. She looked fantastic. Her hair has grown long and curly again. She has the prettiest, old fashioned looking face. Both she and her sister always have men flocking around them. I thanked her again for talking to me that night. She asked me how I was doing with the chemo and I told her it was okay, except for my being so tired. Pat said this is normal. The man she was with, came over to talk to me later. He said he was at her house the night I called her, and that he had been with Pat while she was going through her surgery and chemotherapy. He encouraged me to keep a positive attitude. He said that, that is what will keep me going when times get rough. He was very thoughtful and tender about all this. Pat is lucky to have someone like him giving her his love and support. I envy her that.

September 13, Tuesday

Hello,

Don just called. (I knew you would be interested.) I was right. His ex called him Sunday morning. Once again they are talking through their differences. He would like it to work out, but he says that he is not optimistic. He explained to me more of the details of their relationship and asked me to keep them confidential, which I will, but honest I do not want to get in the middle of this.

I told him he has a new pen pal and that I will get your letter to him somehow, one of these days.

Well, I think I am cured of this attraction. I mean I do have some pride, plus his indecision gets to be a turn off after awhile. Once again, he and I have agreed to just be friends and that sounds good to me.

Today was another support day at Staff Development. I made it through the whole day, but I am exhausted. Hopefully I won't go through this after each treatment.

This really is just a note, but I had to tell you the latest since I was recently raving about Don again.

Bye. Love you,

September 15, Thursday

Dear Lillie:

Our notes must have passed in the mail. Did you get the book I sent?

So the news is no reconstruction? You are so brave and I admire you. You sound very comfortable with your choice.

I am proud of you in so many ways. You have taken what could have been a negative situation, and turned it into a very positive one. In the process of helping other women, you are benefiting. This is the way the world is meant to be, and you are the proof that it can be done.

Sharon had told me about your book being offered through the catalogue. She explained how it came about through your "gortex suggestion" on the mastectomy bras. I say "Yea! And, keep it up!"

So, are you back to work and into the same old routine? And, no one "stole" your position out from under you, right? Like I said before, "They wouldn't dare."

I haven't heard from Sue for awhile. I hope she's okay. Sharon and I talk on the phone once in awhile and also write occasionally. I miss so much being on Prodigy with all of you. Maybe one of these months I'll splurge and go on briefly.

Enough for one night. Have fun on your Florida tour. If they send you to California — call me!

Bye. Love you,

*S*eptember 15, Thursday

Hi,

I really appreciate the "five minute" call. It added even more to this "up" day. Jack's right. I think you do need a break from all this. I've been constantly flooding you with all these letters for what, four months now?

What I need to do is go back to writing in a journal. It's just that it's much more fun writing to you than to myself.

The truth is that I'm sick of the subject too. I think I need a break also. Do you think if I just ignore it, it'll go away? (I guess that won't work.) I know this has to be getting old for you, and the people I work with. Everyone is still great to me, but it's no picnic having someone like me around all the time.

I'll try to write more upbeat letters and talk about other subjects. (There's got to be a life beyond breast cancer.)

Well, your second five minute phone call just now was even better than the first one!

Talk to you later. Are you going to make a third five minute call?

Bye. Love you,

*S*eptember 17, Saturday

Good Morning!

Well, guess who called last night? And, guess who says it's *really* over this time? I explained to him about the boy who cried wolf, and I told him that I didn't believe him. We talked for a pretty good length of time though. I recommended that he find a "wild woman" to play with for a month, or two, to help him get over his addiction. He said he's not into "wild." I suggested that he go out and meet someone else who will sweep him off his feet. (What do I know about relationships, and problems of the heart?)

A few minutes after we hang up, the phone rings. I thought it was you with another "five minute" phone call, but it was Don again. He says, "Would you like to go out for breakfast in the morning?" What am I going to do with him? What am I going to do with myself? Tamsin's right. When it comes to men I'm hopeless. I keep telling her that the truth is that I am quite *hopeful*.

He gave me directions to his studio. I'll drive to his place for a change. I've been very curious to see his studio. I will tell you about it after our date.

And, he got your note. He said he could read most of it, but had problems with something about humility. Are you ready? He took it to work to have an Hispanic friend help him with translating that part. His friend didn't understand it either. (Got me. I have no idea what you wrote.) Oh, except he said that you said you were a woman of "many interests" (which I had already told him.) I said, "She is also a wicked bad flirt." He laughed. He said it's too bad that you have a boyfriend because you and he do have a lot in common. Right, — mainly me. I am trying to stress that point with him.

Actually I already had a hot date with a little man planned for today. I am going to take Nick to feed ducks later this afternoon. So — my datebook is full for the day with my current #1 and #2. Yes, Nick is #1 at this point.

I met a man from Anaheim last night on AOL. We chatted for about half an hour. He goes to the Cowboy, but doesn't dance. He sounded very nice. I don't know if I'll hear from him again. I'm not hearing from any of my new online acquaintances. I'm beginning to think there is a problem with my receiving e-mail. I haven't gotten any although all these people I'm meeting are saying they will write.

I've gotta go and get my car washed.

Bye. Love you,

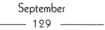

September 17, Saturday

Sharon:

I am so glad you wrote. I needed this letter today. Do you mind if I just talk on and on? I have been overwhelming Rita lately with my problems, so since she needs a break can I pick on you?

First, sincerely I am so glad that you are still writing. Lillie sent me a nice note telling me about her book promotion tour in Florida with the catalogue company. I am so proud of her.

I know how upset you must be feeling regarding the postponement of your reconstruction. Don't these doctors understand that their changes devastate us? It's so easy for them to lead us on, and then re-arrange our lives without a passing thought as to how it all affects us.

Lillie is not going to ever have reconstruction. She has decided to wear the two prosthesis for the rest of her life.

This morning I had another date with Don, my "photographer" friend. He invited me to his studio (nice) and then we went out for breakfast, as he had to shoot a wedding this afternoon. As always I enjoyed myself immensely with him. He is such good company for me. I think we appear to be pretty compatible. It would be great if he could see it that way. He and his girlfriend keep the on again, off again connection going though. I've gotten to the point where I am still attracted to him, but I accept the fact that nothing is ever going to come of us while he continues to hold on to her.

The chemotherapy this time is really tiring me out. Towards the end of this past week I started getting some energy back. Today, I am exhausted again. Even typing this letter is wearing me out.

I do not like the chemotherapy treatments one bit. I know I should be thankful to get this extra precautionary step, but I swear it is not anything to write home about.

Some of the women I have talked to recently, who have done this, say that it's like child birth. Once I get through it, and past it, I will look back and believe that it wasn't so bad. While we are going through it though, it is the pits.

I went on AOL again about two weeks ago. I was e-mailing all these people on the bulletin boards regarding breast cancer, dancing and writing. I couldn't understand why no one was responding. Today I found out there was a glitch and I could not receive mail, but it's since been fixed.

As this letter proves I have really missed writing to you, and today I needed to do just that.

It's a "poor me" letter. Lately I seem to write a lot of them and I don't like that either. Usually I am very up about life. (You can see why I am wearing Rita down with my letters.)

Please don't give up on me. Write me again. Hopefully my next letter will be more cheerful. This is just life that I'm experiencing here.

Bye. Love you,

September 17, Saturday

Hello,

I just wrote a long letter to Sharon with all my problems. See, I'm going to spread them out. This letter to you is going to be short and sweet.

I told you that I would write after my date with Don so here I be. First, though, — my neighbors are moving out today. That is the best news of the day. Finally we will have some peace in the neighborhood again. I am tempted to move next door into the two bath apartment, but I don't think I can handle another change right now.

Okay, on with the story. Here is Don's business card. Now you can write him direct. I also got a picture of him. I think it's adorable, but you will probably say, "What?" If you are curious about him, and promise to mail it back to me, I will send it to you.

His studio is in a very up scale area of Orange County. Rita, his photography is total art. The man is quite talented. I loved every one of his pictures, including the ones of his exes. I even liked the boudoir, and very sensuous, pictures of two exes ago. The man knows what he is doing and should be famous.

The place is decorated with antiques and plants, along with his photographs. It is all done with exquisite taste. He is not a very good housekeeper, as I suspected, but I think when you are that creative some exceptions can be made.

Don said that when he gets an antique toy tractor painted red, (It's now silver and in his salesroom) that he wants me to bring Nick and Dani down and he will do some portraits of them. I'm thrilled that he has even offered to do this.

We checked out his new computer and programs. We even "waltzed" once around the studio. We talked books and family, and then went out to eat. He picked one of my favorite breakfast places. They are a small chain here. We sat out on the patio. As usual I pigged out. I had carrot and raisin pancakes. Yum.

I loved every minute of talking and being with him. When we got back to his studio I told him that I was going to leave so that he could get ready for his wedding shoot at the Ritz Carlton. He gave me one of his incredible hugs, and a sweet kiss. I was surprised once again.

Rita, nothing romantic may ever come of this. I really don't have the strength right now to give him a run for his money, but I do like him a lot. The more time I spend with him, and the more I get to know him, the better I like him. If we just remain friends that would be wonderful in itself.

Now, while I was writing this Tamsin called. She and Nick are moving into my extra bedroom as of this evening!

Well, life is short, beautiful and so unpredictable at times. All we can do is enjoy it.

Love you—

September 19, Monday

Dear Rita,

I have a funny story to tell you, or maybe it's one of those times when you had to be there. I told my dance friend Barbara about it, right after it happened, and we both had tears in our eyes from laughing. One of my regular dance partners was doing a "ducking" type move last night. He is about 6'2" tall. When he came up under my arm his face hit my left "boob." He looked at me and said, "I hope that was as good for you as it was for me." Joe knows I had a mastectomy, but honestly I don't think he realized that what he hit, and what I didn't "feel," other than the impact, was make believe.

I'm enjoying being back on AOL. Once again I am meeting some neat people. The best part is that I can stay in touch with my friends on Prodigy and CompuServe because I can go through the "Internet" gateway. I have an Internet address at AOL and they can write me back at this online service. I am thrilled over discovering how to do this. Now, I just have to get all of their online "addresses."

Also, I am now able to use my fax/modem program. (Do you have a fax number at work? If so, what is it?) Actually, I wish you would get a computer and then we could write through e-mail and have "real time" chats on line.

Oh, and I contacted some book agents, publishers and one movie producer through AOL. The response I'm getting is that they have no need for breast cancer books at this time because the market is flooded with them. The producer said that they recently signed a contract for a TV movie on the subject. (I don't think they realize that breast cancer women cannot read enough on the subject. I have a mini library going at this point.)

I went to the Cowboy for only an hour and a half last night. Don never showed up, but he did say that he might go scuba diving if he could find someone to go with him. On the other hand, maybe he and his ex are back together again. Who knows?

Bye. Love you,

September 23, Friday

Hi,

I feel that I have so much to write you, but I don't know where to begin. See what happens when I skip a few days without writing to you?

Instead of your getting all kids of letters from me, I am getting tons of mail from you. Like #1, #2, and #3 envelopes? Unusual for you, but more like something I would do. You wear me out with all the work you do and the errands you run. This party is getting to be big time already. Bet you'll be glad when it's over, but just think how memorable it will be for both of you. (How is Jack ever going to top this in two years when you turn 50?)

How is your hair now? I hope you are more satisfied with it. Strangely enough I am getting a lot of compliments on my hair. I have no idea why. It seems that since it has thinned out it is much easier to manage and has more softness to it. Also, the last cut that Regina gave me is sort of cute. People keep telling me that I look younger, but I look in the mirror and know the truth!

Actually, I needed to get off that pity trip I was on. I decided that I was sick of complaining about everything and you know what? Now that I've stopped moaning and groaning, things aren't so bad after all.

See, right now I don't have anything to bitch about. Enjoy this letter.

Bridget's shower is on October 16th. I haven't even thought about a shower gift as yet.

We have been having some really beautiful weather here too. When I am on my walks at work it feels so balmy and not hot, not cool, not too windy, but just right. Today was warmer but there was still an ocean breeze.

Our "neighbors from Hell" are out of here. It is wonderful. Last night the lady who lives in the four plex behind me stopped me in the alley. Lois said that she has lived here for twenty-two years and had never experienced anything like them in that time. She said she was feeling sorry for me living next to them. I told her that I would just shut myself in the bedroom and that way I couldn't hear most of their fights.

Yesterday I trained all my former employees on what seems like the most complicated computer system in existence. Out of over 3,500 employees only about six currently use this method to access our e-mail. Last week I trained the Anaheim office (four counselors) and yesterday the Santa Ana office (five counselors). It took me forever to learn it myself so that I could write up a training guide, and know it well enough to teach them. I spent over four hours with them and I think it went really well, but it tired me out considerably.

While there one of the counselors gave me the enclosed pictures. He took them at my farewell potluck. Once again, remember that, that was the day I found out I had to have the open biopsy so I was beyond stressed out.

Today was my Friday flex. I finished cleaning the apartment. I started it last night when I got home from work. Then I had a ten o'clock appointment with Dr. Nielsen. He thinks I am tolerating the chemo extremely well. He brought up the subject of my not being able to exercise until I finish the chemo. I told him about my dancing on Sundays, and also about my two fifteen minute, brisk walks on work days. He was amazed. He could hardly believe that I am doing this.

Then he told me that normally he would tell patients to not eat red meat, but in my case he is recommending that I eat more of it until after I finish the treatments. I told him that I had already started eating filet mignon and he laughed. I asked him to check my cholesterol test results. This is the other thing that surprised both of us. You know how it is supposed to be under 200 to be considered healthy? Mine was 143. Between that and my low blood pressure he said that I may be healthier than him. I am physically in great shape other than this disease.

I have started getting some sores in my mouth. (Not nice) I told him that I am trying to heal them with an old prescription which I had at home. He said to continue using it, but if the sores get worse he will write me a stronger prescription.

We also discussed the constipation. He said it is definitely not any of the chemo drugs, so it has to be the anti-nausea. When I told him that his stool softeners didn't work, but that I got an enema to help, he said that this is probably the best way to go right now. Neither he, nor I, want me to go back to having bleeding hemorrhoids. So, Dr. Nielsen won't be seeing me again for four weeks unless anything comes up that I feel a need to see him about. My exhaustion is normal for the chemo and there's nothing he can give me for that. It's just part of the package deal.

I went from his office to Danielle's open house party. (I'm enclosing her invitation.) It was lots of fun. As usual Danielle knocked herself out for this and, like you are doing on Jack's party, she spent a small fortune.

I finally met her boyfriend. He is a dear, sweet man and I can see why she has been with him for almost fifteen years.

It was great to be with my old staff. We talked a lot, laughed quite a bit and stuffed ourselves. She also had four bottles of champagne. I'm not supposed to be drinking alcohol right now, so I only had about two or three sips of it. Yum. And, then Danielle sent me home with a doggy bag full of food. Want some egg rolls? Nick and Tamsin had some for dinner, along with Danielle's delicious cabbage and chicken salad. (Tamsin was in seventh heaven.)

I am pretty tired. Bye once more.

Love you,

P.S. I have to share this with you. Last night when I came home from work Nick was asleep on the couch. Tamsin was with him reading a book. I came into my bedroom and on my nightstand was the following: a little black rubber wheel from one of Nick's toy cars. Inside it was a tiny bouquet of flowers from one of my patio plants. It was so sweet and delicate and original.

I asked Tamsin, "Did you take Nick out to pick flowers today?" She didn't know what I was talking about. She came in my room and I showed her. She knew nothing about this gift and was touched by it too. She looked at me, smiled and said, "Mom, he loves you very much."

You tell me how a barely three year old could think up this display of love? This little boy just amazes me with himself.

September 25, Sunday

Hi,

I feel like I have so much to write you, and if I don't do it now that I am going to forget half of what I wanted to tell you. I'll have to start making lists soon. I've heard breast cancer women joke that they think the chemo killed off their brain cells. In my case I'm almost convinced of it.

Where to begin? First, I got an appointment card from the plastic surgeon for October 20th. I am so excited. It's like there is a light starting to shine at the end of this tunnel. Of course I have no idea where in Los Angeles this place is, but I'll find it.

Then, did I tell you that I posted a notice on a Bulletin Board on AOL for other breast cancer women to contact me if they wanted someone to talk with, and we could support each other? Also, I am now in an online support group for cancer survivors. They meet "real time" in a chat room every Monday night. The group leader sent me last week's log to download. I read through it this morning and I feel like I know the people in the group already.

I have been in touch with a very nice lady in Oklahoma who just finished her chemo last month. Her name is Deanna. And Sue from Prodigy is now on AOL, and we are in touch again. I have asked AOL to send Sharon and Lillie free software and a free month online. Sharon wants to sign up already. I don't know about Lillie.

Yesterday I got a nice note from another lady who saw my Bulletin Board message. She told me a little bit about her breast cancer, and asked me to write her regarding my disease. I wrote her a long letter about me and told her where I lived and the date of my surgery, etc. She answered last night and said that she lives in Orange County too and works for our newspaper, The Register. I was so surprised and immediately answered her note. I told her that I knew who she was. She is a local celebrity here in Orange County. I've seen her on our news channel, and also read articles in the paper which she has written. About two or three weeks ago there was an article in The Register about her being diagnosed with breast cancer in August. I remembered feeling so sorry for her at the time.

Anyway, she asked me if I would be going to The Race For The Cure today, and she gave me her phone numbers.

I was so tired last night that I fell asleep at 8:15. Tamsin said that Don called at 8:30. But, it was good that I crashed early as I had to get up before daybreak for the race. I got there at about seven. It was a beautiful, yet sad event. (Sort of bitter sweet) I was very emotional. It was incredible to see the thousands of people in support of Breast Cancer Research and Early Detection.

I was touched by all of us "survivors" who stood out in the crowd with our special pink sun visors. The part that got me teary eyed though were the signs on peoples backs. They were pink, and were in memory of loved ones who have died. There were names, and then the relationship, like, "My Mother," "My Auntie," "My Sister," and the hardest one for me to deal with was right in front of me during the walk. It was a lady and her husband. Her pink sign had a name and underneath it she wrote boldly, "My Best Friend." It was beautiful, yet so very sad too.

There were tailgate parties going for different large groups represented, and Orange County Employees had one. We, County of Orange Employees, got our picture taken as a group. Linda, my friend from my old office was there, and two other ladies from work. They are the reason I ended up doing the 5K instead of the one mile fun walk. They were doing the three plus miles, so I decided to try it too. Of course now I'm exhausted and achy and wondering if I'll make it to the Cowboy tonight. I didn't go to church after the race. I came home and crashed out for about fifteen minutes.

I looked all over for my new breast cancer friend from The Register, but there were thousands of people and I couldn't find her. We will meet some other time.

Oh, yesterday morning when I was grocery shopping I got Nick a plastic sword and some more "Power Ranger" cookies. We had had a discussion about both the night before. He was still sleeping when I got home from the store, and I was going out again, so I left them on the coffee table.

When I got home he was playing with the sword. Tamsin said, that he saw it first thing when he woke up and he just kept saying, "Wow. Wow. Wow." Then, "Grandma is my best girl!" She said she cracked up. (I am loved.)

I've gotta go cook some vegetables. Oh, I got the sores on the roof of my mouth healed, but now I've got sores on my gums and they bleed and hurt when I eat. Does this mean I have to start making filet mignon puree?

Bye. Love you,

September 26, Monday

Hi,

I had absolutely no intentions of writing to you tonight. But, as usual, here I am. I got your long letter and I think that I'd better answer it now. Your menu for Jack's party makes me hungry every time I read it. You could not have ordered a catering service, and had so much variety on the menu. It all sounds delicious.

So, Jack thinks what you are giving him tonight is it, right? Tonight is his birthday? I am tempted to call, but in case you are "celebrating," I don't want to be the one who interrupts you!

Today in the mail I received a denial for the disability benefits insurance. I was turned down because of the breast cancer. (No surprise) Tomorrow I am calling the Union to cancel my membership with them. I only joined to get the extra benefits.

Last night I had so much fun dancing. I danced and danced. At one point Allen was standing by my bar stool, waiting for me to come off of the floor. He said, "A guy has to get in line in order to get a dance with you." I laughed. I was pretty popular last night.

Don showed up, and to tell the truth, I really didn't get a chance to dance much with him either. At about six o'clock he came over and said, "Do you want to leave?" I said, "Sure. I'm hungry as usual." He said we could get something to eat. I suggested that we pick up a pizza, and come back to my apartment so that he could meet Tamsin and Nick.

We got a large one and shared it with Nick and Tamsin. Nick was quite entertaining and was in awe over Don. And, Don was quite responsive to him too. He was really good with Nick. He had him laughing and climbing into his lap and playing with his beard. It was cute to watch the two of them together.

Don told me that he wanted me to know that his mind is not in a good place right now for him to start a new relationship. He said he cares a lot about me and doesn't want me to get hurt. I've thought about this on and off all day. I think there is a warning there and I'd better heed it. Also, I keep thinking of something that was in one of the lectures at church. It went, "Insanity is doing the same thing over and over again, and expecting different results." Well, I started thinking how this is reminding me of when I fell in love with Justin. And, then I think, "I don't want to go through an experience like that again." Even the words are starting to sound the same.

So, it's time for me to back up a bit. I am growing too fond of this man.

Even though you didn't ask, I am sending Don's picture. (Please return it.)

Oh, tonight was my first night with the online "cancer survivors" support group. It was fun. The people were great. I joined late as they started before I got home from work. But, I just jumped right in. It gets very busy with so many conversations going on at once. If I get a copy of the log I might send it to you, although I suspect it'll appear to be boring and confusing. It's one of those things where you have to be there to understand it.

I'm out of here and off to bed.

Love you,

September 27, Tuesday

Hello,

I have a letter sitting on my dresser for you right now. Since I'm home from work today I decided to write you another one to go with it. (It's a #1 and #2 mailing day!) Actually, there is not much to write about, but what else can I do when I'm home like this?

I woke up at four-thirty to go to the bathroom and almost fell on the floor. At first I thought that my equilibrium had left me. I had to hold onto the furniture and the walls to get me there. I am better now, but I am still very weak. I don't dare drive into Santa Ana like this. Strange. Maybe my count is really low again. I'll find out Thursday when I get the result of my next blood test.

I've been using the old medicine I had for the mouth sores and it's working okay. At least my gums have stopped bleeding, but they are still very sensitive.

Bye. Love you,

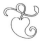

September 29, Thursday

Dear Rita,

Well, I'm having another "vacation" day today. My blood count is lower than the last time (2.0). Earlier this week I figured that it must be real low because of the way I've been feeling. My chemotherapy for tomorrow has been canceled. Betinia says for me to stay indoors, away from people, until at least Monday. I explained to her about my taking so much time off work and that I get worried that I'll run out of vacation time, and then there will be no paycheck. She said that she will leave it up to me to determine how I'm feeling by tomorrow, but I definitely have to stay away from anyone who is sick.

Also, the sores in my mouth are popping up continuously. I just get one cleared up and another comes along. I've asked her for another prescription for medicine for the sores. She is going to check with Dr. Nielsen and get back to me.

Oh, the good part of all this! The chemotherapy will be administered every four weeks (on my flex days) and I will only wind up having six treatments over the six month period. (Versus the original eight treatments.)

People at work are trying to fatten me up too. Yesterday someone gave me a piece of poppy seed cake in the morning, and in the afternoon another person gave me a blueberry muffin. One of the clerical staff from downstairs has called me over two dozen times in the past month with computer questions. She brought me the muffin to thank me. That made me feel good.

I haven't heard from Don since I sent him the e-mail telling him that I was going to back off a bit.

But, I have met another gentleman online. He is from Arizona originally, but is in Northern California working temporarily as a consultant with a Police Department. His name is Stephen, and he is Chinese-American. He sounds like a doll. I gave him my phone number already, and I definitely would like to hear more from him. He doesn't dance, but he does listen to country music.

Did I tell you that Nick plays on the computer? I got a "Disney" program a couple of months ago for he and Dani. He loves it. I have to get more, but they are expensive.

I know you are busy with party preparations and getting ready for your trip to Mexico. I've been thinking about you and Jack a lot lately.

Don't worry about me. I'm not alone like I was over the Labor Day week-end, and also, the low blood count didn't come as a surprise to me this time. I'll be fine.

Bye. Love you,

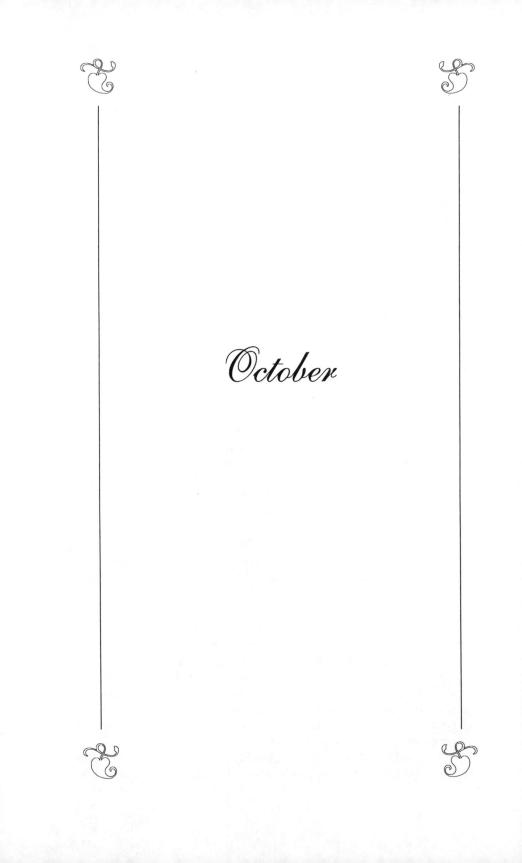

October

*O*ctober 1, Saturday

Rita,

I just know that Jack's party is going to be a huge success. I am amazed how relaxed you sounded on the phone. If it were me I would be a wreck.

What day do you leave for Mexico? You must be excited. Take lots of pictures.

Now, about Don. Yes, he does look like Santa Claus. And yes, I must be attracted to men who look like Santa. I love beards, and I love "cuddly" men. I still like Don, but I have had enough. I need to feel that I am number one in a man's eyes. This will never happen with him. He is still in love with his ex-girlfriend. Anyway, meeting the right man to fall in love with is just a numbers game. I am going through the numbers and have been for almost a year now. Pretty soon "he" will be right here when he is supposed to be. I am not giving up on it happening.

The men I am meeting online have been total gentlemen. I would like to meet them in person some day. I have Stephen's phone number. One of these days I am going to call him. Jim also sounds interesting. Mike I haven't heard from all week, and that happens sometimes.

The women I meet online are all so fun too. Last night one lady from San Diego told me that she met a guy from Florida online. They kept writing, and then they started talking on the phone. Next he sent her airline tickets. She went to visit him and they fell in love. She is now packing up to move there with her two daughters. Wow!

Chris, at work, has met two men from AOL. I don't think she has been real impressed with either one. Like I said, it's a numbers game.

I gotta go. I will be thinking of you at three o'clock your time.

Bye. Love you,

*O*ctober 1, Thursday

Lillie—

This should be short, but I wanted to get a response back to you and put it in today's mail. You wear me out with all that you are doing, flying here, there and everywhere. I'm glad that your Florida trip was so successful and productive. And, it pleases me to hear that you are also participating in the Race For The Cure. I have my blue t-shirt on again today from last Sunday's race.

The good news here is that I am back on AOL, and I can write you through the Internet if you give me your Prodigy address. Sharon is thinking of coming over to AOL so I requested that they send her some free software and a free month online to try it out. While I was doing that I also asked them to send you some. You might want to try it. Sue is already on AOL so we are able to communicate again.

On AOL there is a Cancer Survivors group which meets every Monday night, nine o'clock your time and six o'clock my time. We meet in a "chat" room and it is really fun. The people are very nice. I'm enjoying it. Also, I have met a couple of interesting men in the chat rooms. Last night, since I couldn't go out anywhere because of the chemo side effects, my entertainment was AOL. I joined a party in the "over forty" chat room, and did we ever party. It was hilarious. I think I had more fun there then I would have had if I had gone out somewhere.

Enough for this one letter.

Bye. Love you,

October 6, Thursday

Hola:

You will be in Mexico when this arrives, but I didn't want you to think I had gone on strike or anything.

I am so glad that Jack's party was such a success. And thank you for calling me while it was going on. I felt like I was participating in it with all of you. (You all sounded wasted!) Your Mom was the one who shocked me though. Did she tell you what she said to me? I thought it was you when she said that!

We are getting rain too, but in our case it is much appreciated. I have even gone walking in the rain during one of my work breaks. It felt wonderful.

My blood count is up enough this week to get the chemo tomorrow. Good. I want to get them over, and done with. This time I have a long holiday week-end to get it together after the treatment.

Nick is a cutie, but this little man keeps re-arranging my bedroom; correction — the whole apartment. I just notice it more in my room. He's got a thing for moving decorator items and stuff. Like, my bedroom silk plants wind up in the living room and dresser items wind up in weird places too. (My perfume was in my slipper.)

I have also been busy with AOL. I am writing and having "real time" chats almost every night with Stephen. He is going to get his hair cut today, and then have a picture taken to mail me. I'll let you see it when I get it.

Also, Sharon is now on AOL. Yippee! She and I are both thrilled. We can get back to writing our daily notes. I've missed her since I left

Prodigy.

Rob is on too. He writes me every once in awhile.

I have a copy of the chat log from last Monday night's cancer group. Maybe I'll send it to you, but I don't want you to get the wrong impression and think this is all weird. You probably already do, so what the heck.

Work is okay. I have a new project assigned to me, and I've been learning what it's about so that I can train some clerical staff on the procedure. Also, I have been learning more about that complicated computer system, which I wrote you about before, as I am doing more training for the Work Program staff beginning next week.

I finally put in a full week too. I was getting worried about running out of vacation time.

I'll keep writing while you are gone. You'll have a mini-book to read when you get back.

Bye. Love you,

October 7, Friday

Hello,

You must be all packed and ready to be on your way. I will be thinking about you and also writing you. You can't escape my letters so easily.

Actually, today was chemo day. It's the same routine as before except today I feel cheered up. Stephen, my friend on AOL just sent me the most beautiful bouquet. I almost started crying. A few nights ago when we were online he told me he was sending me something on Friday to cheer me up. (I thought he meant an e-mail.) I am overwhelmed by this. He has my address because, as I told you in an earlier letter, he is mailing me his picture.

And, this morning he left me a note about meeting him tonight at eight o'clock online. (We have a "computer date" here.) Let's hope I have the energy to push the keys by eight o'clock tonight. I took a short nap when I got home from the chemo clinic so maybe I'll be able to do it. Also, now I am very motivated to meet with him again.

I want to get to know this man more. He has just blown my mind with these flowers!

Talk to you later.

Bye. Love you,

*O*ctober 10, Monday

Hello,

As we are sweltering in the heat wave here, I am wondering if you are getting the same in Mexico. I suspect it must be hot there too. Periodically, throughout the day, I will think about you and wonder what you are doing and where you are.

Yesterday was so much fun at the Cowboy. I stayed and danced non-stop for two hours, and probably over did it. Even driving home was hard after that. But I felt like I was very much in demand. I had seen Paul earlier in the day, after church, when I picked up Nick at Sunday School. I asked him if he was going dancing and he said he'd be there. When he showed up I invited him to sit at our table, and introduced him to my friends. Then Allen showed up and I introduced he and Paul. Twice during the evening I had three men asking me to dance at the same time! It was a little overwhelming. Finally I was losing all balance and coordination, and I just had to get out of there before I made a fool of myself.

Eric and Bridget came over last night. She looks wonderful. Her face has that "pregnancy glow" to it, and she is well rested and healthy looking. The only weight she has gained appears to be "baby;" eighteen pounds so far. The doctor told her she could gain up to twenty-five pounds and she only has one more month to go. She can't wait for her shower next Sunday. Also, tomorrow is her twenty sixth birthday.

For her shower I got a baby bath tub and put a lilac (for her purple passion) diaper bag in it. In the diaper bag are: cloth diapers, baby bottles, baby face cloths, a box of baby wipes, 3 onesies, and a pair of matching booties, baby soap, shampoo, oil, lotion and it seems there are a few other things that I am forgetting, but that diaper bag is full. The hard part was trying to wrap this thing. I dislike wrapping gifts anyway so this one was especially annoying.

Stephen has become our hero. My breast cancer sisters cannot believe that any man could be so thoughtful, and caring as to send flowers on chemo day to someone he has never met. They are just as much in awe of him as I am. And, then I also told them that he is helping all Cancer Survivors by donating his platelets on a regular basis. His platelets are used for children on chemo.

He left a message on my machine Saturday morning, but I wasn't home. He has a nice sounding voice. It's very deep and sexy, and he sounded nervous. But, I think that makes him even more endearing.

I am very tired this time from the chemo. I just don't have my normal "bounce." It is going to be fantastic when I get off chemo and I feel energetic again.

I have to save some of this key pushing energy for the group to-night.

Bye. Love you,

October 12, Wednesday

Hello — Hello again,

I am going to try to type this as fast as I can, so please ignore the typos. I have so much to tell you.

First, I love Jack's birthday party pictures and you look great in all of them. Also, I read the article about where you are staying in Mexico. It sounds like heaven. You should have a relaxing vacation there.

Okay, where do I begin? I was interviewed at lunch time by a reporter from our local newspaper. It'll be in Sunday's Register. The article is about "Cyberspace Women On Line."

The reporter called me yesterday. She said that she had heard about me and my online support group with my breast cancer sisters, and the men I'm meeting. She asked me if I would I be willing to talk about it. At first I was hesitant, and especially when she mentioned my picture would be included, but I thought "What the heck." If more women, who need us, can find us online then it's worth it.

The reporter was very nice. The interview took about forty-five minutes and she took lots of notes. I talked a lot and she asked lots of questions. She was laughing over some of my stories. I hope what she writes (and what I blabbed about) doesn't embarrass me. I'll send you a copy.

Then, last night I got a hilarious card from Stephen, with his picture in it. I wouldn't say he is handsome, but I think he's cute. All I know is that he is my hero with his actions and kindnesses. I hope I am able to meet him someday. I told him that I would probably talk about him during the newspaper interview.

I know there is much more to write about, but when I don't stay on top of it, with daily letters, I lose track and wonder if I already told you "whatever."

Bye. Love you,

Later:

Also, I wanted to enclose a clipping of my breast cancer sister who is a news reporter here in Orange County. She writes articles for seniors. She is the one who had the other reporter call me about being interviewed.

Then, while I'm using a big envelope I thought you might want to see a picture of Sharon. She is the sweetest lady and I am crazy about her. I am glad that I've met her and I hope to meet her in person some day.

And, I am not done yet. I figure you probably want to see Stephen too, right? Okay, here is the hilarious card that he sent me and his picture. Now you go find a big envelope and return both to me!

I will send you a copy of the newspaper article when it comes out on Sunday. I am not thrilled about the fact that my picture will be included. I have been avoiding cameras because of my "chemo" complexion, and also my "pinched" face. I asked the man who was taking the pictures if he could take ten years off my face and add ten pounds to my body!

I'm tired. It's been too exciting a day for me. This time, this letter is really over.

Love again,

$$\text{🙰}$$

$\mathcal{O}$ctober 16, Sunday

Good Morning:

I've gotten to the point where I have to make myself notes of all the things I want to be sure to tell you. Actually, I am tempted to call, but I am really busy, and know you must be too after getting back from your trip.

Once more, where do I begin? Enclosed please see what made today's paper. There are some inaccuracies, like the date of my surgery and other bits, which are minor. Overall I think she did a pretty good job. What do you think of the picture? I never like pictures of me so I don't know. I'm just glad it's over with, except for the teasing I know I will be getting from everyone.

Also, here is a laser copy of a picture taken of Ann and I my first day back to dancing. This was one month after the mastectomy. I think I look ghastly, but Ann looks really pretty here.

Yesterday was a fun and busy day. Tamsin and Nick and I went to the park in the morning. I got lots of exercise. After lunch Arthur and Dani and Bridget all came by. The kids play so well together and it was great having all the family here (minus Eric who was, as usual, at work).

After they all left I went over to Paul's house. I had AOL send him some free software and a free month online too, and he wanted me to help him get setup and navigated. (This he could most likely do himself as he is such a computer guru, but I went and had a good time doing it.) I stayed about three hours. He loves it, and now he can't believe it took him this long to go online.

My breast cancer sister, Sue, just discovered a new lump in her remaining breast. Her reconstruction was scheduled for December 16th. She is having tests done on the twenty first. I am practically hysterical over this, but she is handling it so calmly. I hate this damned disease.

Okay, what you really want to hear about is where Stephen and I are at this point, right? I saved the best for last.

We have spent the past two nights on the phone talking for about a total of five hours. We are trying to get to know one another better. He originally thought he would fly down here one week-end. I suggested that we meet on neutral territory, and half way between us. We are talking about meeting in Santa Barbara, but not until I am healthy enough to make a four hour drive.

Do I have a crush on him? Yes I do, but at this point it is a "fantasy" to me since I have never met him in person. He says he really is who he is portraying to me. If that is the case then I think he is dynamite. Then when we meet there may be no chemistry involved. It's hard to know how this will go. What I did express to him is that if this doesn't work out romantically (and what are the chances of that?) that I definitely want him in my life as a close friend. And, he has agreed to that.

Naturally I will keep you posted.

When are you going to get a computer and come online with us? It doesn't make sense for me to keep writing these postal letters ("snail mail") when I could be sending them to you through "cyberspace." Think about it please! Talk to Jack about it. It is the future, and it is fun.

I know there must be more that I am forgetting about, but I've had enough. Don't forget I am online writing to people constantly these days so you are getting a break from the daily mail. Aren't you glad for that?

Love you,

October 18, Tuesday

Hello,

I have really missed hearing from you. I didn't even get a post card. I hope this means that you were too busy having fun. Once you get all settled at home please write so I know everything is okay.

Today is another at home day, and I'm using my vacation time again. I'm just not sleeping good at night. I have fever and chills and also, today I am pretty weak and lightheaded. This is not the third week, where I normally would be experiencing the low blood count, but maybe it is starting earlier since each time I get the chemo my count is lower.

Okay — the juicy stuff. MEN, or I should say singular, Stephen.

Rita, I know I have experienced some weird relationships, but this one is totally new for me. I have a crush on him now, and we've never even met. He is becoming a very close friend, and what I am learning about him I like a lot. I have no idea what it's going to be like once we meet face to face. I was hoping that his video would come today while I was home. He sent it priority mail. I am thinking about sending him the one of Eric and Bridget's wedding. We'll see about that though!

Anyway, we are still e-mailing each other constantly every day, and sending cards to each other, and pictures. Last night was my online cancer group and he IM'd me before it to tell me that he would meet me after my group. (So cyber romantic) I felt like I was back in High School when my boyfriend used to wait for me, and walk me home while carrying my books. I told all my breast cancer girlfriends and we spent more time last night in what is known as "the loft" talking instead of being in the group. ("The loft" is when you are in a room, but do IM's instead.) Sharon was there. This was her first night in cancer survivors and I think she enjoyed it. Then two other breast cancer sisters were Im'ing me. I told them about Stephen and my "hot" online date after group. I got teased bad, but I think they are really happy for me.

So, I met Stephen and we chatted for over an hour, until my stomach was growling so loud I thought he could hear it through "cyberspace."

Rita, I honestly don't know about May. I am using so much vacation time for chemo effects and I have the surgeries to do which will involve a lot of time off work also. I have my appointment in Los Angeles Thursday morning with the plastic surgeon. I should know more after that.

Paul is enjoying being online. I knew he would. We e-mail each other often. Next week-end he is going to a dance festival in San Diego and is entering a Jack and Jill competition. This is his first one. I'm really excited for him and proud of him that he is doing it. Those competition days are over for me. They were fun, but nerve wracking.

I was teased at work, but I also received a lot of compliments regarding the newspaper article. What did you think? And be honest.

I keep eating because my weight went back down to 103 pounds. A Sarah Lee cheesecake is waiting for me now.

Bye. Love you,

*O*ctober 18, Tuesday

Stephen,

I can't believe I am doing this but, here is one video tape that maybe you can see me in. It is my youngest son Eric's wedding tape from two years ago. I do not like it of me because I was operating on only four hours of sleep, and I was stressed beyond the max. The original site in this huge park, which my daughter in law, Bridget, had reserved turned out to be taken over by a school's athletic event. We found out that morning, and I was having chairs and a wedding cake delivered to that site. So, my ex-fiance and I went to the park. I was in baggy, around the house sweats,— and thinking I would just be there a few minutes and come right home to get myself ready. WRONG. Everyone else had other stuff to do so I wound up at the park putting things together.

Then I had to rush to my oldest son, Arthur's, house to get my grand-daughter, Dani, who was the flower girl. After that my brother, his wife and son were arriving at my apartment from San Francisco, and it was just way too hectic.

Added to the stress was having three ex-husbands and a fiancé at the wedding. (You try coping with that.) See why I don't think I look so hot here?

My son and his wife are so cute together. They have been married two years and are still like honeymooners. They are the perfect couple. And, they will have their first baby in less than a month.

Okay — if I can explain the people here. . . and introduce you to my family, and my extended family, which includes exes and ex-in laws.

Me — in the baggy sweats earlier, and later in the blue silk dress. My hair was short and sort of colored golden brown. (I was constantly having a grandchild in my arms throughout the day.)

Eric, my youngest son (27) and his wife, Bridget (26). . . the bride and groom

Arthur, my oldest son (also 27 until November 8th — the boys are 10 ½ months apart) was the best man and the jokester. They are always playing jokes on each other, and everyone else. He really made me feel good when he did the toast and talked about Eric being more than his brother, but also his best friend. The cute little blonde girl, who was the flower girl, is his daughter Dani.

Tamsin, my daughter (23) is in the short white skirt and black top. She was with her boyfriend at the time. The cute little boy in blue coveralls is her son, Nicholas.

The older couple in the gray suits (and he was the minister) are my Uncle George and Aunt Dot. They are wonderful people. He is my mother's younger brother.

My first ex husband, also named "Arthur," was the thin man in the navy blazer, red tie and eyeglasses. He sat with me up front during the ceremony. He was my High School sweetheart, and is the natural father of my two sons. He flew out from New Hampshire, but his wife, Darleen, couldn't make it.

My second ex-husband is Tom. His wife was with him in a floral dress. He is the only one of my exes who doesn't like me much, and we do not have a continuing friendship. Tom adopted my sons, and he is Tamsin's natural father. Confused yet? And there is still more if you can find everyone on this tape.

My third ex-husband is, again, an "Art" and he is the handsome, taller man with the dark beard, and the dark tweed jacket with a blue shirt. You can see that the two Art's get along great. They were talking with each other for a good part of the day. This Art came down from San Jose with his fiancee and her two girls. She is the pretty Filipino lady. Art is an electronics engineer. He and I remain very close friends.

My fourth ex-husband, well — you are spared. He was not invited. We were only married for one year, and he did not bond to my kids like the other "father's." He and I are friends though and his current wife and I get along okay. I see them out dancing and he e-mails me on AOL. His name is Rob.

More: My brother Bud, his wife Lynn and son Myles came from San Francisco and we were filmed at my apartment prior to the wedding. She is the blonde lady and he is the handsome, white haired gentleman with a mustache and lots of smiles. I hope you can find him here.

My ex-sister in law, Ashley, caught the bridal bouquet. She and my ex-mother-in- law, Laura were also at the wedding. My boys' best friend is the one who caught the garter.

Whew. There were other friends there, but honestly the majority of the people were Bridget's family, which is huge.

I'm done. I hope you still write to me after this. Thanks.

Love,

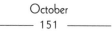

October 20, Thursday

Dear Rita,

I just tried to call you but no one was home. I'm leaving in a little while to drive up to Los Angeles for my plastic surgery appointment. I am excited somewhat. This letter will probably be finished tonight when I have more to tell you.

Hey, you are getting a break. Stephen is taking over for you. I swear he is helping me through the chemo effects, just by being there. He causes me to be motivated and happy when I am really being dragged down by what feels like lead in my veins. I think I am falling in love with him! Is it possible to fall in love with someone that you have never met face to face? Actually, he is going through this feeling too, and he has both feet firmly planted on the ground, which is another trait of his that I admire.

Yesterday I got the video tape of him. I have only watched it *four* times so far because Tamsin is making fun of me. Stephen is cute, and has a baby face. I'm going to look like an old lady beside him. He says he likes older women. Hmm. I told him that at least no one would mistake me for his mother.

Danielle said, "DO NOT send that tape to Rita until I have seen it!" Chris is upset because I mailed his picture to you before she saw it. I am taking the video tape into work so she can see him. I think I told you, or maybe not, that I have introduced Chris and Stephen online. When he and I were on the phone the other night he was "chatting" with her, while he was talking to me, and relaying messages back and forth between us. Chris is the one that you thought was Karen, in the picture I sent from our meeting in the park. We have known each other professionally for almost twenty-five years. Chris said that she told Stephen that he is doing wonders for me, and she is so glad that he is in my life right now. She said that she told him I come into work exhausted, but smiling and happy because of the sweet things he does for me.

Yesterday I was just beyond weary while at work, but I kept going. I was glad I was there as I got lots of e-mail regarding the newspaper article, and people were calling me. They all made me feel so good, and said many complimentary things about the picture, the article and me. The women said that I am totally an inspiration to them. The men are cute too, and everyone is following this online romance.

I hope all is okay with you, and that you are just very busy. I have not heard from you for so long. Please write or call and let me know how you are.

Love you,

October 21, Friday

Rita,

I finally got two long letters from you. I am glad that your vacation was so perfect. I'm looking forward to seeing the pictures. These pictures of Cape Cod are beautiful. (Sigh)

Well, I can't wait to send you the video of Stephen. I took it to work

yesterday and showed everyone. I heard comments like: "He is so cute."
"He is a teddy bear." "He is so young looking." "He is a saint." and on
and on. . . . and I heard, "Go for it!"

I feel so lucky to have met him. I am falling in love with him. We
were online last night for I think four to five hours, just chatting and
discussing, are you ready — sex. (I'm ready.) He made me cry last night.
When we were joking about sex, I told him to get serious for a minute.
Then I said, "What about my missing breast?" He wrote me some beautiful notes, and I was so touched. In the end he said, "All the more
pleasure for the one remaining." I love this man!

We don't know when we will meet, but maybe in mid December.
This is a rough time for both of us, between my chemo, the new baby
coming, his buying the new house, his involvement with so many volunteer activities, and an upcoming conference. And, of course, the holidays.

I wish I was healthy and strong for him, but he is so understanding
and so gentle. He is a truly beautiful man. I want him! I can't wait for
you to meet him on the video. I will mail it Sunday.

My plastic surgery appointment: Not quite what I was hoping to
hear, but not bad. My doctor is a very nice Vietnamese man. He won't
do the surgery until at least three months after the chemo. He is looking at April, or May, depending on his schedule. He will not remove
my remaining healthy breast, so forget that idea. Plus now Stephen has
me motivated to keep it, right? Then, he really doesn't want to do the
abdominal surgery. He says I don't quite have enough tummy right
now. He said, "I can make you a small one from it, maybe." I said, "No
thanks — I'd prefer them to be the same size."

He said I would have two scars from an abdominal implant, and it
would probably cause me to have back problems from the removal of
the abdominal muscle, and I'd be prone to hernias. Also, I would be in
the hospital at least four days, and off work for four weeks after that.

So it looks like I'll be getting a saline implant. I will be in the hospital one day over night and off work for two weeks. Then I will go back
to him some time later and he will adjust the implant and lift the right
breast so that they match in size and shape. At that time he will remove
some tissue from under the good breast, and part of it's nipple to graft
over to the left breast to start an areola and nipple there.

I told him that I have lost weight, and worry about one boob growing while the other stays small. But, I guess if I'm not fat at this age of
my life then it probably won't ever happen.

There's got to be more to tell you. I just know there is, but I feel
mentally wasted lately. I have an oncology appointment in four hours

and I want to clean the house and answer some AOL mail between now and then, so I am out of here.

Love you,

P.S. I cannot wait for you to see Stephen on this video. Wow!

October 21, Friday

Hello,

Two letters from me in one day means you are home from vacation, and I'm up to my old tricks again. Actually, I just got off the phone with Elaine. I want to write to you before I start an e-mail to Stephen, and possibly end up online.

My oncologist walked in to the exam room, looks at me and says, "You still have hair!" I said, "It's thinned, but I still have hair, and I am ever so thankful for that." Then he read my article from the newspaper. My chemo nurse, Betinia, saw it Sunday. They have it hanging on the chemo clinic bulletin board. Anyway, he starts reading it and says, "I can't believe you are a grandmother. A mother, yes, but not a grand-mother." That made my morning because I was feeling about seventy years old. (It's been a really bad week for energy.) We discussed my sleeping problem and he gave me another prescription for that. It's Elavil, a mild anti-depressant. I don't think I am depressed, but he says I could be and not realize it. (I can fall asleep, but I wake up at two, three or four and I can't go back to sleep. This pattern is supposed to be a sign of depression.) I told him that I am incredibly happy these days and that I have a lot going for me.

And, we also talked about Stephen. He is impressed that Stephen does Apheresis and gives his platelets to chemo children. Betinia is "wowed" about this too. (My hero)

Dr. Nielsen also said, "Your prognosis is excellent." I already know that, and am so grateful for where I stand in this whole process. I think he wanted to reassure me since I was bragging about grand-kids and Stephen to him.

Then I checked my e-mail and guess what? A publisher contacted me via AOL and said to send them a query letter and one chapter as they may be interested. I immediately wrote the letter, packed up five chapters, our picture, a copy of the newspaper article and took them to a Postal Center. They should have it by Tuesday. I am thrilled that some-one will at least read it and, hopefully, give me an honest opinion. Step one here.

My aunt and uncle sent me the nicest letter regarding the newspa-per article. Then, Elaine called tonight as she got her copy. She loved it and is Xeroxing it for some breast cancer women she knows. Also, I sold Elaine on AOL. She is going to get a modem and I am going to request that they send her software. Pretty soon she and I can write via e-mail. When are you going to join us?

Stephen got my video. He says I'm not so bad looking as I am making myself out to be. Of course he isn't going overboard about my looks either. He is an honest man.

I'm glad you are there.

Bye. Love you,

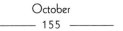

October 22, Saturday

Hola,

I just got the package with all your vacation pictures. They are beautiful. But spiders, bats, lizards, moths— and you call that a vacation? Yuck! Also, I'm looking at you climbing up those ruins, and I don't normally have a fear of heights, but you do — and I'm getting dizzy. Honest, I don't think I could climb them they are so steep. I am proud of you!

Nick is waiting for me to take him to a Pumpkin Patch, but I wanted to mail this while I was out so that you will have the pictures to show others.

This morning I got a teddy bear, wearing a big red bow, from Stephen. (Explanation: Stephen asked me what I wanted for Christmas this year and I told him I wanted *him*, with a big red bow. Then I had told him about Marvette's comment that she thought he was a "big teddy bear," and I said that I agreed with her.) The teddy bear was sent to hold me for now. It came with another cute and funny card.

Well, I was going to end this, and you called, so guess I really don't need to go any further since we just covered every available topic.

Bye. Love you,

October 26, Wednesday

Good Morning,

All is wonderful here. I am sleeping really good lately and eating lots. I've gained three pounds and I'm loving it. Stephen is back from Lake Tahoe, but just for one day. He and I chatted online last night for about an hour.

Stephen is so busy. I don't know how he does it all. He volunteers for everything. This week-end he is assisting the School District with a 10K race to raise money. A few weeks ago he was the bartender at some other city function. He makes me tired just listening to all he does.

Oh, and he accepted an assignment in Nevada, but he will be staying in Lake Tahoe while he's working there. On his days off he will drive home to work on the new house which he bought! (It's a four hour drive.)

Remember Jessica, the lady who I talked to the night before I had my mastectomy? She had her mastectomy about two years ago and had a really rough time of it. Anyway, she called me a week ago to ask about the vacant position in Systems, which will fill Bruce's spot. I talked to her for about an hour telling her all about the job, and the working conditions and how much I enjoy being here. She said she was intimidated by "Systems," and she felt that she didn't know enough. I told her she knew more than I did, because I didn't even know what a screen saver was when I got here.

Anyway, I must have done a pretty good sales job because my Manager said Jessica put in a memo to transfer, and hers was the only one received. (People are afraid of PC's because it's all new to them.) So, Jessica may get the job. That would please me immensely because I like her a lot. She is about my age and is a tall, sexy blonde with a great sense of humor. It'll be fun if she joins our team.

Bye. Love you,

$\mathcal{O}$ctober 28, Friday

Hello,

That is so strange about the mail with my article in it. Did you get a picture of Ann and I? If not then I think it was in the same envelope. My breast cancer sister Deanna didn't get hers either. She called me the other night. I hadn't heard from her online in over a week and was getting concerned. Deanna called to say that she was going through withdrawal because her computer broke, and she hadn't been able to come online and join us. She said she was calling because she didn't want us to forget about her. (Like we could. . . NOT.) I sent her a second copy of the newspaper article also.

What was a coincidence was that Sharon and I were getting very worried about Sue because we had not heard from her for awhile, and she was having the mammogram on her other breast for the lump that was found. Last night I finally got e-mail from her and she said that her computer got a virus. She couldn't go online, and she was going through withdrawal and missing us. I know exactly what they were going through.

Other breast cancer sister news: Sharon starts her reconstruction next Friday. She is very nervous about it and asked if we could meet her online the night before the surgery to give her support. I am going online after I write this, and find out what time, and where we are going to meet, and if she wants the other breast cancer sisters there too.

I haven't heard from the Publisher about the book, but I am told it takes up to two months to get a response.

Are you sending me vegetable cards because of all the steamed vegetables I was eating? Actually I am burned out on them. And, I am eating chocolate again! Yea! As a matter of fact Stephen and I talked for about two hours on the phone again last night. He says that there is a box of gourmet chocolates and cashews in the mail to me. (My Trick or Treat) I think that he is trying to fatten me up. Actually, what he is doing is spoiling me rotten, and I love every bit of it.

I got a cute Halloween card yesterday with another picture of him in it. In this one he is wearing his eyeglasses. He got back Thursday night from Tahoe and we e-mailed each other pages. Then we got on the phone last night, and we only got off when we did because Tamsin needed to use it.

I don't know how he does everything. He has so much energy. Stephen was thinking of coming down here next week-end, and I do want to see him, but I get chemo on Friday, and I'll be pretty wasted until at least Sunday so I told him not to bother. The next week-end is his conference. It is getting harder and harder on the both of us. And, he is feeling exactly what I am feeling. This is not just one sided here.

I took the video tape to the Work Program yesterday so Danielle could see him while I was doing my training. She and Chau, and the others all watched it and not just once, but several times. They studied every bit of him. (Poor man) The verdict was, again "Go for it." I'll be curious to hear what you have to say about him.

I am incredibly happy these days Rita. I cannot tell you how much I appreciate Stephen and all the kind and thoughtful things he does for me. What a difference from some of the men I have dated in the past. This man is — well, he is like you and Danielle. I guess you could say he is a good friend and also, I am attracted to him physically.

People at work tease me. They say that if they just mention his name I beam all over. They think it's wonderful, and of course they are pretty impressed with him too.

Last night he said that he saves every e-mail I write him. I told him I have every one of his. He said we could write a book. I agreed, but told him that that book has to wait until ours is finished!

Okay, I think this letter has gotten quite long enough.

Love you lots,

Good Evening,

Here I am getting back into the once a day letter writing routine again. Actually, NOT! But, I was thinking about you and decided to write a short note. (I think it will be short anyway.)

I forgot to tell you that Nick got his Halloween card and loves it. He pretends it's a mask and peeks out the eyes of the pumpkin. So what are your plans for the Holiday? I bought about five bags of candies today for the trick or treaters. Nick has an adorable gray mouse costume, and Tamsin is going to take him around the apartments as it's pretty safe here.

Monday night is usually my online Cancer Survivor's group, but I may have to skip it to give out the candy.

Last night when I was reading some books to Nick I realized that he has never been on a boat. I told him I would take him for a boat ride today. Tamsin, Nick and I went to Balboa and took the Ferry back and forth from the Island. Then he rode on the Merry Go Round.

After that I went out by myself on another shopping spree. I bought a lot more Christmas gifts and tons of clothes for me. I really did a number on my VISA, but it felt great. I got three dance skirts to wear with my new lace up Roper boots. I hope I can dance in these boots. I've gotten very used to moccasins and dance shoes.

Tonight I got e-mail from Don. It seems like it's been ages since I've seen or heard from him. He is back with his girlfriend again. He had one of my church's tapes that I'd given him laying around, and she asked him where he got it. It turns out that she goes to my church now too!

Stephen is working his butt off today getting everything prepared for the race tomorrow. Then he has to be up at four-thirty to make sure everything is in place

I feel so wonderful this week, except for the hair that keeps falling out everywhere. I have more energy now than I have had since the chemo started. This morning I was complaining about all the hair falling out and Tamsin heard me and said, "I know Mom. . . I had to clean it all up in the bathroom today." (It was her cleaning week.) Actually I try to clean it up, but there is so much of it that I must have missed some. But, fortunately I still have plenty left on my head!

Once again this got longer than I suspected it would.

Bye. Love you,

November

November 1, Tuesday

Rita,

Eric and Bridget just left. She looks incredible for someone about to give birth. She is beaming, and is in really good shape physically. The doctor said she has dilated to two centimeters and the baby is going to come soon.

Bridget is going to write and tell you this, but I'm beating her to it. She saw the same Disney Babies print, which you sent them, at the mall last month and told Eric she wanted it for the baby's room! She is thrilled with it.

I got the longest e-mail today from Stephen. He is up in Lake Tahoe and getting to know his new roommates. His job sounds dangerous to me, but he says it's not as dangerous as the other's since he does the technical end of it usually. (I still worry about him though.)

Stephen said he was wearing the shirt from the "Cowboy," which I had sent him, and his roommates asked about it. He told them "his lady" sent it to him. Then he told them about me and showed them my picture. I got a compliment from one of his roommates. She told him that she thought I was pretty.

His letter was a joy to read. I am tempted to mail you a copy. He describes how beautiful it is in Tahoe, with the pretty and light snowfall. He also talks about his love for me. (He told me in this letter that he loves me!) I know he misses me, and I miss him tremendously.

I got a phone call from Don. He always surprises me. He teased me while we were on the phone about when am I ever going to meet Stephen. I told him what was going on, and he said that he was glad for me, and that I deserved all the good things which are happening in my life right now. I feel bad for him though. He keeps going back with his ex, and he sounds so depressed all the time. It just doesn't sound like the type of relationship a person would want to be in. But, I can't judge any one on his/her relationship, right? My current one must be the strangest one of them all.

I'm enclosing some Apheresis information for you, which Stephen had sent to me. It explains what he does regarding donating his platelets. What did you think of the tape?

Jessica is getting the transfer to Systems. She'll be on my team. I like her a lot. I was teasing Bev, who's office is down the hall from mine and who also had breast cancer, that we can start our own support group on the sixth floor of Administration soon.

Bev said that her manager was asking her how I was doing with my chemo and Bev said she answered, "Marilyn? Oh, Marilyn is doing *just great. . .* She's got hair on her head. She got her picture in the paper, and she got a new boyfriend. And, she might get a book published!— All I got was a sick tummy and a bald head!" I cracked up. Bev always makes me laugh with her funny stories. She had her breast cancer about three years ago, is younger than me and is the cutest lady you'd ever want to meet.

I know I must have more to write, but I want to write Stephen one more note tonight.

Bye. Love you,

cNovember 5, Saturday

Dear Rita,

I am weaker today than I was yesterday, and just super tired and shaky, but I have a long list of things to do. I asked Tamsin if she would go with me in case I need her assistance. I'm so glad that she moved in as she has become a big help to me.

Enclosed is the note that the breast cancer sisters got last night (e-mail) from Sharon regarding her surgery. I tried calling her, but she wasn't home from the hospital yet. I sent her an online note in case she was able to log on, and then I kept checking to see if I got any e-mail from her. I can put my mind to rest now that the surgery is done and I know that she's okay.

Also, yesterday afternoon I got another beautiful bouquet, with a sweet note, from Stephen to celebrate my being over half way through the treatments. See why I love him so much? Then last night he called on his lunch time, and we talked for an hour.

At nine this morning I am calling the airline to try to get a flight for Reno for November 18th and I will stay three days. Stephen will have that week-end off. I would have preferred the Thanksgiving Day week-end, but he has to work, plus that is the busiest time of the year for flights. I just hope and pray that my blood count is up. I want this time with him to be "quality" time.

Stephen has what turns me on the most in a man. He is very intelligent, and, he also has a huge, kind heart. You know these have always been a priority with me — more so than looks. On top of all this he's funny too!

I have much to do, but I wanted to get this ready for the mailman.

Bye. Love you,

November 5, Saturday

Dear Lillie:

I want to answer your letter tonight because if I don't do it now I don't know when it will be finished.

As usual your whirlwind life just exhausts me. How do you do it all? I am normally a high level, energetic and compulsive organizer. Lately, I have to push myself to get through a routine day!

We miss you. Did you ever get the AOL software? Try it and write us, or if not then send me your prodigy address so that I can write you once in awhile through the Internet.

Thursday night a group of the breast cancer sisters went online and held a one hour support group for Sharon. She was very worried about her reconstruction surgery on Friday. We gave her so much love and support that she was laughing, and then crying tears of happiness in the end. We all got notes from her on Friday night that the surgery was a success. She is in some pain, but the new "lump" now forming under her surgical dressings makes it worthwhile. I am so happy for her.

And my love life is flying! I am falling in love with the man who was mentioned in the newspaper article. We have exchanged pictures, videos, cards and gifts, and spent hours on the phone, and send each other e-mail daily — multiple letters daily that is, plus we do some online "chatting." I am flying up north to spend forty-eight hours with him in two weeks if my blood count is high enough for me to make the trip. We are both so excited about this. Wish us luck! (All the AOL breast cancer sisters are already planning our online wedding!)

My daughter and grandson moved in with me about six weeks ago and it is working out great. She has been good company for me as I struggle through the chemo. I am more than half way done with it now. Only two more treatments to go!

Lillie, don't lose touch, and I hope to see you on AOL with us some day soon.

Love you,

November 5, Saturday

Rita,

Another two letter day! What are things coming to around here?

I had to let you know that I got my plane reservations. I will leave on Friday afternoon, and come back Sunday afternoon, so it'll be about forty-eight hours with Stephen. Please send me good thoughts that I will be strong enough to do this and enjoy our time together.

I did more Christmas shopping, and lots more "Marilyn" shopping. Tamsin and I went to a lingerie store and she picked out a delicate, off white, Victorian lace teddy for me to take to Reno. I wrote to Stephen telling him that I think he and Tamsin have been talking!

When we got home there was a message on the machine from Don. I called him, and he wanted me to bring the kids to his studio tomorrow morning so that he could take their pictures. He also said that he would do one of me for my "sweetie." As it turned out I could hear that he had a cold, and we decided it may not be a good idea for me to come there this week-end after all. That's good because I called Arthur to see if he can get Dani next week-end so she can go too. Don is such a good photographer that I would hate for her to miss out on this opportunity. Oh, and he and his girlfriend are off again.

Next I logged onto AOL to see if Stephen had gotten my message about the reservations. He had written me a two page letter. He was so excited and ever so cute. I let Tamsin read it. We don't know who is more excited about this — him or me.

In the mail today I got a letter from Lillie. She still hasn't come onto AOL with the rest of us, and she is so busy. Lillie finished the last chapter of her book. She just gave another speech at a dinner for 400 people for the American Cancer Society, and she has been asked to join a new breast cancer research group in Pittsburgh. (Whew!) *Plus*, she has a heavy duty, stressful job as it is. Lillie amazes me. Her one comment about all that she is doing is: She has the need to do it all *now*, because she has faced her own mortality. I understand where she is coming from.

And, here is Sharon's note from today and her progress. I am so pleased for her and cannot wait until I have my own reconstruction. Today I went to the prosthesis store and bought another bra and ordered two Velcro backs for my prosthesis. I always have to take the time on Sunday nights to wash both when I get home from "sweaty" dancing. This will give me extras.

Tomorrow should be another busy day. I am trying to get a lot of Christmas shopping done while I can, because I know there aren't that many "good" and available days left for me.

Good night.

Bye. Love you,

Hello,

I have a letter for you from yesterday which is sitting on my dresser. I am having a very difficult time typing so I hope that I can catch all the typos. This has probably been the sickest day of my life. I don't know what I would have done with out Tamsin here with me. She has been so wonderful. All day she has been picking up after me, and laundering my linen and nightclothes. She's asked me a couple of times if I want to go to the hospital. I tell her that, "This too shall pass."

But, in the meantime I lie in bed and think that I don't want to continue with the treatments. I've had enough. I want them to STOP! I don't want to play this game ANYMORE! Of course I will continue them, but this is how I think when I feel so rotten. Obviously I won't be going to work tomorrow. I just hope I feel better. I can't imagine going through another day of this. Then I ask myself — "If this is the mild stuff, what can the strong stuff be like?" (I hope to never find out.)

I am so weak, tired, lightheaded, and sort of dehydrated. My butt is sore from going to the bathroom so much. I am nauseous and in pain. I had saltines and a root beer float for dinner, and immediately had to go into the bathroom. (Grrr)

I was reluctant to have Tamsin move in with me. But Rita, it is great that she is here. I must make this day up to her somehow! I so appreciate all the help she is giving me. She even went online and sent Stephen an e-mail to let him know I hadn't forgotten him. He checks for letters periodically through out the day and I didn't want him to worry. I wanted him to know that this was a "down" day, and I wouldn't be online much.

But, I did check my mail a couple of hours ago. He was glad that Tamsin had written to him to let him know what was going on. He is so compassionate and understanding. Rita, I believe he is the most beautiful man I have ever met. Whether he is in my life romantically, or platonically — I want him in it!

Sharon sent me a note and said that the reconstruction surgery is much more painful than the mastectomy. (I think you said that Linda's sister said the same thing.) But, Sharon did say that it's worth it in the end. She keeps peeking inside the surgical bra and there is definitely something there. She is such a sweetheart. I also told her about the lace teddy, and how it felt like something was missing. (You know like, "What's wrong with this picture?") She said that since her mastectomy she has tried on numerous teddy's and night gowns — for a more sexy look, but she gave up trying to find one that made her look normal. I can't believe I am going to wear it, but Stephen is so reassuring that I think I'm going to feel okay about it.

Well, as I was lying in bed it seemed like I had all kinds of things I wanted to tell you, but my mind is kaput too. Plus, I have to write Stephen a little note before I crawl back into bed.

Thanks for continuing to be there for me throughout this ordeal.

Bye. Love you,

November 8, Tuesday

Hello,

I am tempted to call, but since we talked for an hour yesterday I am going to just write. The baby is on it's way. Eric has called twice from the hospital and I've called once to see how they were doing. Bridget's water broke at home at one o'clock this morning. They both sound wonderful. The baby is in position, and the nurse has felt it's head already.

Tamsin is getting ready and then we are going to the hospital. It may be awhile yet before the baby is born, but I want Bridget to know that we are giving her lots of love and support. When I talked to her on the phone she was telling me that when the contractions started she began crying, and they gave her some pain medicine to relax her, but they also slowed down the contractions. I started crying while talking to her. I told her to rest up because she is going to be working a lot harder later in the morning. (It's only eight o'clock right now.)

I called Arthur and naturally he is thrilled! Today is his 28th birthday. What a present to get. When Eric called me at six o'clock he asked, "Mom, is a Scorpio hard to raise?" It's a little late to be concerned over that I guess.

Today I am feeling much better in regards to the nausea, but I woke up with bleeding hemorrhoids again, and a very sore butt. I should be able to go back to work tomorrow.

Last night's online Cancer Survivors support group was so much fun. We can only fit twenty-three people in a room and within the first half hour it had filled up, so I left early. (I had planned to anyway.) We had two new members join us, and both were quite young. One was a teenager. (Sad)

One of the men in our group is coordinating the up loading of all our pictures so that we can see what we each look like. He has only loaded one picture so far, and it was mine. It was like a magical thing to click on the screen, and there I am smiling back at me. I immediately forwarded it to Stephen, my Boston Buddy, Paul and some of my breast cancer sisters. My hair was long and curly in this picture.

This morning I got e-mail from Sue and she wanted to know if I would like to be in a documentary about breast cancer. I told her to send me the producer's number. I just might do it.

I miss Stephen and wish that he were here with me now.

Love for now. . . and, I probably will call later and leave a message when the baby is born!

November 8, Tuesday

Rita,

I just know that I am going to finish typing you this letter and you will return my phone call. What a fantastic day! Grandbaby number three is beautiful. Tyler DeForest, born one day after his parent's second anniversary.

The details: Tamsin and I got to the hospital at ten o'clock. Bridget was in hard labor with contractions every couple of minutes. She was so brave though, and not crying out or anything. She was being so strong. We stayed for about forty-five minutes, and then I told Eric we were going to do an errand and would be back in about an hour.

We went to Knottsberry Farm and I got a little Christmas gift for Stephen. I got flowers for Bridget, a little stuffed rabbit for the baby and some cards, and then we had lunch.

We got back to the hospital at about twelve o'clock. Bridget had been pushing for at least a half hour at that point. She was already exhausted. She was in a birthing room, and both she and Eric said that they would like me to stay for the delivery of the baby. I was thrilled, and surprised too, but ever so happy that they wanted me there.

Bridget just worked so hard and was tiring herself out. Eric was an incredible coach and remembered all the right things to say to help her. I was so proud of the both of them. During every contraction I was saying, "Push. Push hard." When the contraction had passed I would collapse onto the rocking chair at the foot of her bed, thoroughly exhausted.

Oh, and then they told me that if the baby was a girl they were going to name her "Madison Ruth" after me. (Ruth for my middle name.) I was very pleased and honored about that too.

At about one fifteen the doctor came in and decided that Bridget, and the baby needed some help so she used a suction apparatus to help bring Tyler into the world. He was born at one thirty, and is a big and beautiful baby. He is 8 pounds 10 ounces, and 20 ½ inches long. His hair is dark and curly like Eric's and he has very handsome features already.

The nurse let me hold him before anyone else. Again that surprised me, but the kids agreed. Then Eric held him, and next he laid Tyler down across Bridget's chest for a little while. Bridget started crying happy tears, and then we were all crying and laughing and telling each other how much we loved one another. It was quite emotional and beautiful.

I went with the nurse and Tyler to the nursery. Tamsin, Bridget's best friend and Nick got to see him through the nursery window. The nurse explained to me that Tyler's cord was wrapped around his neck as he was coming through the birth canal, and when he came out he didn't cry much compared to other newborn babies so they wanted to watch him closely for the next day or two. Also, his color was quite purple. Well, I stayed pretty close to that nursery for the next hour and he was screaming his little lungs out way before I left. (Good sign) And, of course, then he started turning a nice pink color. The nurse said his blood sugar was low from the stress, but she was going to feed and bathe him and then take him back to Bridget.

I think Tyler is going to do just fine. I told Nicky today that now Grandma has "two best boys"!

Now I'm worn out. I know I will sleep good tonight, but what a boost after this past horrendous week-end. It's a nice tired feeling that I have tonight. Tomorrow it's back to work and the regular routine.

Rita, I am so incredibly happy. Each of my kids, now has a child of his/her own. I can see how each of them parents and I'm proud of them. Arthur is a wonderful Dad. Tamsin is a good Mom to Nick. I see her with him every day and know it's not always easy being the Mom, but she and Nick have a wonderful relationship. And, now Eric, — he's already the proud Daddy. He and Bridget will be great parents too.

November 10, Thursday

Hello,

It was great to talk to you last night. I didn't mean to cut it short, but I had so much to do, and I was tired. Today I am feeling better, and I have much more energy. I hope this continues and that I am really strong by next Friday the 18th.

Stephen called. He is so good. He told me that he did not want me to feel that I was obligated to do anything I did not want to do that week-end. I said, "No, that was what I was going to say to you." He had me laughing again. We are both so excited about this. I told him that I am probably going to stick to him like glue for the whole time I'm there.

It seems like I had more to write about, but shoot. . .

Bye. Love you,

November 12, Saturday

Hi,

I think I have one letter already sitting out at the mailbox, but before I started doing the errand circuit I wanted to write you another note.

Yesterday I went to Eric and Bridget's. I got to sponge bathe Tyler, and dress and feed him. They have a good baby there. He is already sleeping five hours at a time, and usually if he cries it is because he wants to eat or be changed. He is content to be held and loved.

Then I went up to Los Angeles to an Eddie Bauer outlet store, and got a winter parka to wear in Reno. And, I bought some heavy sweaters and turtlenecks. Stephen keeps telling me that it is freezing up there. I think he will be able to keep me warm though. He is counting the hours. . . until we are together, and then the actual hours that we will be together. And, he keeps telling me about all these wonderful places that we have to go to for meals. My kind of guy!

I just hope I have the energy. No matter what I do lately it wears me out. Just climbing my stairs gets my heart pounding like it is going to come through my chest. Last night I was worn out, beyond exhaustion and finally I just crawled into bed with reading and writing materials.

When I was talking to you last week about whether you had any menopause type symptoms after your hysterectomy it was because I am experiencing some from the Tamoxifen now. I get hot flashes almost daily. I never know when they are going to come on. They're not too bad. I mean, I'm always so cold that even though they are uncomfortable, and can put me into a sweat, I don't mind them too much. Also, I think the Tamoxifen may be making my eyes worse. The prescription on my bifocals needs to be changed, and I need stronger reading glasses to wear over my contacts. I am going to wait until after I finish the chemo in case this is just a residual effect from the chemo, and not a result of the Tamoxifen.

The lady who works for the Publisher, the one who read the manuscript, has been corresponding with me online. She told me to not get my hopes up too high as the Publisher gets hundreds of manuscripts and only selects a few.

I asked her if she was familiar with anyone with breast cancer. As it turns out her family has a history of it and she gets her mammograms yearly. It must be worse to have that threat hanging over your head, as opposed to my being diagnosed with it out of the blue.

I'm almost done with my Christmas shopping. I am going to mail your package today.

It seems like I have more to tell you, but as usual lately, the memory isn't quite all there. Write me a long one.

Bye. Love you,

$\mathcal{N}$ovember 13, Sunday

Good Morning!

I feel so up, healthy and happy today. What a day yesterday was. It is going to be one of those days that I remember for the rest of my life. All of the kids were here with their "significant others" and their little ones. My life is WONDERFUL!

I forgot to tell you that yesterday morning when I was out running errands I had to stop by the prosthesis store again. The lady who owns the store had more time to talk, and she said that she didn't realize until after I'd left her store last week that the newspaper article said I was a grandmother. She said that when she thought about it later she was shocked. I really do feel like I look my age lately, but I guess I am still a young grandmother.

She and I also compared notes on chemotherapy. She had to have a year of the same kind of chemo as me. Yuck. Anyway, she made a comment which I love. She said that now that she has been through chemo she feels that she can handle anything. Her treatments were maybe ten or more years ago. She said that whenever there appears to be a problem in her life she just says to herself, "I've done chemo, I can deal with this too." I feel this way too. It's like there's nothing else that can happen to me that I can't overcome after this experience. But, we'll see.

Bye. Love you,

$\mathcal{N}$ovember 14, Monday

Hello,

I really don't have a lot of time to be writing, but I had to write to you with the little bit of news that I do have.

Arthur is going back to New Hampshire for the Christmas holidays to be with Arthur and Darleen. If possible he would like to see you, and maybe Lisa for one of the days. He wants to do some skiing, and probably some snow boarding while there. If you have the time let us know when he can see you.

When I got home from work tonight there was a card from Allen mailed from Buenos Aires. Once again it had some very nice sentiments. I think he has an easier time expressing his feelings to me in the written word versus the spoken word.

Jessica started in our office today. Since Bruce was at the Comdex show in Las Vegas, I was assigned to give her an orientation, and take her around our building to meet people. We also did a little bit on the computer. She is pretty excited now that she has come to Systems. I hope she enjoys it as much as I do. I think she will.

It is also great to be able to talk to her about breast cancer. We share some of the same issues, such as the side effects of Tamoxifen. She has had the hot flashes and the problem with diminishing vision too. Also, we discussed our upcoming reconstruction surgeries. She has to have the abdominal surgery since she first had radiation with a lumpectomy, and then later had to have a mastectomy.

Laura called tonight. She and Ashley will be spending Thanksgiving with us whether I cook or we go out for dinner. I am glad. It will be fun for Laura to be around her step great grand-kids.

Oh, I just remembered. This was funny. Tonight Tamsin said something to Nick about his "breaking" her rules. He looked at her and very adult-like he says, "If your rules are broken then why don't we try mine?" This kid is so advanced for his age. I don't know how he thinks up the stuff that he comes out with.

Love,

November 17, Thursday

Hello,

I am soaring. Tomorrow I will be in Reno with Stephen. I'm excited and he is too. I cannot even imagine what our first eye contact is going to be like. That scenario has been playing over and over in my mind. All I know is that first I want to have his arms wrapped around me. After that, everything else will be extra.

My weight slipped down to 102 pounds with this last treatment. I have been eating on the hour for almost every waking hour. Maybe I will be up to 103 or 104 soon. I keep trying.

Stephen said that he's going to have munchies stocked in our room. I told him that I might be too nervous to eat anything though.

Last night my friend, Wendy, from the online support group called.

We have become pretty close over the past couple of months. She wanted to wish me lots of luck, and fun for this week-end. It was so wonderful hearing her voice, and matching it to her picture which she sent me last week. She is another wonderful breast cancer sister.

Jessica and I talk almost every day regarding our breast cancer. Yesterday she had a cold, so she stood outside my office door in the hallway talking to me. She, for one, understands the importance of my not getting any germs.

And, my hair: Last night I was in the bathroom coloring it. Tamsin came in and I was moaning and groaning about how thin and limp it is. She very nicely reminded me that, at least I have hair. I thanked her for that.

I must go. Tonight I am getting the Chinese love songs tape from Danielle that she made for Stephen. But, actually he listens to country and jazz.

Bye. Love you,

November 21, Monday

Hi,

Everything is so right in my world. What about yours? My week-end was perfect. Stephen was lots of fun. We totally hit it off from the moment I walked off the plane.

Let me back up and then give you a more complete week-end accounting.

Thursday night right after I had collected e-mail and responded to all of it, my AOL program crashed. It would not let me in to do anything. I was bummed out. I called their office in Virginia and they said it was a problem with the version of AOL which I had installed. They are sending me a new diskette with the upgraded version. I hope it comes today!

In our afternoon meeting on Thursday my boss, Bruce, told us that a week ago he found out that he has a benign brain tumor. The Monday after Thanksgiving he is going to be operated on, and he will probably be out of work for about two months while recovering. I almost started crying when he told us. He is so young and this seems so unfair.

I canceled my oncology appointment for Friday morning as I didn't want to rush around before leaving. I was glad that I did because I was rushing anyway. My flight from Orange County was a half hour late. Then I had to change planes in San Jose, and that airport was so crowded that it was sitting room on the floor only. And then, that flight was forty-five minutes late too.

As I was flying into Reno I could see that there was lots of snow. It was very pretty. I was extremely excited, and nervous. When I got off the plane I was looking through the crowd of faces. Then I came around a corner, and there was Stephen. I recognized him immediately. He said that he had no problem recognizing me either. We hugged, and hugged each other. I almost started crying again. (I'm extremely emotional these days.) And, he had a red rose for me.

It was as if we have known each other forever. I wasn't shy or uncomfortable after all.

We went to the hotel/casino. Stephen had checked in earlier and had already put his stuff away. I unpacked while we talked. Oh and we had little gifts for each other.

He also had a bottle of champagne on ice. (We never did get around to opening it though.)

We went downstairs to dinner and then gambled in the casino for a few hours. He hit one jackpot on the slot machines. I didn't win any money. My gambling luck was off all week-end.

Next we went upstairs to our room. I'm not going into detail, but I'm just going to say that Stephen is a wonderful lover too. He was so good about my missing breast that I wasn't self-conscious at all! He made me feel quite normal and desirable. I love him for this.

The whole week-end was fun, but it went by too quickly. I ate lots, and got very little sleep. Being with him was just as I imagined it would be. Leaving him was very hard to do.

When I got home last night I went to sleep at quarter after eight. There was a message when I got up this morning that Stephen had called at ten to nine. I slept about ten hours and I would have kept on sleeping except for the alarm going off.

Tamsin said that Don called on Friday night. He must have forgotten that I was going to Reno for the week-end. She said that Paul called Saturday morning. . . guess he forgot too.

I honestly don't know what will become of Stephen and I. I love him and he loves me too. We have some obstacles which may, or may not be surmountable. Right now there is my health. There is also our age difference, and of course the racial difference. These do not worry me too much. What concerns me are two other issues. The first is the geographical distance between us, and we don't know where he could wind up in the future with his job. The other is that he says that he is a confirmed bachelor. I'm still thinking that, knowing me, I will want to get married again some day. Stephen has never been married, and at his age he isn't sure that he ever wants to do that.

We have decided to take it day by day, and that's okay with me for now.

Well, I made it to work. Jessica was in my office as soon as I got there to ask about the week-end. While I was talking to her my phone was ringing constantly. Others were calling to ask how it went. People are curious of course.

What are you doing for Thanksgiving? If I have the energy I am going to grocery shop later tonight. If not, then it looks like we'll be going out to dinner. Whatever we do I think it'll be fun. I hope yours is a good one.

Bye. Love you,

P.S. We went to a Chinese restaurant Saturday night for dinner in Reno. Stephen taught me to eat with chopsticks. It was fairly easy, but slow going, and I like eating fast. I got kind of impatient and went back to using the fork. At least Danielle will be pleased with me for learning. Oh, the best part was when he fed me with his chopsticks!

*N*ovember 22, Tuesday

Hi again,

I just wrote to you yesterday, but I have to write again today. Actually yesterday I was pretty tired and I can't remember what I wrote about.

Everyone in the world called, or came by my office, and I returned some week-end calls. It turned out that a few friends (Barbara and Ann) were actually worried about me going to Reno. They said they didn't want to tell me how concerned they were because I was so excited.

I also called Sharon to ask her to let the online Cancer Survivors group know that I had a wonderful week-end, but that my AOL was not working. I didn't want them worrying about me too. Sharon was really happy for me. She wasn't concerned, because she has met Stephen online.

Then I called Don. He said he called because he wasn't sure which week-end I was going to Reno. He said he wanted to come by my office some day to do lunch. He asked me if I was in love with Stephen and I told him "yes," and that I was very happy. We talked awhile and he said that he might be coming down with another sore throat. I told him that I didn't want to be around him if that was the case. But, I let him know that I am doing the turkey dinner this year, and if he didn't have a better offer that he was welcome to join us. I also let Ann and Barbara know that they were welcome, but I believe that they both have family plans. What's nice is that I feel that Don and I are becoming just what he said we would be, "good buddies."

I returned Paul's call. I told him about my crashed AOL, and he offered to put his software in his mailbox for me to pick up this morning before going to work. I got it and I am going to install it and get back on tonight. Anyway, I also feel like Paul and I have become good, "platonic type" friends. I am resolving all the relationship type problems with the men in my life.

And last but not least — Stephen called me at work yesterday afternoon. He was starting back to work last night. He said he misses me. I know I am missing him.

Oh, I forgot to tell you that when I was in Reno. . . I asked him if he was disappointed. He assured me he wasn't, and said that he was "in heaven." He also complimented me by saying that he thought I was better looking, and younger looking, than in my pictures and video. That made me feel good.

Today is Bruce's last day. He is taking care of last minute details and he remains cheerful and positive about his new health challenge. Juanita will be our acting supervisor until he comes back to work the end of January.

Well, I am going to be busy through Thanksgiving day. I have tons to do before then.

Have a wonderful holiday.

Bye. Love you,

November 23, Wednesday

Dear Lillie:

Your long, and informative letter is greatly appreciated. I am going to send it on to Sharon as she is always asking about you. I try to tell her all that you are involved in, but I can't seem to keep up. Where do you find the time and the energy? Slow down some, because you are wearing me out!

Seriously though, I admire you so much and all that you are doing. I think each of us, in our own way, is trying to educate people about, and hopefully some day eradicate, this disease.

Sue just facilitated a breast cancer workshop for her school district employees. Also, she and I may be in a documentary for PBS regarding breast cancer issues. It goes into production in January, and the producer seems interested in both of us.

The lady who was assigned to read my book liked it and wrote a positive report to her boss, but the Publisher decided that the material was not in line with their publications. She has encouraged me to continue writing the book, and to try to find someone else to publish it. I am not disappointed, as just hearing her compliments has motivated me to continue.

I like your idea about the Mothers of Daughters with Breast Cancer Support Group. Your pamphlet is great. One of our breast cancer sisters, Wendy, attends a Cancer Support Group for Athletes. (She is a runner.) Wendy would like this to become a nation wide support group someday. She is a wonderful lady and I will put you in touch with her when you get logged onto AOL.

I'm home sick today as I woke up with a sore throat and my blood count feels sluggish. Tomorrow I am doing the Thanksgiving dinner for everyone, including my ex in laws, so I hope I'm feeling better by then.

My week-end in Reno with Stephen was beyond what I had hoped for. He was just as wonderful in person as he has been online and over the phone. It was very difficult to leave him Sunday. Today I received a beautiful, autumn bouquet for Thanksgiving from him. We plan to continue our relationship, and be together when we can, as we can. It is not easy since we live so far apart.

Lillie, I am so glad that you continue to stay in touch with us. I hope to see you on AOL soon. Please take care of yourself. Don't try to be a Superwoman. Have a wonderful Thanksgiving.

Bye. Love you,

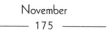

November 25, Friday

Hello,

I just woke up from a nap. I have a nasty sore throat and it has turned into a head cold, so this letter might seem spaced out. But, then that is nothing out of the ordinary these days, is it?

I've heard from a lady who is willing to critique the manuscript. She contacted me through AOL because of the notice I have on the bulletin board in the Writer's Forum. She teaches at the University of Michigan, and also has some published works. She had a close encounter with what she thought was going to be breast cancer, so she is interested in learning more about this disease.

My Thanksgiving was perfect. I came down with the sore throat Wednesday so I didn't go to work. I was able to do a little preparation for Thursday, but mostly I rested. Thanksgiving morning I slept in. When I got up my achy throat was still with me, but not too bad. I was able to cook dinner and it turned out pretty good. Laura, Ashley, Eric, Bridget, Tyler, and later, Arthur came over. We ate continuously throughout the day. Laura and Ashley brought the dessert.

Little Tyler is getting cuter each time I see him. He has such a perfect little face and body. We all took turns holding, feeding, and rocking him throughout the day.

It thrills me with how well my kids are getting along. All of them are currently doing great. The other thing that makes me very happy is the fact that they love each other's children as if they were their own. The three little ones can't help but thrive with all the love they get from this family.

Nicky was acting up some in the beginning of the day. I think he was just hyped up over all the company. Tamsin kept putting him in their room and he was throwing little temper tantrums. (Not so nice.) Later he calmed down and was okay.

Did I tell you that my weight is up? I've gained three pounds over the past two weeks. I'm at 105 pounds again. Other than this cold, and sore throat, I feel pretty good. Having everyone here yesterday helped me to keep going. The only one who was missing was Stephen!

Don called on Wednesday night to say that he wouldn't be coming for dinner yesterday as he still has his cold. He sounded terrible. Once he and I are both healthy, and available, I am taking the kids down to his studio to get their pictures taken.

Ann came by today for a short visit. She didn't want to get too close to me though as she keeps catching colds. We think the radiation treatment she had last year for her Thyroid Cancer destroyed her immune system. Anyway I made her sit through Stephen's tape and she thought he was cute. She said the same thing Arthur said, — that he looks more Hawaiian than Chinese.

Well, I am glad I am having this cold over the long holiday weekend so that I am not using up more vacation time from work. Wednesday is blood lab day, and then Friday more chemotherapy. I hope I am healthy enough to do it. I want to get this over with!

Write me a long newsy letter soon.

Bye. Love you,

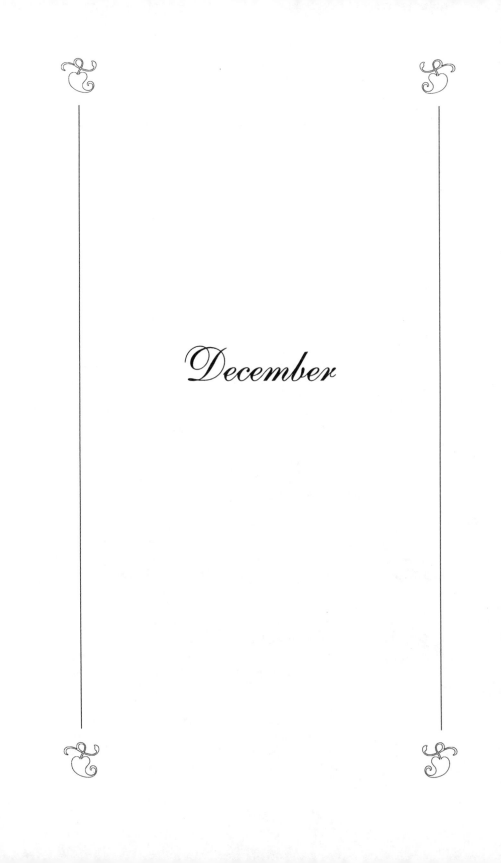

December

*D*ecember 1, Thursday

Hello,

Here I am again . . . feeling like it's been forever since I've written, but I have been really busy. Yet I'm also also trying to get rid of this cold by getting rest too. (Juggle. Juggle. Juggle.)

I am waiting for replies from the two ladies who volunteered to critique the book. Grace I already wrote you about. Janette is an animal Behavioral Scientist (Ph.D.) at the University of Oklahoma. Janette goes into the field in Africa. She has published scientific work, and is thinking of writing her own book, which would be a compilation of her letters to family and friends while in "the field." This morning Janette sent me a picture of one of her subjects. . . an ape. I downloaded the file and checked it out before going to work. Cute — you would have loved it.

I met both of these women through my notice on the Writer's Club bulletin board on AOL. I continue to meet, and make new friends online. This past week I met a man in Pennsylvania. He lives on a rural mountain top. It's just he, and his dog. When his last relationship broke up, about eight years ago, he sold his house and bought a ten acre mountain top. He cleared it himself and built a house there. He is sort of a recluse, but proably not really. Actually he seems like a pretty nice man.

One of my breast cancer sisters, Wendy, e-mailed this week-end that she had a 101 degree temperature. On Monday night I found out that her doctor had put her into the hospital to monitor her, and to run some tests. I called Sloan Kettering Hospital in New York twice on Tuesday trying to reach her. The first time I called the hospital I got her roommate, and she said that Wendy had gone for tests. The second time I got her boyfriend who said that she had just been taken away for more tests. He did say that Wendy was okay though. I sure hope so. I know that once you have cancer and any little pain or illness comes into your body — the tests begin.

Don called last night. He asked how my online romance was going. I told him it was wonderful. He said that he is finally over his ex, and that he even got the phone number of a lady he met at the Cowboy. He is thinking of asking her out. Then he said that if I'm feeling okay after Friday's chemo maybe we could get together this week-end for brunch.

Tyler has been over almost every day this week. Tamsin and Bridget swap babysitting. Yesterday Tamsin went to the local community college to take her entrance exams. Bridget watched Nick for her. The night before, Eric and Bridget had a work seminar so they left Tyler with Tamsin. Every time I see him he looks like he has grown . He is going to be one big boy! Tomorrow Arthur is keeping Nick over night so that he and Dani can have some time together.

My hair is falling out by the handfuls lately. This past week has been especially bad. I think I have lost about 50% of my hair since the chemo started. I hope I don't lose much more. Every morning when I wash my hair it just comes out in my hands. And I'm talking about quite a few strands at a time. Then when I blow it dry and brush it, more falls out onto my shoulders and the bathroom floor, sink and counter. I have to clean it up about twice a day. My bed has strands in it. . . my plates of food. . . my keyboards. It's everywhere but on my head!

It doesn't seem possible that it's December. I'm still wondering where summer went. Next year I am going to make up for this year big time!

There probably is a lot that I am forgetting to write you, but I guess this is it for now.

Bye. Love you,

P.S. I will let Arthur know what you said about available times for him to visit with you.

*D*ecember 2, Friday

Hello,

And what are you up to tonight? I got your long letter about New Hampshire and all the secret Christmas shopping you all have been doing. Your Thanksgiving sounded very dangerous though. How is your ankle and also your knee? A turkey on the floor sounds like a very interesting meal, but I'll pass.

We got word from Bruce's wife that he is doing wonderful. It sounds like he has some serious things to work through before he is going to be back to normal though.

I should be in bed sleeping as I am really exhausted. (Chemo day here.) I've been having some fever with sweats, and then chills, and I feel lousy — but I couldn't sleep. So, I got up and logged onto AOL one more time to see if I had any e-mail from Stephen. No, but — Lillie, the last of my breast cancer sisters from Prodigy is now on AOL. I was so thrilled to get her note. I hope she is going to love it as much as the rest of us. Also, she is going to be in the PBS documentary with Sue and I for "Woman to Woman." Maybe we three will get to meet. I think it is only fitting that Sharon also be on it, but I doubt she would agree since she is a very private person.

Okay — so no mail from Stephen. I answered Lillie's note and wrote
a few other e-mails and decided to pick on you again. I gathered up all
kinds of stuff to fill this envelope. Here's a picture and an article about
Wendy from my support group. The article is about her Cancer Support Group for Athletes. She is another incredibly nice lady. I am very
fond of her. I am also worried about her since I haven't heard from her
in a week, and that is not like her. I am e-mailing her and not getting
answers. I may try to call her again tomorrow. I hope she is alright.

Also, here are four post cards that I received from Allen from his
South America tour. I don't know what to think about him, and the
way he feels about me. It gets confusing at times, but I think we really
do just love each other as good friends and dance partners.

Well, speaking of men again, and talk about confusing: Tonight I
got an e-mail from Don. He says he has been thinking about me a lot
and is going to call tomorrow. . . and he said other stuff, which only
confused me more. I think that I am always going to be mixed up when
it comes to men because I just don't understand them.

This is it for tonight's letter.

Bye. Love you,

December 3, Saturday

Hi,

I almost called you tonight. I was kind of upset, but I'm okay now.
Today I mailed you a letter. In it was the picture of Wendy. She called
from the hospital tonight with some bad news. The breast cancer, which
they thought they'd gotten all of, is now in her lungs and bones. I am so
upset by this news. Wendy said that she cried all day yesterday when
she got the results of the test, but now she has it under control. She is
being so brave and so strong about all this. I, on the other hand, got off
the phone with her and broke down and cried.

She is the most wonderful lady. Whenever we get someone new to
our Cancer Survivors group, Wendy is right there being ever so supportive. Wendy just turned forty in October. She has been so happy
with the way her life has been going. She has a great career and has
been running marathons again. Everything was going her way and
now this. I do not want to believe that this is happening to her.

Wendy said that Monday they will start her on Taxol which is a
heavy duty chemotherapy compared to what I am doing. She will lose
her hair again, but she doesn't think this form of chemo will make her
really sick and tired like the other treatments. But, she probably won't
be able to work. Also, she has not asked her doctor for a prognosis as

she doesn't want to know. She said that she is really good at denial. I am heartbroken for her. Please send some of your good wishes and thoughts her way.

Sorry about this. I cannot even think about other stuff to write about at the moment, but I had to tell you about Wendy's call. It was write this, or call you, and I thought it would be best to just write it down on paper.

Bye. Love you,

*D*ecember 7, Wednesday

Hello,

Look at the enclosed headline from this morning's paper. One of the nation's most affluent counties just filed bankruptcy! Things have been pretty hectic here. They say we will get our paychecks on time though. They also say that our retirement monies were not involved. What I haven't heard them say yet is what happened to our Deferred Compensation. I have about $12,000 invested in one program and about $8,000 in another. According to what I am hearing it sounds like the County Deferred Compensation was part of the investment fund that lost 1.5 billion dollars. Our Treasurer just resigned. He made some very risky investments, and the result is that we have all lost a lot of money.

No one has heard from Wendy. I have a feeling that she is still at the hospital. I need to call and find out, but it is so hard to call from work, and then by the time I get home, after running errands, it is too late (her time) for me to call. I don't want her to think that she is alone through all this. I am really worried for her.

Oh, and Sharon does want to be in the documentary with us. I hope it's not too late. I thought she wouldn't want to do it because of her privacy. But, when I told her that Lillie, Sue and I are all doing it she wrote back and said she wanted in too. I am so glad that she is going to do this.

Both Grace and Janette, who have read the manuscript, have been in touch with me. They both feel that it is worthwhile. Maybe someday we will really have a genuine book here.

It looks like Stephen will be down the week-end before Christmas. That Friday I will be with my doctors and the blood lab all morning for a six month check-up. Stephen will be flying in to Orange County that afternoon. On Monday he will fly home.

That is the last week-end to see Arthur and Dani before he goes back to New Hampshire, so sometime in there we will be doing the gift exchange with them.

Paul called me on Saturday. He wanted to know if I was interested in going to his house to work on computer stuff, but I told him I was heading to bed. I was pretty chemo exhausted. He was going to try to get to the Cowboy early Sunday so we could dance, but he got there right after I left. Ann told me that later Barbara danced with him and then said to Ann, "Why did she let this one go?"

Don and his girlfriend showed up at the Cowboy after I left too. They are back together again.

I went out to one of our district offices this afternoon to do a training. There were people there that I haven't seen since before the mastectomy. They all told me how great I looked, but honest I don't think that I look so hot lately. My hair is very flat because it is so thin. I don't like it, but then I still feel thankful that I have any hair left — period.

Saturday morning Sue sent me e-mail. She was so excited because she was going to the hairdresser to get her hair trimmed. This was the first time in a year. I was thrilled for her.

Well, I have e-mail to answer, but I wanted to be sure I wrote you a long one for a change. I thought you might be missing lengthy letters.

Love you,

December 8, Thursday

Hi,

It's becoming a one letter per day again. So much keeps happening that during the day I tell myself that I have to remember to tell you. . . whatever it is that is going on.

I called Wendy today. She is home from the hospital. It was great to hear her voice. She is pretty down about what is happening right now with her disease. That's very understandable. I just wish that there was something I could do to help her. Now I can understand how frustrated you were feeling being "there," and wanting to help me "here." She said that she talked to her boss, and told him she will probably be out of work for at least six months. He told her not to worry and that her paychecks would continue. I don't know the man, but "God Bless him!"

I asked Wendy if she still had her wig. She said that she did, but when her hair grew in after the last chemo it grew in curly, and the wig has straight hair like her old hair. Now she wants a curly wig.

And, we received your large box of Christmas gifts. Thank you. But, one gift, which looks like a book, says, "To Jack from Rita." Now is this mis-named or do you want me to mail it back to you, to put under your tree for Jack? Let me know.

Also, I got two very long letters from you. Yea! They were newsy and I enjoyed them from beginning to end. I love the picture of the Mt. Washington Hotel, with the snow covered mountains and blue skies in the background. I am going to take it to work with me tomorrow to put up in front of my desk. This is definitely a picture which you could enlarge and enter in a contest, or peddle to a shop in New Hampshire. It's beautiful.

I'm enclosing three more post cards from Allen. He has been home for a week now, and I am still getting cards from his South America trip.

Stephen and I are quite excited about his visit. It looks like it will be a four day week-end. He said he will even go to the Cowboy with me — never mind that he doesn't dance. And yes, I picked up on the fact that even you also are willing to go two stepping with me. Trust me — you will love it. And the guys will love you!

Well, the County is in an uproar. Our Director is sending us e-mail through out the day as he learns what is going on. We have been told that our retirement monies were not affected. . . but, the paper says part of it was. Also, this morning he said that both Deferred Compensation programs would be affected. I immediately took a break and walked over to our payroll office to dis-enroll and stop my deduction. Then this afternoon he e-mailed us that the second Deferred Compensation program was safe and had not been invested in the county pool. I'm still canceling the deduction until the dust settles, and we know what is what.

We have implemented a hiring freeze as of December 5th. All business trips have been canceled until further notice. (Unless they are made with special permission.) There is no ordering of supplies unless they are mandatory to our work functions. Even "post its" are out. The world has news reporters camped in our Civic Center. It is nuts here.

Actually I am doing quite well so far with this last chemo. I am pleased as I expected it to be a pretty bad one. I have fatigue, and of course the hair loss continues. My hair looks horrendous lately. There is nothing I can do about it. Jessica and everyone else assures me that it will grow back, and will be prettier than ever. I hope so.

I got e-mail from Lillie last night. Emily, from the Owl Poke production company, has already made plans with her to interview she and her family next month. She is still hoping (as am I) that they will bring Sharon, Sue, Lillie and me together for an interview.

Tonight I got an e-mail message from one of the publishers that I recently sent the manuscript to. He was acknowledging it's receipt. So, now I sit and wait and see what he has to say about it. This is all kind of strange. Here are all these people reading my letters to you! My life is right out there in the open these days.

I am very tired, but I wanted to get this written tonight. Thank you again for the gifts and pictures.

Love you very much.

December 10, Saturday

Good Morning!

It's about seven o'clock and I have been up and doing for almost two hours already. You know I will be taking a nap this afternoon. I wanted to be sure to have a short note ready for you when the mailman comes.

We had just been talking about going two stepping, — well, read this article from yesterday's newspaper. It's the second time they have mentioned that on Sunday afternoon's you can find the best dancers at the Cowboy. And, I am one of them. The fact is that the regulars (myself included) have always known this, and we've been going there for years; way before "country" dancing became the fad.

I just packaged up a turban to send to Wendy. I had gotten two last summer and I've been fortunate in not having to use them. Of course at the rate I am losing hair I may still need one of them. Please ask Clara (and anyone else) to include Wendy in her prayers. My neighbor, Lois, has included her, and Lillie has too. I don't do a lot of the normal type of praying, but I do positive affirmations.

Speaking of positive. . . this is probably going to sound negative, but I really mean it in a positive way. Today's paper is all headlines again about our financial condition here in Orange County. It is worse than they had stated last week. Well, I was thinking this sure hasn't been my year for health and wealth — but I still have lots of happiness. I'm not really down about what has happened. I realize that many positive events, and some wonderful people have come into my life this past year.

I cannot thank you enough for being here with me through all this. I really and truly appreciate all that you have done, and been for me.

Bye. Love you,

Rita—

*D*ecember 12, Monday

I am so glad you were home yesterday when I called. I think I was in a state of shock actually. I'm still thinking to myself, "Is this real?" Well, is it? I mean — I think — maybe this man, the Publisher, is some kind of an online kook, and he is just pulling my leg and playing a joke on me. When the contract comes I guess I will know more and be more believing of it.

Stephen is thrilled for me, but as is his nature, he is encouraging me to be cautious. We were talking online last night and I said, "It's a good thing I told Rita you were a great lover, huh?" He wrote back and said that he was laughing and blushing.

I called Danielle and Jessica and told them. They are both pleased for me too. Pinch me so that I'm sure I am not dreaming. Then I told everybody I know at the Cowboy. Later on I thought to myself that they must think I make up half the stories that I tell them.

Oh, and I was in the kitchen after I called everyone, cooking my dinner when I saw my neighbor, Lois, at her kitchen window across the back alley. I have never done this before, and I must've sound like an old Boston fishwife. I opened my window and started yelling, "Lois! Lois!" She had her window shut, and she lives alone. I could see her looking all around her kitchen. . . like she was freaked out. And, then she saw me, started waving and opened her window. I told her by yelling it across the alley.

I heard from Wendy. She is extremely tired, and dealing with the mouth sores from the chemo. I wrote back and told her about the dental paste that I have been using and how it has helped me a lot. She said that she will ask her nurse about it today.

When I went dancing last night I gave Allen his Christmas present. He opened it and put them on. He dresses "swing," not country and I found the greatest pair of red Christmas suspenders. They looked really cute on him.

Last night I was raving on and on to Tamsin that I was nervous about Stephen's visit and I said, "What if he thinks our whole family is nuts." She cracked me up. She said, "Mom — we *do* put the "fun" in dysfunctional." And, did I tell you that one day I was going on and on about something else that was going on in the family and she said, "Well, you know the family motto Mom — 'Shit happens'." I think all my kids missed their calling.

Oh — just speaking of funny things the kids say (you know how I can ramble once I start) — Tamsin told me last night that the last time she was over at Arthur's he asked her if I was doing "computer sex" with Stephen. Then he said to her, "You know what I mean. . . like, let me pull down my 'file menu' and maximize my icon." (Dirty minded kid.)

I really have to end this. Write and tell me how Jack is doing. I'm enclosing a wallet sized picture of the whole family. Also, Jack's Christmas gift from you is being returned. My excuse lately for the strange things I do is chemo — what's yours?

Bye. Love you,

December 13, Tuesday

Hi,

This one really is going to be a short one, I think. These are my famous last words. My friends online were teasing me about my "short" notes because they just don't exist.

Wendy came to the group for a little while last night. Everyone was just so loving and supportive to her. She sounded good and stayed until she was too tired to continue. Wendy mentioned that she is planning a trip to Boston soon to see Deepak Chopra. I told her to look you up while she is there.

Later in the evening Sharon e-mailed me that Wendy shared with her that the cancer is also in her liver. I cry every time I start to talk about her to anyone. Please keep her in your thoughts.

Well, I have told the world about the Publisher's call on Sunday. I'm still going around thinking it's a dream and maybe I've gone off the deep end fantasizing, but the contract came.

I called Bud and told him that I was faxing him a copy. He said, "Oh the famous authoress." I said, "No, I am *just* a letter writer." Who knows this better than you???

Yesterday afternoon Danielle came by my office to bring me some Christmas gifts and a pair of chopsticks. I tried to use them, but I've already forgotten how. She had only been gone about five minutes when the receptionist called and said there was a surprise for me. It was a bouquet of daisies in a basket. I have one very thoughtful and romantic man here.

I may not be writing for a few days as I have a lot to do before Stephen arrives on Friday afternoon, and then I know I won't be writing while he is here. I just don't want you to think I have forgotten about you.

Bye. Love you,

*D*ecember 14, Wednesday

Rita—

Do you believe this? I tried to call you again today, but got Jack. Nothing major but I just wanted you to share in my excitement.

Remember when I moved back East, and bought the house down the street from you? After we left the bank with my loan approval, we got in your car and looked at each other, and screamed at the top of our lungs? (Thelma and Louise we ain't!) That's how I feel today. I wanted to scream "We did it!" But, I called from work so it was just as well that you weren't home.

There is so much happening here. My blood count is down and I am dragging, but yesterday, as bad as I felt, I made it through the whole work day. When I got home the phone didn't stop ringing. And, there were so many things needing to be done. I was feeling a little overwhelmed. But, I'm compulsive and got through all of it, and crashed about nine thirty.

People are teasing me constantly. Then when I tell them they are in the book they go "What did you tell Rita?" You are famous my love, and I hope everyone still loves *me* after this.

Oh, also enclosed is a picture that I got in the mail from my "Boston Buddy." He kept telling me that he was going to send one, and it arrived yesterday. Even though we live close to each we have never met in person. We talk on the phone, and now that I have convinced him about how wonderful AOL is, he has signed on and we are e-mailing each other again.

Two more days and Stephen will be here. Every time we think we are making plans for activities during the four days, something comes up and the plans shift. I have no idea what we will actually be doing until he gets here and we do it. Originally we were going to Disneyland Saturday, but Dani and Arthur are coming over for the gift exchange. Then I talked to Karen yesterday and her party is that night. I had forgotten. Did I tell you all this already? If so I apologize, but honestly I am pushing my limit to the max lately. So, we may wind up going to Disneyland on Sunday instead of to church and the Cowboy. Who knows? — I'm just the hostess and the tour guide.

I know what I wanted to tell you, but I kept forgetting. Remember when I was first diagnosed and I became obsessed with looking at other women's boobs? Well, now it's hair. I just notice women's hair all the time. It must drive people nuts. I go around complimenting everyone on their hair.

I can't wait to have LONG, DARK, CURLY **HAIR** again. Isn't there an old hippy song about that? I'll have to find a copy for Wendy and myself.

The other night when I was talking to Stephen I told him if he loves me this much now, — can you imagine how much he is going to love me when I have two boobs, long hair and lots of energy! His answer was that he is worried about the "energy" part after our week-end in Reno. He says I might need a younger man than he.

My lunch hour is ending. I have to go. Sorry if I sound somewhat manic. It's probably because at this point — I am.

Bye. Love you,

December 15, Thursday

Dear Bud and Lynn,

How are you? And thank you so much for your help earlier this week. It has been a hectic week in every area of my life. Do you believe all that is happening? I am being teased radically at work, but it's okay.

I called Rita last night to discuss the contract and the book. When we were talking I told her that now I have two concerns. The first is that the style of my letters to her will change over the next four to five months, just because I know that they are going somewhere other than to her. She cracked me up. She said, "I can see it now. 'Dear Ms. Pelrine'."

Also, I was a little concerned about family, co-workers and friends feeling uncomfortable talking to me anymore for fear of what I will tell Rita ,and then you know where it will wind up eventually. But, so far that isn't happening.

Yesterday I was in a meeting. One of our Staff Development Trainers was at the meeting. When he heard about the book, and that just about everyone else in the meeting was in it, he asked if he was in the book too. I thought a second, and then I said that maybe he was in one sentence. Everyone roared.

This has to be a short one as I have so much to do tonight. Tomorrow Stephen will be here. This will be the first time he and the kids have met. My life is pretty exciting in all areas lately.

Enclosed is a copy of my currently most favorite picture. It is a first, but hopefully not the last. All my children, and their children, and me in one beautiful, and happy as you can see, picture. It was taken last month right after Tyler was born. You can see Tamsin's friend Teharu's "bright light" shining down on us from the mirror behind! We didn't stop to think about his and the flash's reflection showing up in the picture.

Love you both a lot.

*D*ecember 15, Thursday

Hello,

This better be short. I can't believe I am writing to you and my brother while I have all kinds of other things to do. I really am addicted to writing letters. Do you think they have a twelve step program for people like me?

I just walked through the living room and our Christmas tree smells so good. It is the best smelling tree that I have ever had in California. It smells as good as the ones back East. And, it is also beautiful.

Today my new office roommate, Chris and I threw an early morning Christmas "open house" at work. Chris did the decorations and I did the food. We did a great job of it too. Then we e-mailed all of the Systems Division and Human Resources staff to come by to get in the holiday spirit. Our office got thoroughly "warmed" and it was fun. I think everyone who came enjoyed it. Chris and I took a ton of pictures so be prepared.

I told our Manager, Sandi, that it was probably dangerous putting Chris and I in the same room. She and I have been plotting fun things to do.

And, for next week's "social activities" we have started organizing for all of the Systems Coordinators, including our Manager, to Christmas carol on the four floors of Administration. Not everyone in "Sysco" is happy about this. (I am not a very good singer and I asked if I could be in the middle of the group, and have someone tall stand in front of me.)

The rehearsal is at lunch time on Tuesday. On Friday we will serenade everyone. I personally think that this will be a great thing to do. There is so much glum news coming out daily about the County's financial situation. This will hopefully lift people's spirits. But, on the other hand if we don't do too good a job of it they may be throwing tomatoes at us.

You know how we were talking last night about people being afraid to talk to me now? Well, today was also our Sysco Christmas luncheon. We went to a very nice restaurant. There were about fourteen of us. Anyway, we all were joking about everything, including the book. The people I work with are so funny! I wound up having pains in my stomach from laughing so hard. Every time someone would say something funny I would pretend that I was taking notes. All in all I think most of my co-workers are pleased that they are going to be in "The Book."

What was nice, and kind of different, was that at one point my friend, Rick, was teasing me about how I couldn't go on talk shows and speak in front of groups because of my past history with Agoraphobia. He said he would go with me, and he would stand behind me. I could just put my hands in my pockets while he stuck his arms out as if they were mine. He would do the hand gestures, and while I moved my lips, he would do the talking. Rick said, "Of course people will wonder why you have such a deep voice." I looked at Jessica, who was sitting across the table from me, and I said, "I'll just say it's a side effect from the Tamoxifen." The others laughed, but only Jessica, my breast cancer sister, really got it. She and I went hysterical.

Okay — all small talk aside. Tomorrow is a big day for me. I keep trying not to think about it. All the breast cancer women have warned me that I will get nervous about these check-ups. This is my six month one, and I think they will be checking me over pretty good. I know they will never find more cancer, but then I remember that I thought initially that they wouldn't find any. So, I am trying to think positive and yet, there will probably always be that little doubt in the crevices of my mind. It's just part of this whole experience.

Enough. . . I have to go as I have a lot to do before Stephen comes tomorrow afternoon. I did the mega grocery shopping tonight so there would be plenty of food for the next four days. And, yes, I plan to cook. Actually he said he would do it if I was feeling low in energy.

Please let Jack know that I am sorry about his father's death. I felt awful when I got off the phone with him on Wednesday, and realized I hadn't said anything to him about it.

Love you,

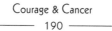

*D*ecember 20, Tuesday

Hi,

I have the feeling that this is going to be a ten pager so grab a cup of tea and get comfy. It's going to jump around some, and I'll probably not finish it all at one attempt. There is so much I want to tell you.

First though, I am so glad you called Saturday morning (not once, but twice—?), and that you and Stephen got to meet. Even if it was just a meeting over the phone, I am pleased that you got to talk with him. What did you think? Deep, sexy voice, huh?

Also, enclosed are a ton of pictures. I debated on whether to send all of them or not, but what the heck. You might be interested. If you aren't don't force yourself to look at them. I understand. There are some from Thanksgiving day with the whole family (minus Dani). The others were taken last Thursday morning when Chris and I did our Christmas party.

Some people you might want to note (and who's who is written on the back): Jessica, my breast cancer sister who recently transferred here from the Districts. Also, there is Newton from Human Resources. (He is the one who's wife had breast cancer three years ago.) There is Chris my long time work friend, and current office roommate. Juanita is one of my team members and she is currently filling in for Bruce as our supervisor. Rick, is my friend that I worked with years ago in Quality Control, and he got promoted to systems a few weeks after I transferred here. He has the best sense of humor. There is never a dull meeting when he is present. Oh, the lady covering up her head is our Manager, Sandi. She had just gotten into work, and did not have her make-up on yet. Marvette, in the picture with me, is the secretary that I went out to dinner with right after the mastectomy. Remember her back surgery story? (Sad) Then I joke with Jessica and Juanita (both about six feet tall) that they are the "amazon" women. . . see the picture of me in between them. Jessica was leaning up against my desk so she doesn't look quite so tall here. Now you have met my new work family.

Oops — be right back. I just remembered that I have to call Betinia at the chemo clinic. WARNING: This letter is to be continued.

Damn! I just got off the phone with Betinia, and we were talking about my blood count which showed as very low on Friday. I got the results yesterday afternoon and had already done so much all weekend around people, including twelve hours on Sunday with thousands of people at Disneyland, that it was too late for me to be taking any precautions. Anyway, we were talking and I said something to her about December 30th being my last treatment. She said I still have one more treatment to go after that. (I almost started crying again.) I told her that I had discussed it with Dr. Nielsen on Friday and he agreed that this would be the last one. She said that it's supposed to be at least seven treatments over six months. I said, "No. I was told when I went to every four weeks that it was only going to be six treatments." I don't think I can make my mind accept the fact that there will be more. I've been looking forward to December 30th as being the last of the chemo, and have already been celebrating it. I've been feeling great about starting the New Year chemo treatment free. I hope that she is wrong. She is going to check with Dr. Nielsen and let me know what he says when I go for my next treatment. If they tell me there is more I might just refuse it. I know I am being a wimp, but my mind is not adjusted to this new development.

Okay — where was I? (Back to Friday)

I did the medical appointments and got home just in time to shower and change before going to the airport. I took Nick with me. Honest I was just dragging my butt. I knew my count had to be low. But, when Stephen walked off the plane, I became re-energized. I think falling in love with a man like him is definitely the cure for chemo side effects. A spoonful of sugar *does* makes the medicine go down.

He and Nick hit it off. And, he remembered to bring Nick some airplane peanuts. Nick has now added "Steben" to his list of people he loves. Oh, and I think you are a good candidate for that list too.

My Aunt Dot called around six Saturday morning to let us know about Uncle George's death. I in turn called the kids to let them know. Eric, who never takes time off work, cried so hard, and for so long that he couldn't stay at work.

After breakfast Stephen and I went to Seal Beach and we walked on the Pier. I also showed him my favorite little beach. It's the one I showed you and Jack too. Then, we picked up two large pizzas on the way home.

Just as we got back to my apartment Eric, Bridget and Tyler arrived. A few minutes later Arthur and Dani came too. We had the pizza for lunch, and opened gifts involving Arthur and Dani. I gave Stephen one of his gifts so that he wouldn't be feeling left out.

The kids stayed until around five. By then Karen and Bob's Open House party had already started. I was too drained of energy to make the long drive out to their new house. We stayed home, and watched TV and pigged out on pie and ice cream.

Sunday we went by Little Saigon to have "Dim Sum." Unfortunately it was nine in the morning and the restaurant wasn't open yet.

We got to Disneyland just before ten. The first ride we went on was a new one for me. I was hesitant to go on it because I thought it might be too rough, but it was great. I want to go on it again some day. It's called, "Star Tours" and is sort of like using virtual reality in that you almost believe that you are flying through the galaxy. It was exhilarating.

We, as Stephen called it, "ate our way" through Disneyland for twelve hours. We stopped and splurged on all kinds of snacks and also had hot dogs, then later a real lunch, and in the evening we had dinner at a nice restaurant in New Orleans Square.

We saw the Lion King parade which had some great music and dancing, and we saw Santa Claus, and had our picture taken with him. Our last event before leaving the park was to see the new "Fantasmic" laser light and water show. It was incredibly awesome.

Needless to say we didn't go to church or the Cowboy, but I told Stephen, "next time." Monday was for visiting, and meeting work friends. We went to the Work Program and he met Danielle and the others. Since all of them had seen his video tape they recognized him right away. Chau made me feel good when she told Stephen how lucky he was to have me.

Next was my current office so he could meet the Systems staff. First we came into my office, and Chris got up and gave him a hug. That made me feel good. She told me today that she felt like she already knew him since they had met previously online. Also, when we went into Marvette's office she looked up, grinned at the both of us and said, "Oh, the Teddy Bear." Stephen and I both cracked up. He met a lot of the people who are in these pictures. It was a very pleasant visit and I was proud of him and my co-workers.

I took Stephen for lunch at Maxwell's on the Huntington Beach Pier. It was nice, and something different for us to experience together. It is a very old restaurant that is romantic and elegant, yet you can dress casual there. I've heard that it is going to be torn down soon. It has been quite the landmark here.

After that we went by my church as I wanted him to see where I spend my Sunday Mornings. When we got home I found the message from Betinia about my low blood counts on Friday.

We got to the airport an hour early. There were strolling Victorian Christmas Carolers to entertain us. (Nice touch.— Orange County might be down right now, but we are not completely out.) As soon as he got on the plane, and I turned around to leave I started going through Stephen-withdrawal.

I got home and kept busy catching up on stuff around the house. Then I went online for my cancer survivors meeting. About ten minutes later Stephen, who was by then home and on his PC, came into the group.

Sharon was there and she asked Stephen if he was taking good care of "our Marilyn." His response was that I was the one who had spoiled him all week-end. He always says the right things.

Oh, I forgot to tell you that Saturday night Tamsin and Nick took my car and went to the movies. I fixed a filet mignon and champagne dinner by candlelight for Stephen and I. Very nice except by the time we ate I was in plaid flannel pajamas. What can I say? Also we exchanged our Christmas gifts.

I received two turtle dove ornaments. (On the second day of Christmas my true love gave to me...) He is such a romantic man. Then I got a gift pack of Jessica McClintock perfume, soap, lotion and gel. I love it and I keep smelling my wrists. This is Stephen's and my favorite perfume. He also gave me a beautiful silver picture frame.

I know there must be more for me to write about, but I feel lately as

if the faster I go the be hinder I get. I'm used to being organized, and
having everything caught up. I feel overwhelmed when I have more
on "my plate" than I can almost handle. (Notice I said "almost" because, I still pretty much get it all done.)

Bye. Love you,

December 21, Wednesday

Me again-

I probably won't be writing much until after the Holiday, but I remembered the little things that I forgot yesterday.

Yesterday at work we had our first "Sysco Christmas Carolers"
rehearsal. It went better than I had anticipated it would. Most everyone was resistant to the idea, but we had so much fun that they want
more rehearsals before our actual performance. The only Coordinators
who didn't show up were the guys from both teams. This morning I
sent them all an e-mail that said, "Real men" for the subject of the mail.
. . and then in the text, " sing Christmas Carols." I guess that ought to
get some of them irritated with me. We are not professional singers,
but in a crowd we all sounded good. It's true that there is safety in
numbers.

I love these people in Systems. We laugh and have fun. The laughter is definitely good for helping me be healthy. Between you, Stephen,
the kids and the people I work with I laugh a lot, and I am loving all of
it.

Oh, I keep forgetting to tell you that my weight is just about normal now too, and I am very pleased. I think all the eating I've been
doing over the past six weeks, and also the contentment I am feeling
from being in a relationship with Stephen, has me putting on the pounds.

Jessica and I continue our breast cancer support talks. Whenever
we feel like it we can just talk about our concerns, and I always feel
better afterwards. It is wonderful having her in Systems. She is pretty
excited about the book, and said that this is the type of book she was
looking for before she started chemo, and there wasn't one to be found
in any of the bookstores. Her concern about the book though is that
other women will read about all that I am doing while on chemo and
wonder why they can't do it too. But, then on the other hand it could be
a motivator.

Jessica is amazed that I am doing almost all of my normal activities. . . and falling in love. I've thought about it a lot. I know I am compulsive and organized, but I think that when a person wants something bad enough then she just does it. I want to dance so I do. I want to

spend time with grand-kids — so I do. I wanted a special man in my life — and here he is. I think other women will do what they want, and have what they want most too.

I assured Jessica that I am not always as "up" as they see me at work, and that you are the one who gets the brunt of my down times. I don't want them to think I am perfect when in reality I cry all over your shoulder as needed.

Last night I thought more about Betinia's comment yesterday regarding at least one more treatment after the first of the year. I have made up my mind that I won't accept any more. I don't think I will regret this decision. If the chemo that they have given me so far can make my blood count go so low, and have my hair falling out — then it has to have worked, and accomplished the killing off of any stray cancer cells. Since you are going through this with me — do you agree with this decision?

Time for me to get on with other things.

Love you,

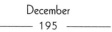

$\mathcal{D}$ecember 23, Friday

Merry Merry Christmas to you and Jack and the kids,

This may be my last note prior to then, so I want to get my wishes in now. I know it will be a great Christmas for all of us.

Actually, I am going to try to make this short (joke, right?) — but, I have pictures to send you from Stephen's visit and other miscellaneous ones taken this past week.

Yesterday I was telling one of my former Quality Control analysts about Wendy and I started crying. I almost cried again last night when I read a letter she sent me. She is such a beautiful person. In my mind I "will" her to be healthy. It is so frustrating to not be able to make her all better because I want it to happen so badly.

Wendy is so appreciative of your offer to stay with you and Jack. I gave her your address and phone number and mailed her a picture of us today. I hope to be back there one of these days to meet her in person. Actually, I would like to meet all of my online Cancer friends.

Well, today should go by quickly at work. We have our Christmas caroling at ten o'clock and today is the Western BBQ lunch.

Oh, Arthur called me and told me about his not being able to see you and Lisa. He is really disappointed. He didn't realize that Arthur and Darleen had already made commitments for those days. Next time I guess.

Love you,

*D*ecember 26, Monday

Hi,

Are you working today? I forgot to ask you when I talked to you yesterday. I hope the rest of your Christmas was everything that you hoped it would be. Mine continued to be wonderful and magical. The whole holiday was that way this year. Every part of it was perfect.

You know what else I got? (I forgot to tell you this too.) When I got home from work Friday there was a huge bouquet of two dozen long stemmed, lilac Sterling roses from Stephen. They are the most beautiful bouquet I have ever received.

When my co-workers and I caroled on Friday we got a very warm reception from the Executive Managers and all others in our building. But, the best part was that we had fun doing it.

I think I told you that I've talked with Blaine on the phone again. (The younger man that I met through Prodigy.) Well, last night, after the kids had left, I went to the Cowboy to dance. Blaine showed up, and was watching me dance. I didn't know he was there. When I came off the dance floor he came over to give me a hug and he commented about what great dancers we all were. He was sort of amazed at the quality of our dancing. I said, "But, I told you I was a 'dancer'." He seemed intimidated by us and he left about two minutes later. I hope I hear from him again, and that he didn't get scared off. I tried to tell him that I thought his Country Swing was a fun style, but he didn't want to do it.

This is it. Even though I have today off work I have lots to do.

Love,

*D*ecember 28, Wednesday

Hello,

I got your letter and it made me chuckle when you talked about all the shopping you did for yourself. That's not selfish Rita. I take great pleasure these days in buying and giving to myself. In the past I would feel guilty, but not anymore. My breast cancer sisters understand this too. We deserve all the pleasures we can get, and I am including a universal "we" — so that goes for you too! Life is too short, and we must enjoy it to the fullest.

Yesterday I called Bruce to see how he was doing and to wish him a Happy Birthday. Then when I got home last night I had this thank you note in the mail from him. I thought it was nice so I'll enclose it for you to enjoy too. He is doing wonderful. Bruce said that his doctors say that he is their "miracle." Right now he has some problems with his equilibrium, but he is walking and getting exercise to bring it back. He is doing amazingly well considering what he just went through.

Did you have any surprises from Jack on Christmas? Did you get your watch? Boy — what a snoop! Only kidding. I know you just "happened" to find everything by accident.

Remember Jacqui, the clerical supervisor who was learning line dancing, and had called me before the mastectomy? She is now on AOL. Jacqui joined our Monday night cancer survivors group. I am really pleased. She called me last week and said that she should be mad at me because she spent the whole week-end on AOL and didn't get much done because of it. I think she is as hooked now as the rest of us.

My bobbed hairdo, which I had styled two weeks ago to make my hair look thicker is growing in and I like it more now that it is a wee bit longer. Also, I am thrilled as I am at a normal weight for me. I'm still on the thin side, but this feels much healthier. I hope I am able to keep it on after Friday's treatment.

I looked at my calendar today. How about meeting in San Francisco on May 20th or 21st? We could probably stay until the 26th or 27th. I am trying to give myself driving time to and from there too. Think about it and discuss it with Jack and let me know. (And, yes he should come too.) You will love Sonoma. It is so historical and romantic. I'm looking forward to going there again.

This is it for today.

Love,

*D*ecember 29, Thursday

Dear Aunt Dot,

Thank you for this wonderful letter. I know you must have a lot of notes to write so this is extra appreciated. It was so nice to talk with you on Christmas. I am glad that you have so many loving friends around you at this time. You are very much loved by a lot of people.

I know you miss Uncle George, but his spirit will always be with you. He was a most wonderful man, and dearly loved by all of us here.

Tamsin said that when Nick climbed into your lap during the service she was afraid at first that he was annoying you. When she saw that he was giving you comfort she was relieved. Yes, he is a very sweet little boy. It is my pleasure to have them staying with me at this time.

Take good care of you.

Love,

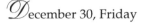

*D*ecember 30, Friday

Happy New Year!

Soon we will be in 1995. It hardly seems possible. Where did 1994 go? Whatever your plans are I hope they are fun, and please drink a glass of champagne for me. It's chemo week-end so I know I won't be imbibing.

I have a confession to make. This past week I have had about one cigarette a day. Also, for Christmas Eve and Christmas Day I had one glass of champagne each. Yum. Actually I don't really feel guilty about the cigarettes or the champagne. I'm not over doing it on either.

Guess what? I am getting fat. My jeans are actually tight. I had a hard time zipping them up today. I now weigh more than I did before the surgery! But, I guess, I'd better not over do it. I could get used to eating like this and "grow" to like it.

Monday night when I was in my cancer survivors group Kris, from Massachusetts and I were talking. I mentioned your store and she knows it. I encouraged her to drop in one of these days and say "Hi" to you. I didn't think you would mind. She lives in Watertown, and she grew up in Jamaica Plain not too far from where I lived.

Wendy sent me the most inspiring e-mail yesterday. She said that this week's treatment did not hit her as hard as the last one. She is out and walking around New York City. On New Year's Eve she is going with friends, in her mother's wheel chair, to the Marathon which she thought she would be running in again this year. Her friends, who are running, are going to push her in it. She will get to participate after all.

Well, I've got my jug of water out and have started chugging it down for the last time. I am so excited that there are no more treatments after today. I will have to send Mary, from my online group, a congratulations too. Today is her last one also.

I'll bet Tamsin will be happy about two months from now. Today she is "shaving" the bathroom floor again. She teases me about it. Too bad we couldn't be recycling all this hair. But, — soon it'll have stopped falling out.

One last item. Yesterday Jessica brought me a newsletter which she gets from a breast cancer group in San Francisco. I really enjoyed it and sent off my subscription payment immediately. It was interesting, but there was one article that had me concerned. The writer stated that the American Cancer Society does not give out accurate statistics regarding breast cancer mortality. It said that 50% of women who have breast cancer will die within ten years of their diagnosis. There was no footnote to show where these new statistics came from. But, it kind of shook me up. I sure hope the author of the article has her facts wrong!

Okay, time for me to get my show on the road.

Love,

December 30, Friday

Dear Dr. Trung:

I have given much thought to my upcoming reconstruction surgery. Could we have another interview to further discuss the type of surgery I will be having? Today is my last chemotherapy treatment and now I am of course looking forward to the next phase in this breast cancer experience.

I am aware that you felt that I did not have enough abdominal tissue to have this type of implant. Since our talk in October I have conscientiously been eating to gain weight. I am now over what I was prior to my mastectomy. Hopefully I have gained enough to be able to use my abdominal tissue. Could you re-think this option? If you feel that this is not something you would like to do, then could I speak with another plastic surgeon who has done this type of implant?

This is so important to me that I do not want to have regrets later. Please contact me regarding this request.

Thank you so much.

December 31, Saturday

New Year's Eve Morning — 12:08AM to be exact.

What am I doing up? (That is the big question.) I am feeling, for the last time here, LOUSY. I am chilled and feverish and nauseous and miserable, but you know what? I don't care! I know this is the end of it, so it's not that bad. And, I have my computer to keep me company. I just wrote to Stephen and now it's your turn.

I sent him an e-mail that says, "Misery Loves Company" as it's title. He is so sick Rita. And, I am worrying myself sick over him. It's been a full week and he still has the flu and strep throat. His fever has gone really high and he can't eat. He's on antibiotics and losing weight.

Enclosed is a copy of the letter which I sent to the plastic surgeon this morning. Obviously, I am still hoping to be able to get the abdominal tissue implant and in March or April.

Tamsin picked up Arthur at the airport tonight. She said he had a wonderful time and he did a lot of skiing. He brought me — two "Sky

Bars" . . . great son! And, he also brought me a health and energy stone. It came with a tiny bag and I've attached it to my key chain.

Tonight Tamsin was just briefly reading my 1995 horoscope. It said that I was going to grow my hair really long. (They got that right.) And, she read some of the 1996 horoscope which said something about my "uniting" two households. Hmm — wonder who it will be with?

Bye. Love you,

January

January 1, Sunday

Hello,

I am excited that we are starting a New Year and that there is so much to celebrate in it. And I am not complaining about 1994, because what with all that did happen it was still very good to me. No more chemo treatments! Yes, Benitia was mistaken when she thought there was at least one more. (Fortunately, I didn't have to make that decision, as to whether to continue or not.)

The sun is shining and it is like a warm spring day. I started the day off at church and it was wonderful. Reverend Michelle was the main speaker and she talked about "What's New?" I was already in a positive mood and her talk only reinforced all the good feelings I was having. She reminded us to see each day as a new beginning. For those who are doing resolutions, we were encouraged to take baby steps instead of promising to do all of whatever it is, at once. This reminded me of you and I, and this past year, and how we have taken it day by day and step by step.

Tamsin and Nick went to the mountains yesterday with Teharu. Afterwards, they stayed over night at his house. Tamsin called last night, and said that they had fun playing in the snow. Nick was leery at first, but then he joined right in with their snow ball fight.

I took advantage of having the apartment all to myself, and got some things done. One biggie was that I organized all of my paperwork for the past year. Boy, did I spend a lot of money!

When I got home from church, I cooked a steak dinner and had a glass of sparkling cider with it. It seemed like I should have been doing this with Stephen or someone else, other than by myself, but "next year."

I just got off the phone with Ann and she told me about the New Year's Eve dance party last night. Everyone was there. She said that Allen even showed up with a date. (Good for him!) I told her that next year, hopefully, I will be there with all of them too.

Stephen is finally out of bed and feeling better. I have been so worried about him this past week. It was frustrating to not be close to him, or to be able to contact him. I wrote him e-mail last night to welcome in the New Year, and told him that even though it seemed like we should have been together, it was probably better that we weren't. Misery might love company, but we would have been too sick to enjoy ourselves.

So, what did you do last night and today? I hope 1995 will have all of your dreams coming true.

Love you,

P.S. I just realized that I don't have any three cent stamps. I guess this will have to go with two twenty-nine cent stamps.

January 3, Tuesday

Hi,

It was wonderful talking to you this weekend. Please keep me posted as to the status of your's and Jack's relationship. It did kind of depress me some. I love you both, and so it is sad hearing news like that. I think you understand. If there is anything that I can do to help, please let me know.

I did go dancing New Year's Night after all. It was very crowded. We are spoiled. We regulars are used to having the dance floor to ourselves on Sunday afternoons. Since the Cowboy didn't open until later in the evening, the club filled up fast. But, it was fun and I saw people that I haven't seen since before the mastectomy. I was at the bar getting a glass of water, when an old friend saw me and said, "Hey, I saw your picture in the paper!" I also saw the newspaper ad guy. I didn't think I would ever see him again.

Allen was there and we danced a lot. The dancing was a struggle for me, since the floor was so crowded. I was kind of weak and using up even more energy than normal, due to the volume of people. Finally, after less than two hours, I knew I'd maxed out and had to leave.

Yesterday, I had "to pay the fiddler" for all my dancing fun. I was completely worn out, so I stayed in, rested, and ate high protein foods. And just because I wrote that note to my plastic surgeon, I lost two pounds with this treatment! (Grrr)

My online support group was in the evening. It is so strange to know, and love, so many people that I have never met in person. We have become so close, yet we only chat and see each other's pictures. Last night was extra special, because Lillie joined us for the first time. She was a big help. One of our members comes because her mother has cancer, and she passes the chat logs on to her. Lillie has so much experience, what with being an oncology nurse, dealing with her own cancer, and recently helping her mother-in-law, who died of cancer. She was able to answer a lot of questions for this member.

Stephen is still pretty sick. He was able to get out of bed yesterday and to go out for a walk, but then he collapsed into bed when he got home. He has lost twelve pounds and still has a sore throat. He said he will call his doctor again today. Everything is still great between us, but it is hard for me to be so far away from him.

I put in my vacation request for May. As soon as I hear from you I will call my brother to ask him to save the townhouse for us.

We have started our January "monsoons," and it makes for dangerous driving. Southern Californians are not used to driving in inclement weather.

That's it for now. I still don't have any of the new thirty-two cent postage stamps, so the Post Office is sure making out from me when I double up on the old stamps.

Love you,

January 4, Wednesday

Hi,

I'm home from work again today. I did get up and dressed, and then I asked myself, "Why am I doing this?" I had a rough night with chills and then my stomach is still acting up. So, I called Juanita and said that I wouldn't be in. I just keep reminding myself that this is the last time I will have to go through this.

It's probably just as well that I stayed home, as it is pouring out and Tamsin had an appointment with a counselor at the Community College. She would have had to take Nick with her on the bus. I dropped her off, came home with Nick, and then picked her up when she was done.

It is always wonderful to get your phone calls. Naturally, I am a little upset about you and Jack splitting up. I love you both, and it is hard to think of you as no longer being a couple. Then I start worrying about you and money. It will be rough at first. If you feel that you can't afford the May vacation let me know.

We were so busy talking about other things, that I forgot to tell you how much I like your new hairstyle. It is beautiful and it looks so soft and silky. My day will come too. Also, the pictures of you and the kids are the best you've ever sent. Are you going to have wallet ones made? If so, please put me on the list for receiving one.

Now, your birthday is coming up soon. I hope that it is a good one for you, even in the midst of all your changes.

I'm not in much of a letter writing mood today, but I had this lone picture, which I forgot to return in yesterday's mail.

Take care and it is my turn to be here for you!

Love you lots,

Hi,

January 5, Thursday

I'm home using up more vacation time and hating every minute of it. This is my second day in a row. My stomach has calmed down quite a bit, but now it's the weakness and fatigue. My heart has been banging fast and furiously since I woke up. I managed to eat and shower and then I had to go back to bed. But, I keep telling myself that next month I won't have to go through this. I will be gaining strength and energy—and hair too!

Even though I have one letter sitting on my desk to mail, I had to write a note to tell you about the storm yesterday. Once again, I think someone was looking out for me and I was glad that I had not gone into work after all. You must have heard about how bad it was here.

First, Bridget called last night. She, Eric, and Tyler were in their new car taking Eric to work, when they got stuck on a flooded street. All of a sudden the water was up to the car windows. They couldn't open their doors. Eric went through the window and pulled Tyler out after him. As the car was filling up with water and floating down the street, Bridget also climbed out through the window.

A Good Samaritan with a truck came by and helped the kids. He drove them to Eric's work, where Bridget's Dad came to get her and the baby. Next, Eric walked back to the car. The flood had receded some, so he pushed the car back to their apartment, which was about two or three miles.

Everyone is fine. My concern right now is that Eric might get sicker. He has been fighting the flu. Bridget said that he was only wearing a wind breaker and tennis shoes, and naturally he got completely soaked.

Their car is covered by insurance, so that should be taken care of. Right now, it is a dead car that is filled with water and debris.

Then Arthur called and said that he and Brian had taken Brian's car to work. They were wishing they had Arthur's four wheeler jeep Cherokee on the way home. The flooding was past the headlights on the car, and it took them two hours to drive home in the evening.

All night, there were police sirens going off around us, and my own car alarm went off twice, when the trash can lids flew onto it.

Today, the sun is shining and everything is clear and bright. Strange weather we have here in Southern California.

Love you,

January 6, Friday

Hi—

This will be short but sweet, as I have good news all around.

Stephen called last night, and he is going to come down again in February. He is feeling much better, except for a lingering cough.

I am feeling much better too, and I think that I am now past the worst of the chemo.

Oh, and we got e-mail today that the County Deferred Compensation program will only show a ten percent loss for it's members. A $1,200 loss versus $12,000 sounds good to me. And, although there is nothing in writing, the word is out that the other Deferred Compensation program did not suffer any loss, as the monies were not invested in the county pool. So, once again bad news is now sounding like good news.

My weight is down again and I am only weighing 105 pounds. But then again, I haven't heard from my plastic surgeon yet. Maybe I will gain the weight before he gives me an appointment.

I hope you are feeling better. Keep me posted as to what is happening with you and Jack.

Bye. Love you,

January 10, Tuesday

Hi,

I'm sitting here and looking at all your pictures for about the third time. The one of you and Jack is going into my wallet. The one of your family, taken when you were a little girl, goes into your album. The picture that you took in Mexico, and had enlarged and framed for Jack, is so beautiful that I almost can't stop looking at it. Your photography only gets better and better. Thank you for sharing all of these with me.

Have you heard about the flooding in Sonoma and Napa? The rivers in Northern California have flooded over into the towns. Today, we have a new storm coming and it is supposed to be worse than last week.

Bridget called last night and said that their car is totaled from the last storm. Their insurance company is paying them the blue book value, but it doesn't cover the balance of their car loan. Now they are out looking for another car.

My brother called and confirmed that the townhouse is ours for the May vacation. You know what I'd like to do for that week? Rest. This will be my first real vacation in almost two years, and I am ready to just relax, read books, and eat, and sleep lots. How does that sound to you?

My latest project is getting a group of committed dance friends together to go back to Club Dance in Knoxville, Tennessee next autumn or winter. This has been one of my goals since the cancer diagnosis. Everyone I called yesterday said, "Yes." I think we may wind up with about a dozen people. The next step is to write for the tickets, and then start making hotel and plane reservations.

I told my online support group about this goal and one of my breast cancer sisters, who is a ballet teacher in Georgia, said that she and her husband would meet us there!

I was talking more to Kris and she still plans on coming by your store to say hello to you. She is one of our younger members. I forget what type of cancer she has, but it is not breast cancer. I've seen her picture in our group's collage and she is a cutie. Oh, and she is a writer. Kris does articles for the newspaper back there. I think you will enjoy meeting her.

You are always in our chat logs lately. I should start sending them to you. Last night, Wendy said that she won't be going to Boston, but to Toronto instead. She will be checking out their alternative cancer treatment, which involves large doses of vitamins and some mild chemotherapy. She doesn't know yet when she is going, but she asked if I had any friends in Toronto that she could stay with. (She was teasing me.) When I answered in the negative she then asked if you could move there so that she could stay with you. (Joke)

Wendy had e-mailed me earlier this week. She has an appointment with her lung specialist on Thursday, as she is having problems breathing. This is not good news, but throughout all this Wendy is keeping her spirits up, and continues to cheer the rest of us on while we go through our own struggles. She is not running of course, but continues to get exercise by walking around New York City.

Stephen has become a regular in our Cancer Survivors group. He comes as my support person. I am glad that he is meeting my friends.

Well, guess this is enough. Now, I have to find a large envelope to return all of your pictures. Write me, as to how things are going with you and Jack. I trust that you will make the right decision.

Love you,

January 11, Wednesday

Hello,

This is going to be one of those letters where I am just bouncing information off of you, as a way to talk to myself. I'm still in a quandary about the reconstruction, and trying to come to a decision. The more questions I am asking lately about the various types of implants, the more I learn, and the more I feel a little bit in control of the situation.

I had asked our cancer group leader, Jane, to tell me about her reconstruction, as she used her abdominal tissue and is very pleased with the results. Jane is forty, married and lives in Michigan. She was diagnosed with breast cancer when she was in her early thirties and had a lumpectomy. A year ago, she had a recurrence in the same breast and had to have a mastectomy.

Jane explained the two types of abdominal tissue implants to me better than any doctor or reference book has. I'll try to translate it for you.

The first type is a "TRAM" flap, with micro surgery. This is the type that Jane had. There are a lot of requirements for being qualified for this implant. One of them is that the patient must have a lot of abdominal tissue. The tissue is removed from the abdominal area, along with a small portion of the long muscle at the very lowest part of the abdomen. All of this is then reattached micro surgically to the breast area. The tiny blood vessels from the abdomen are then attached to the pectoral muscle in the center of the chest, and to the large triangular muscle in the back that covers the shoulder blade. Next, the portion of the long muscle is attached in the same way, and is used to support the tissue which will construct the breast.

The other type is the *tunnel* type of "TRAM." This is probably what my plastic surgeon was referring to, as he mentioned removing my complete abdominal muscle for the implant. The muscle is removed from the opposite side of the breast being rebuilt, and is tunneled up, and "flapped" over to the chest where the mastectomy occurred.

Jane said that she is extremely pleased with the results of her TRAM, but the recovery process was not so wonderful. She spent at least two weeks using a walker to get around. I have heard this before from other breast cancer women. It takes quite some time to be able to walk standing up straight.

There is an additional bonus, (to go along with the new breast) in that this type of surgery is like getting a tummy tuck. But, on the other hand, another disadvantage is having a scar which runs from one hip bone to the other.

Mary, who is also in my cancer survivors group, said that she had her implant done at the same time as her mastectomy. She chose the silicone implant, as she had heard too many horror stories about the saline implant, and the constant needs for fill ups due to leaking. Some women told her that the saline breast gets all wrinkled when it deflates.

Based on all this information it looks like, even though I have once again gained back lost weight, that I still won't qualify for the TRAM. And I don't think I have an option with my plastic surgeon regarding silicone versus the saline.

After my appointment Friday, I will know more and write you what I learn then.

I have one letter already waiting to mail to you, but I am out of stamps. When the rain stops I will get to the post office. We have been having continuous storms. There has been so much destruction caused by the flooding. Stephen is on his way, as a volunteer, to help a Search and Rescue team. His home town in Northern California is under a state of emergency.

Tamsin and Nick both start school next week. She is finishing up the last of her registration requirements today. When she had her orientation earlier this week Nick went to his new preschool on campus. He loved it. This should be good for the both of them... and me too!

I'm out of here for this one.

Bye. Love you,

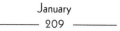

*J*anuary 14, Saturday

Hi—

How are you? Once again, I am tempted to call since I feel like a long letter is coming on, but writing will do. Also, I wanted to send you this book on Primates from my friend Janette. She took some of the pictures in it. I thought you would enjoy reading through it, since this is one of your many interests. Tamsin and I both read it and agreed that it was hilarious. You can share it with Lisa, but please return it to me someday.

Another storm is coming, so I am going to take advantage of a no rain day to get some errands done. I'm going shopping for a birthday present for Stephen. (February 8th) He won't give me any clues as to what to get him, so I'll just have to guess and hope that he likes whatever he winds up with. I have some ideas. Men do like toys. Women like clothes. Maybe, I will satisfy both of us and get one of each!

Well, yesterday was the appointment with Dr. Trung, my plastic surgeon. I am satisfied that I will be in good hands with him. We talked to some length regarding the various types of implants. He checked my "tummy" and said I probably had enough now to do the abdominal implant. Dr. Trung does not do the micro surgery TRAM. If I had insisted on this type, I would have to change doctors and go to the clinic in Woodland Hills. That is quite a distance from where I live. He said that not too many doctors are experienced in this type of reconstruction. Dr. Trung also told me that, occasionally, the tissue dies from this surgery and then the woman is left with no breast and without part of her abdominal muscle.

We talked about the tunnel TRAM. He could do this implant, but I would lose all of my abdominal muscle, and it would interfere with my dancing. Since I am not willing to give up my dancing for a boob, I decided to not go that route.

Oh, what was funny was that Dr. Trung does ballroom dancing. While we were talking about dancing, he said that he had the best dance teacher on the West Coast. I said, "There is only one 'best' dance teacher and his name is Phil Adams." Dr. Trung laughed and said that Phil was his dance teacher. I told him that Phil was my third dance teacher, and that I used to be on a dance team, which he choreographed for. Small world!

Okay, back to the surgery. Since Dr. Trung does not do silicone, I will have the saline implant after all. He showed me pictures (before and after) of many of the women he has done. They all looked good to me. Once again, he fitted me and explained the procedure. Dr. Trung said, that he will have me looking like a teenager again! I can live with that.

My next blood test for my oncologist is Valentine's Day. Dr. Trung will also be checking the results of this test, in order to determine if my count is going up. Once my count is high enough, he will do the surgery. It could be as soon as the end of February. He said, I will then be lopsided for about six weeks. The left breast will be firm and high compared to the remaining good breast. I'm probably going to be wearing vests and baggy jumpers again for awhile.

After six weeks, I will go back and at that time he will do the, as Jane calls them, "decorations." When he does the nipple and areola grafts from the right breast he will also work on it, so that I will have "Twin Peaks." (My words, not his.)

I think I will have about two to three months of no dancing. But, the good news is that I should be pretty much through with the reconstructive surgeries, other than the tattooing, by the time we meet in Northern California. And if the roads are still closed from this winter's storms, I may just fly to San Francisco myself and meet you there. We can rent a car to get around.

There has been a lot of destruction in Sonoma and Napa from these storms, but Stephen said that since Bud's townhouse is in the downtown area it is safe. Mostly the vineyards were damaged.

Nick got his preschool physical and shots Thursday. He and Tamsin both start school on Tuesday. She will be going full time, and we are all excited and pleased that she has made this decision about returning to school. As yet, she hasn't picked a major and will be taking only the basic requirements until she decides. Nick will be attending the on campus day care full time.

Bridget and Tyler were over again last night. Tyler is huge. He's a regular "chubby cheeks" baby. One of her Dad's friends asked her if she was feeding him bricks. Stephen is doing okay with his latest assignment in helping with the disasters in Northern California. He is mainly working indoors and has plenty of assistance. The blood bank called him. A child receiving radiation is in need of his platelets. Stephen explained that he is still on antibiotics and asked them to hold off for one week, so his health will be better. I am so proud of him.

Lillie just finished her design for a breast cancer awareness pin. She has signed a contract with a jeweler. The profits from the sale of the pin will go towards funding her new support group, for Mothers of Women With Breast Cancer. She is such a go-getter. Also, she was recently asked to do another speech in October at her local mall. They will be sponsoring this year's Race For The Cure.

Do you think you would want to do the walk in your area this year? Maybe you, Linda, and Lisa could do it together. Think about it.

Oh, one last item. There are two AOL parties in Orange County the weekend that Stephen will be down. We may go to the one at the Waterfront Hilton, here in Huntington Beach. The newspaper reporter who interviewed me may be there also. I would like her and Stephen to meet.

This letter really got kind of lengthy, but I wanted you to hear the latest on my next phase of this experience.

Bye. Love you,

P.S. No, guess it's not over yet. I asked Dr. Trung if I could talk to some of the women that he has performed this surgery on. He gave me the phone numbers for two of the women. One is out of the country on business, so I couldn't talk to her.

I did reach the other lady, Mary Beth. She is a nurse with my HMO and works in Los Angeles, even though she lives here in Orange County. She was so helpful and we talked quite awhile. Mary Beth is extremely pleased with Dr. Trung's work.

She was diagnosed with breast cancer in November 1992, and finished her chemo (the same kind as me) in June 1993. She waited six months to have her saline implant done. The following year—this past September, she had the nipple and areola added.

She said that she looks so good that it is hard to believe that she once had the missing breast, and the big mastectomy scar. Mary Beth takes out her "before" picture every once in awhile, to remind her of what she used to look like. She feels that what Dr. Trung did is like a miracle.

I cannot wait!

*J*anuary 15, Sunday

Sunday, Another Happy Funday-Sunday here!

I wanted to write you before I went to church, as I am going to stop at the Post Office on the way. Enclosed are some of Arthur's New Hampshire pictures. He brought them by yesterday, when he and Dani were over. He looks like he was freezing.

Here is a picture of Stephen and I for you to keep. It is the one that I am mailing in for the Cancer Survivors Group collage. I like it of both of us—his great smile and also of me, except for my being so skinny and pale.

Want to hear a sort of funny story? Well, I have been shaving my legs every day for about thirty five years, except when I wear pants. Last night, I realized I hadn't shaved my legs for a week because I had been wearing pants, or skirts with tights, to work because of the rainy weather. I thought I'd better shave them for church and dancing. Well, there wasn't anything to shave! Maybe a little bit, but I have I lost most of my hair there too and I didn't realize it. Jane from my group said that she lost all of her hair from the eyebrows down. She had the same chemo as me. And, here all these months I've been routinely shaving just skin!

Yesterday, I went to the Crazy Horse Steak House and Saloon to make dinner reservations for February 10th, for Stephen and I. I want to take him out for his birthday. They are going to put balloons around our table and save us a table in the Dance Hall for after our dinner. There will be a live band. Even though Stephen doesn't dance, I think he will enjoy it. Do you remember going there when you were out here?

While I was at the Crazy Horse, I bought him one of their black jackets. Then, I went to Brookstone and got him a travel clock. He is my "gypsy" and is always going from one place to another, so this seemed like a practical gift.

Also, I got him all kinds of little Valentine's gifts and put them in a big, red gift bag. Saturday night, we will be going out to dinner again. He is taking me out for Valentine's Day. After dinner, we will go to that AOL party at the Waterfront Hilton. It is an appetizer buffet and DJ dance to raise money for The Make A Wish Foundation.

It is so nice to be able to make plans and know that I am going to be able to follow through on them! I don't have to say, "I'll see how I'm feeling."

I bought this tape for Stephen, as it has a song on it that reminds me of him. Well, parts of it do. ("Wind Beneath My Wings") But, I was listening to it while I was out doing my errands and the song, "Old Friends" reminded me of you. There are other songs on it that I thought you would like, so this copy goes to you. I will pick up another one for Stephen today. I hope you enjoy it. The singer comes to my church every once in awhile, and she gives me goose bumps when she performs. Let me know what you think of it. ("Old Friends" might be a Kleenex type song. It brings tears to my eyes anyway.)

I have to get dressed and out of here soon.

Bye. Love you,

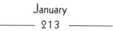

January 17, Tuesday

Good Morning,

It is cold here, but the sun is shining and the ground is finally drying up. I had four days off and now I feel rested and caught up, even on my magazine reading which was getting months behind. I am feeling stronger and healthier with each passing day. I'm in love with Stephen and with life. Does it get better than this?

And how are you doing? Any progress in your decision making? Let me know what is going on.

This morning Nick and Tamsin started school. The bathroom became a mad house. Tamsin and I were doing the "ten step" in there. Maybe, I should have taken the two bath place next door. If it becomes available again, I might just do that.

Sunday, I went to the Cowboy and stayed for three hours. I think just knowing that there is no more chemo is giving me spurts of energy. I had a great time. Don showed up and was alone, but he seemed to be doing okay, as he was hanging around one lady in particular. We only got to dance two dances together. I asked him if he was ever going to be happy again and he answered in the affirmative. I just feel so bad for him. He is too fun a person to be feeling this melancholy all the time.

One of my regular dance partners, Ray, was commenting about how he goes out on weekend nights and there is never anyone to dance with. (We are spoiled on Sundays.) I told him, that now that I am off of chemo, I will be going out more on the weekends. We agreed to meet

Saturday night at In Cahoots. He is an incredible dancer, so I know I will have fun.

Oh, and I have twelve people wanting to go to Club Dance at the end of this year. Karen called last night, and said that four friends of hers and Bob's want to go too. I told her that I had already written for twelve tickets, but I suspect that when the time comes, some people will back out.

Yesterday, was like a free day for me. It was a work Holiday and I had no "to do list" planned. I took Nick to the large mall that has a Merry Go Round. Then we went to two candy stores and four toy stores. It was a "Nicky" morning. When we got home, I cooked a regular dinner. When Tamsin came home from getting her nails done, we did more shopping. All day I was out spending money and having fun doing it.

Enclosed are our pictures from Christmas. There are some great ones of Nick and Tyler. Lately, my camera has been having problems with rolling the film, so I never know what pictures, or film, are going to come out.

Stephen will try to come down when I go in for my reconstruction surgery. He asked if I wanted him to be with me. At first, I was hesitant. I know I will be out of it and in quite a bit of pain—plus I'm sure I will look ghastly. But, the more I thought about it, the more I realized that I would really like it if he could be with me. It will depend on if he can get that time off though.

Last night, our Cancer Survivors group got a bigger room in the Health Forum. The room we have been using could only hold up to twenty three people. For months now we have been begging and pleading with AOL to recognize us, and give us a Forum type room, which holds forty three people. After we had been in our group for an hour, we all entered our new "home" together. It was pretty wild in there with so many conversations going on at one time, but the jokes that we shared last night were hilarious. It's almost like we are trying to outdo each other with one liners.

I told Stephen that I think I would like to write a book called, "Love and Laughter," and have excerpts from our weekly chat logs in it. There is sometimes pain, but much love, and we do laugh a lot too.

Write me.

Bye. Love you,

P.S. Another post script. I seem to remember more as soon as I end a letter. I really am okay about the saline implant, as the more I have thought about it the better I feel. I think I just needed to get more information, in order to weigh my options. It is another decision, made by me, that I know I can live with. I do have peace of mind over this step.

January 19, Thursday

Hi,

I haven't gotten a letter from you for some time now. Of course, I wonder how you are and what is going on back there. I am tempted to call. Maybe, no news is good news?

Tamsin and Nick are enjoying school. She had a very full day yesterday. She had classes all day and then one in the evening. I drop Tamsin and Nick off at school on my way to work, and they take the bus home after classes. Last night, when I got home from work I drove her back to the campus, came home to babysit Nick, which included getting him dinner and giving him a bath. Then we went back later in the evening to pick her up.

Nick was so tired from his long day that he, on his own, crawled into my bed at eight o'clock and fell asleep. I felt so bad, waking him up, and taking him out into the cold at 9:30 at night. Tamsin is getting a parking pass, so that she can take my car in the future, and Nick won't be disturbed from his sleep.

Obviously, we are all proud of her and the new choices she is making.

Wendy was kind of confused after her trip to Toronto. Did I already write and tell you that she doesn't know whether to get her hopes up, or consider the doctor there a quack? He told her, that if she followed his program she would be in remission within eight weeks. That is a challenge which is hard to turn down.

Yesterday, Jessica and I were talking more about reconstruction and we were comparing notes on the implanted breasts, which some women have shown us. One interesting point, that we both agreed on, is that the women are not modest about the reconstructed breast. I had given some thought to this in the past and Jessica and I came to a similar conclusion. We think that maybe sub-consciously the women don't consider the implanted breast as part of themselves. It's like, "Well, I can show it to you, because it is not really 'me'."

I know that I am a very modest person, but since my chest has healed I don't feel shy about showing the mastectomy scar to other women. I don't think I will be modest about showing off the new "boob" either. I mean, I will be pleased to have it, but since it is not a real body part then what do I care?

Work is busy. For awhile there, things were slow, as so many projects have been put on hold due to the financial crisis. But, I now have a new assignment, which involves helping to write a more formal Training Guide for the complicated system that I had trained the Work Program staff on a few months ago. Since our budget has been cut, there won't be new PC's for a lot of our line supervisors. They will instead use their mainframe terminals to access our current office system. It is very complicated and messy, but I guess it is better than nothing. Our team expects that our Help Desk calls will increase, once all the new users are trained and using e-mail.

Ray called the other night. He was confirming our dance plans for Saturday night. Later, I started thinking that I really do have the best of all worlds right now. I have Stephen as my boyfriend, which is a nice secure feeling, but since we don't see each other that often, I still get to have a form of leading the single life too. I mean, I get to go dancing with other men—as friends. I think I have it made. Once again, lucky me!

Okay—I have no real news either, but I wanted to let you know that I miss hearing from you. Write me soon.

Bye. Love you,

January 20, Friday

Hi,

I am being spoiled rotten by Stephen. He is so incredibly nice to me Rita. I cannot believe my good fortune to have met him—especially at this period in my life. Yesterday, the receptionist called me and said there was a surprise for me. More flowers—more daisies. They are so beautiful. It is a mixture of white daisies, colored gerber daisies, and other types of flowers and greenery. Then he sent me e-mail last night that said I have to wait for April or May for the lilacs! Man—I have never ever had it this good in a relationship before.

After work, I went by the See's candy store and ordered some truffles to be sent to our two cancer group facilitators. When I mentioned that I had gotten some for myself, while out shopping on Monday, both of them said that they love them too. Mike is in Virginia and Jane is in Michigan. I sent them each a pound box. They both do so much work to keep our group going, and we all love and appreciate their efforts. (Mike is also the one who uploaded our pictures into the computer.)

Also, last night, I called a new member who lives close to me. Her name is Peggy, is forty six and lives in the next city from me. She has not had a recurrence of breast cancer in over six years. That is great to hear. We were talking last night that we need more women to speak up—the ones who had breast cancer years ago and are now cancer free. Peggy and I are hoping to get together for lunch one of these weekends. Oh, she also helped out with the Race For The Cure last September.

We are expecting more rain over the next four days. Enough is enough already. Stephen is driving back to Lake Tahoe today, but he may get called back if the flooding starts up again. Also, he will continue to do the Apheresis weekly for the child who is undergoing radiation. He will be flying back and forth every other week for that too.

Today, I was "counting my blessings" again. Every once in awhile I do a sort of mental type of inventory. The final analysis is that my life is perfect. I have all good people and events occurring in my life right now. I love my family and friends. I have the best boyfriend. I love my job, the writing I do on the side, and my dance life. My body feels healthy and strong. My home life is great. And I have all the material goods that I could ever want. What more could I ask for?

I'm still waiting to hear from you though, and I hope that you are able to count all good things in your life too. Write me—please!

Bye. Love you,

January 21, Saturday

Rita—Hi!!!

I had no intention of writing to you, but today I got one very long letter, one note card, and a box of clothes from you! I am in heaven here. I love all of them. And, you think you are selfish? I'm keeping the two dresses too. One for around the house—slinky look—when Stephen visits and the short one for dancing. The silk blouses are great too. Thank you again and again.

This was a bonanza mail delivery day. I also got some leggings, which I had ordered through a catalogue, the information for the Club Dance tickets, the enclosed from Lillie, and a package from Stephen. His package had an Apheresis t-shirt for me, this cute boot stamp and a "hug" pin. It was like Christmas all over again!

I have to start getting ready soon, for the dancing I'll be doing tonight with Ray. I am looking forward to it. This will be my first Saturday night out dancing since before the chemo, and he is such an excellent dancer.

Today, I made reservations for Stephen and I to stay overnight at the Waterfront Hilton when he comes down. This is the hotel that Eric and Bridget stayed at on the first night of their honeymoon, two years ago. Every room has an ocean view.

Allen called me at work yesterday. He wants to borrow a Laura Schlessinger book from me, which the stores are sold out on. He also said that he is going to meet me at church tomorrow. This will be the first time that I've seen him at my church. He usually attends the Seal Beach or Fullerton churches.

Now, because of all the new socks you sent, I feel compelled to clean out my sock drawer. Thanks, I think. (Hmmm)

Love you lots,

P.S. I am so glad that everything is going so well for you, and that you got spoiled on your birthday. You deserve it!

January 22, Sunday

Good Morning!

It's Sunday... this has to be my favorite day of the week. I can sleep in—go to church to get nourishment for my mind and heart, and then there is the great dancing in the afternoon.

Speaking of which—I had the best dance time last night. Ray and I danced for three hours. His lead is so precise that I just glide into whatever move he wants. In my opinion, we were the best dancers on the floor. I love dancing with this man. He was totally a gentleman and good company. I hope I have future opportunities to meet him on weekend nights.

Yesterday, I was thinking more about your letter. You lose five pounds and gain it back. I gain five pounds and then lose it. Neither of us is ever satisfied!

I'm mailing Wendy the first page of your letter. She will appreciate your sense of humor, and Lord knows she needs some good laughs these days. I think this is why we joke so much in our cancer survivors group... laughing heals.

Well, there really isn't a lot to write about, but I finished "Slow Waltz In Cedar Bend" by Robert James Waller. I know you enjoyed "The Bridges of Madison County," so I wanted to mail it to you today when I stop by the Post Office. I enjoyed it. It is very different from his last book. Today, I am going to start a book that I have been wanting to read for aeons. It is "Men Are From Mars, Women Are From Venus." Have you read it?

Oh, and Lillie's book will be out in six weeks. When it hits the stores, I will get a copy for you, if you'd like to read it.

Stephen called yesterday. It is always so wonderful hearing his voice. I miss him! He is sending me an earthquake kit, to put in the trunk of my car. He said that when he is down next, we are going shopping for a kit for the apartment. I appreciate so much his concern and loving ways. I think the earthquake in Japan has him worried about us and the big one due down here.

Have to go.

Bye. Love you,

January 26, Thursday

Hi,

How is everything? This is going to be one of my briefer letters (right), but I had to write while things are still fresh in my mind. All is well, but there is more news regarding my job.

Yesterday, was a full meeting day. The morning meeting was the one that had all the news. After the meeting, I told my manager that it was a good thing I had started smoking again—or I would have started smoking again! (I will quit again before the next surgery. I know how important it is for me to stop before a surgery like that.)

Okay. The news is that our agency has to cut our budget even further to help with the money that was lost. Sandi said that there are going to be layoffs. (The rumor I heard later was that 20% of our employees will be laid off. This comes out to about 700 people.) She said that Sysco will be hit hard, especially the team that I am on. Naturally, it is more important to keep "case carrying" staff.

The way it will work is that they will start at the top. People will get layoff notices from their current positions. They can rotate to another position within their classification if there is an opening, or demote to the next lower step if there is an opening.

Also, eventually we might get a five percent pay cut.

All of the movement will involve seniority with the county. I have over fourteen years this time around. I will not be out on the streets. The worst case scenario for me is that I will go back to being a line supervisor. But, I don't think this will happen. The next could be that I will wind up rotating to the Districts as a Program Assistant, which would be supervising line supervisors. The most likely change for me will be that I am transferred to the mainframe team.

Three new Program Assistants on the mainframe team have already been unofficially told that they will lose their promotions, which were effective just before the bankruptcy.

We all went around the conference table giving our hire-in dates, as we all were curious as to where we stood. For the current team, I am about fourth with longevity. We think the team may be reduced to two or three members, so that is why I am speculating that I may be reassigned to fill one of the vacancies in mainframe. Of course this is all guess work at this point.

On February 10th the proposal will go to the Board of Supervisors. Once they have approved or denied the proposal we will know more. After that, it will probably take a couple of months for all the movement of personnel to be completed.

I am not worried. I still feel very thankful to have had this position while I was going through my health challenges this past year. I also feel that a change again would not be bad. This position was also wonderful in that I learned so much while I was here. Whatever comes next will be alright too.

Yesterday, I got a huge box from Stephen. It was a backpack filled with the earthquake preparedness stuff for the trunk of my car. Can you believe I have finally met a man who is this thoughtful? Again, I feel lucky to have met him.

Mike, from my support group, uploaded the Cancer Survivors collage into the AOL Health Forum files. Last night, I downloaded it. There is Stephen and I smiling away, along with many of the other members. It is so great to put faces to people I have grown to love.

Tamsin and Nick are still enjoying school immensely. Tamsin is really into her classes and studies and that pleases me to no end.

Eric and Bridget got their brand new Toyota Tercel. She came over last night with Tyler. He is so big and alert. I was holding him, and talking to him, and he was gurgling back at me. (Actually, he was mostly absorbed in a Care Bears video that Nick was watching.)

My life is good. I hope yours is too.

Bye. Love you,

January 27, Friday

Dear Rita,

It's late. I just got home from an evening out with Laura, Ashley and Joan. I have been anxious to see Joan. She is here on vacation and I only get to see her about once a year. Recently I had given Wendy Joan's address, so that she could write to her regarding the alternative treatment Joan received in Mexico after her breast cancer. Joan has been cancer free for over ten years.

If it wasn't so late your time I would call Wendy tonight. Instead, I just e-mailed her a lot of information. I hope she is able to log on tomorrow and can make the phone calls. I'm enclosing the letter I got from Wendy yesterday. Rita, she is not doing so good. I am very worried for

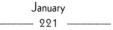

her. I try to hold it in, but as I write to you the tears start again. There must be some way to help her.

Joan explained the Tijuana clinic to me as best she could, and I relayed that to Wendy, but Joan wants Wendy to call her soon so she can talk to her. Also, she gave me the clinic's phone number so that Wendy can call the doctor on duty, and explain her situation to him, and ask if she can fly there for a consultation.

I am trying to stress to Wendy that Joan is a very beautiful and credible lady. She is well educated, world traveled and holds an extremely responsible position within a well known company. Joan believes in this place and the miracles that she saw occur while she was getting treatments. Not only do they have the Laetrile, but they have traditional radiation, chemotherapy, and a healthy diet to strengthen the immune system. They can also administer an alternative treatment known as "live cell." This involves taking fetal cells from the organs of animals, that are then injected into the diseased organs of the patient. She said that their treatments have helped many people from all over the world. The clinic is modern and clean and the staff are wonderful. (It is not how we picture Tijuana.)

Before, I did not believe a whole lot in some of the alternatives, but for Wendy to get better I would encourage her to try anything. I want her healthy and running again soon!

Stephen knows how worried I have been for her. He has met Wendy in our group meetings. Two days ago, he asked me for her address so that he could send her flowers. That is what she is talking about in this note.

I'm enclosing one of Lillie's designs for you to see what she did with it. She used the original breast cancer symbol of the pink ribbon. I am going to order a pin as soon as she gets them. Would you like one too? .

Today—was what would have been a chemo day... but I am done! I got up early and started cleaning house... even the dreaded "wet rooms" (bathroom and kitchen—ugh)—with a song in my heart. It was "no more chemo... no more chemo..." Throughout the whole day and night I have been singing this mantra over and over. You cannot imagine how wonderful it feels to know that I am done!

I am working on cleaning up a book that I wrote over fifteen years ago, when I was in the worst of my Agoraphobia. I have never let anyone read it, as it was for myself. It has since helped me get through rough periods, because it gives me comfort. I compare where I once was to where I am today. I thought I would send it to the publisher if he is interested.

Also, I have started the other book, "Love and Laughter." I enjoy our online chats so much that I thought there must be cancer survivors out there without computers who might enjoy some of our conversations. This will be a time consuming process, but it will keep me out of trouble. (These are both in the dream stage as yet.)

Oh, Joan said that she lives right near your store and she will call you or come by someday to say, "Hi." Do you remember her from when she lived down the street from you, when you lived in Needham? I think that you will like her.

I went to Nick's day care today to pick him up after school. It is a really nice facility. I am so pleased he has the opportunity to attend. He and Tamsin are at Teharu's for the night—so I am home alone.

One last thing—Ray called and we are going to meet again tomorrow night to dance. I am so lucky. I have the best boyfriend and now the best dance partner. This is the life!

Love you,

January 29, Sunday

Hi—

I have Nick here with me. He's jumping on the bed, so it's questionable if I will be able to think what I want to write about. He also has a cold. I hope my immune system is strong enough now so that I don't catch it.

Today is like a summer day. I even have shorts on. This morning I was in wool pants, turtleneck and a sweater for church. (Talk about "hot flashes.") Allen showed up at church again. He invited me to have some coffee with him, but I begged off.

And, I just got back from taking Paul to get his car. He went to a computer swap meet and somehow left the keys to his car in his roommate's truck. Paul took a cab home to get keys and asked me to give him a ride back to his car. It was nice, being able to talk with him, as it's difficult inside a dance club.

This shouldn't be lengthy, as I need to get ready for dancing. I met Ray again last night and had fun. He really is a good dancer and I enjoy every dance with him. Last night was a wee bit strange for me. When I was going into the club someone started honking at me and calling my name. It was Don. He said that he was meeting a date for dinner.

Also, Bob and Karen were there. It was wonderful to see them again, and they invited Ray and I to share their table, which was nice. Last week, it was so crowded that we had to stand between dances.

After a couple of hours, Don came into the club by himself. I introduced him to everyone and danced about four dances with him. I explained that I was there with Ray to dance. (Ray and I do dance with other people, but I felt somewhat awkward.)

I was telling Tamsin about last night and she said that rumors will be flying soon! Oh, and yesterday I was talking to her about something else in my unpredictable life. She said, "Mom don't tell me about all your neuroses. I have enough of my own." I cracked up.

Bye. Love you,

January 30, Monday

Hello again,

This is just an update, and I'm on break at work, so it will be written in haste.

I called Wendy on Saturday and left a message on her answering machine asking her to read her e-mail. As of last night she hadn't read it yet. This makes me wonder if she went back into the hospital after sending me the note about the flowers which Stephen sent her. If she doesn't show up at the group tonight I will try to call the hospital tomorrow. I also put in a request for my church to do daily prayer treatments for her.

Also, Bruce is back at work today and he is looking fit and healthy. Of course, he has a new "punk" hairdo, but it's cute on him. He said that he is back to normal. Whew. He went through a lot.

Nick and Tamsin are both home from school today, as Nick now has a bad cough. Poor baby. He has that hang dog look about him.

Yesterday at church, our minister was talking about the way we "pray" and do our "spiritual mind treatments." She made a couple of points that have really stuck with me. She talked about creative visualization. Do you know anything about this? I have been using it for years and she made the point, "What you give your time, love and attention to expands." This is so true for me. Later in the day, Tamsin and I had an interesting conversation about how thought manifests itself into form. It is like magic.

Last night, I went dancing—Super Bowl and all. The regulars showed up and I had a great time, but between two nights of dancing I was beat. I slept ten hours last night!

I warned you this would be short.

Love you,

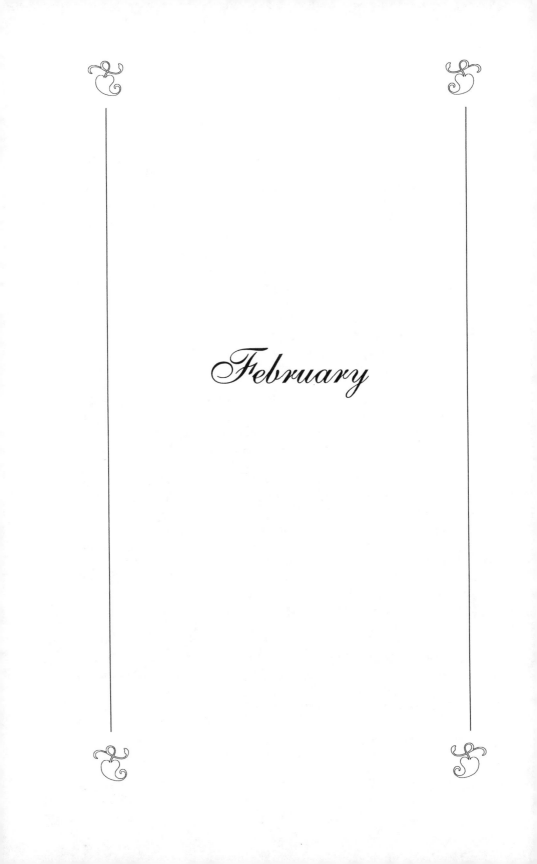

February

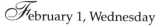February 1, Wednesday

Hi—

Boy, a few weeks ago I was saying, "Write me." You have more than made up for it. Now I can't keep up with you. Your other package arrived with two tons of photos, trouser socks and the top for Tamsin. Again, we thank you. And now I have about three letters that need answering to. See if I say that to you again!

These pictures are great. You look terrific and Lisa is so pretty. Michael, as always, is a cutie. I like the room that Jack built—especially the French doors. The house, with all that property in New Hampshire, is gorgeous. They are all wonderful.

So, you are dieting again? Well, I am now above my pre-mastectomy weight and loving it. My face is fuller and has color to it. I even used hair conditioner today for the first time in months! Yea!

What? No wine??? But, we have to sip some of the wine and also go to the Champagne Cellar in Sonoma. I hope you aren't going to be allergic to all that.

Yes, I read an article about Huntington Beach being the safest place to live. I feel very safe and secure in my little apartment. My area especially, has no crime according to the Crime Watch newsletter for Huntington Beach. Further more, I live at the end of a cul de sac. I like it here.

I did my taxes last night. It looks like I am getting a refund from both Federal and State. That's good. I can pay it on my outrageous VISA! And, yes the framed waterfall picture on my living room wall is the one I took when I was in Oregon. It is a favorite of mine. What else? (I'm trying to answer all your questions and letters here.) No, I'm not jealous that Jack is writing you poetry. I am incredibly happy that things are much better now for the two of you. Is Jack coming to Sonoma? Say yes. Stephen is going to meet us there for a few days. Oh, and one of my cancer group friends in that area may meet us one day too. He is a fox! (He does modeling and bit movie parts for a hobby.) Don't get all excited though, as he has been happily married forever.

Wendy did not choose to go with the Toronto treatments. Taxol, I believe, is a form of chemotherapy and no, it's not the same as Tamoxifen. I called the hospital yesterday to see how Wendy was doing. She was asleep. I spoke briefly with her sister-in-law, who is a doctor, and is spending time with her. She said that Wendy is doing much better, but is very tired. Would you like her address so that you can drop her a note or send a card?

Tell Jack I take all those vitamin supplements now. I also eat lots of fresh vegetables with Beta Carotene. And, regarding garlic...I eat garlic toast with dinner about five times a week, so I guess I am covered there too, or doesn't that count?

I read an article in this morning's paper regarding a new study completed, which concluded that women with high levels of estrogen are more prone to being diagnosed with breast cancer. This totally ties in with what I have been thinking since last May. The reason I felt there was a connection was that two years ago I was having some menopausal symptoms. Since I haven't had periods in twenty years, I had a blood test administered to determine if I was going into menopause. The nurse told me that the results showed that I still had a lot of estrogen. Then, a year later, I find out that the cancer cells were feeding on the estrogen in my body!

It makes sense to me anyway. My breast cancer sisters and I are always trying to find the common denominator. A couple of months ago, I was in the ladies room at work and Bev was there. She stopped in the middle of drying her hands and said, "Marilyn—what do you think caused this to happen to us?" She said, "I keep thinking that maybe because I use so much bleach around my house that that could be it." I just shook my head and said, "No Bev. I don't use bleach." (Blew that theory.) We do this all the time. We are constantly analyzing, and questioning what is causing breast cancer in so many women. What I read today makes me believe that it is connected to higher than normal estrogen levels.

Rita, I am not getting the silicone implant. That is the one that has the poor reputation. I am getting saline and it is not dangerous if it leaks. Don't worry on that!

Yes, I am extremely happy lately. Stephen continues to spoil me. Yesterday, I got another big box from him. In it were two boxes of chocolate truffles. One box is filled with heart shaped truffles. Also, he sent down his "boom" box for me to use, since Tamsin took off with mine when she moved in. (Now I have to get myself one of those tapes, which I sent to you and Stephen.) He sent down the tape back up, which he bought for my computer and miscellaneous other things... oh, and a little stuffed Koala bear for Nick. Is he unreal or what?

I guess this should be enough for today. I bet that after I seal the envelope I will think of more, but if I do I'll try to hold the thought for the next time I write you.

Love you all,

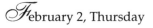

ℱebruary 2, Thursday

Hello—

You would love it here. The weather is like a warm Spring day. Yesterday, I wore a heavy sweater to work and it was way too hot! Today, I'm "layered" and much more comfortable.

Tamsin wore her Valentine's top to school today. She loves it. Thanks again.

Last night was my babysitting night. Nick was so good. He still has a wracking cough though. I am Howard Hughes type paranoid. Every time he wanted to kiss me I'd have him do it on my cheek, then I'd go in the bathroom and wash my face. He is so loving that it's hard to say, "No—don't kiss me." All we need is for me to get sick and then give it to Stephen when he comes down. I'd probably never see him again, since he got so sick after the last time he was here.

Ray called last night and we are going to meet Saturday night for more dancing. He's a nice guy! Ray did say that he has an eye infection, so it depends on whether that has cleared up or not.

I was so tired last night that I went to bed and fell asleep about 8:30, right after Nick did. Ann called though and it woke me up. She and I wound up talking for over a half hour. She loves being in the dance scene and is continuing her classes, and making very good progress too.

I told her about Wendy and I almost started crying again. We got on the subject of cancer and dying. (She is the one who had the thyroid cancer a couple of years ago.) Ann says she still has not gotten back a healthy immune system since she had radiation. She said that she is afraid if another cancer, or bad illness, got into her she would not be able to survive it. I told her that if I ever got to the point that my chances were slim for beating any cancer I would prefer to just have quality days left without going through the really strong chemo. We both agreed that we would choose to die gracefully and with dignity, and leave it at that.

Club Dance is not returning my calls. I've left three messages over the past couple of weeks and "nada." If I don't hear from them by Saturday, I think I will fax them a letter asking what's going on. People keep asking me about the plans, but I can't firm up anything until I know we have reservations made.

When Arthur called yesterday I asked him where he went skiing in New Hampshire. It was Waterville Valley and Attitash. Do they sound familiar? He again stressed that he is not interested in ever going there again in the winter, as it was way too cold for him.

I had uploaded that book that I wrote fifteen years ago to Stephen through AOL. Since he hadn't gotten back to me on it, I finally asked him what he thought about it. I got the response this morning. He said, very tactfully, and truthfully that since it's written in prose form, and that is not something he is interested in, this book did not hold his interest. (Oh well.) Now I'm even more embarrassed that I sent it to my Publisher.

I keep wondering why I love it so much. Maybe because it is so personal and I just identify with all the weird thoughts I had back then. I'll still keep it for myself to enjoy.

Tuesday, I called Sharon to see how she was doing with her arm problems. She hadn't come to group on Monday night. She had an MRI done and they could not find anything wrong. She has to go back to the doctor to discuss where they go from here. It is still painful and the simple act of opening a door sets it off. Sharon also said that every time she gets a fill up on the expander she is in pain. Her reconstruction was in November. I look forward to getting a new boob, but I am dreading the pain of it.

This is my long week at work—and I am pleased that I did not have to call in sick. It's a nice feeling after the past six months.
All is well here.

Love you.

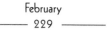

February 3, Friday

Hi again!

I can't believe we talked so much last night. I could have gone on talking, it's been so long. I've put in my request for the week of May 29th, instead of the prior week. Now, I have to wait to see if the change is approved. If so, I will probably fly to San Francisco on the 27th and fly home on the 4th of June. If you come to Southern California for an extra week I really don't have the nerve to ask for that week off too. Between the two weeks I'll be off for the reconstruction and then doctor's appointments and the second surgery—I'm chicken. We are still waiting to find out where we are all going to wind up once the layoffs start. I could be working anywhere by May. I'll leave it up to you to decide what you want to do with the extra week.

Last night, I forgot to tell you that the boot Valentine card is a riot! I have hung it over my desk at work. The wall in front of my desk is becoming a collage of miscellaneous mementos. (I like it.)

We are due for another day of record setting 90 degree weather. This is nice, after all the rain we had.

I'm still laughing and saying to myself, "Rita is taking two step lessons!?" Hilarious!!! Enjoy it. It gets in your blood and then watch out!

Okay—this is my "big" letter for today. Since we talked so much, I probably won't be writing for a few days.

Love you,

February 7, Tuesday

Hi,

I just wrote to Stephen and told him it's a good thing he's not here tonight. I am in a foul mood. (It will pass.) But, I if I had a dog...this would be a dog kicking night. (Only kidding, so calm down...you know I could never do that!)

The day started out poorly and just got progressively worse. Yuck!

I got to work fifteen minutes early. There was e-mail from my boss to come by his office. When I went got there, he shut the door. (Not a good sign in our agency.) So I jokingly said, "Am I in trouble again?" Since Bruce got promoted he has chewed me out twice and I'm not used to being in trouble at work. Anyway, he said, "Yes." And it just went downhill from there. What he confronted me on was mild compared to what goes on at work, yet no one else has been confronted. I told him that I felt like I was being singled out, and said how I resented the last two times too, and asked him, "Why me?" He told me if I had a complaint to take it up with the Union. (Right. He is big in the Union.) I could not believe the conversation we were having.

Then I said that I was resentful of the way he talked to me...like I was some lowly clerk, instead of the professional that I am. (Actually, I should have said "child." If I was a clerk I still would have resented being spoken to like that.)

Anyway, the long and short of it is, I said I was ready to rotate back to the Districts. (I think I've over stayed my welcome here.) He said, "fine" and then I put it in writing.

Well, that is moot now. Later in the day, we got a message from our Director saying that our budget is being cut even further. A lot of people in work are depressed and anxious. Rumors are flying that there will be 50% lay offs. I find this hard to believe, since we would be in dire straits trying to issue benefits and services to the public. Also, the other rumor going around is that they are going to do away with all Program Assistant positions and that we will be demoted to Supervisors.

So—that was my day. Is this a crummy letter or what? Sorry. I thought about not writing you all this, but this is what is happening here.

Actually, I know me and I know I will bounce back right away, and trust that everything will work out for the best. I'm glad that we got to talk on the phone so much this weekend. It was great. I know I have more to write, but obviously I am not in a letter writing mood!

Oh—yes, I just remembered one other thing. I put in my request to change our vacation week and my boss is holding it until we have a meeting tomorrow. Maybe he can't approve any vacations right now, while our jobs our pending. I'll let you know, when I know what is going on there. (Double Yuck.)

Here I am bitching about me, and Wendy is on my mind a lot too. I think that is so wonderful that Jack got her a card. I know she will appreciate it. She wrote me this weekend and is home from the hospital and feeling better. They gave her Neupogen to raise her blood counts, and antibiotics for her fever, and drained fluid from her stomach. But her scans showed that the Taxol isn't working on eliminating the cancer in her liver. She is now in search of an alternative treatment. She may go back to Toronto after all.

Then Sharon's doctor has decided that her arm is so messed up that she has to go in for another operation. It will be done on February 13th and the doctor warned her that it is very painful. She will be off work for at least another two weeks. Poor thing!

See? After writing all this stuff I already feel like my problems are minute. I need to count my blessings again, and know that things aren't so bad after all for me. I already feel better. I guess just writing it down helps once again.

I will write more when I am feeling up to it.

Love you,

February 9, Thursday

Hi—

I'm writing on a fifteen minute work break, so this will be another short one. Also, since Stephen comes tomorrow morning I probably won't be writing again until next week. Oh, and your birthday card for him arrived yesterday. At least, I assume that is what is in the envelope. I was teasing him last night and I said, "You've got mail here, so does this mean that you are moving in?" Now he is really confused as to why he would get mail from anyone to my address. I didn't tell him it was from you, naturally.

I'm fine about work and the situation I wrote you about. I figure, that once the County knows what they are doing regarding downsizing I will have a new job anyway. All of us are pretty stressed out and anxiety ridden. It's the not knowing and not being able to start making mind adjustments that is the hardest. Like anything else, the waiting for the unknown can drive a person crazy.

Yesterday, in our meeting, Jessica suggested that the County get some kind of psychological counseling for the employees. I mean, it must be even worse out in the Districts for the line staff. We heard this morning that someone took down a picture of one of the Board of Supervisors, smashed the glass and tore his picture. Now, that is scary. It depicts the violence which some employees might be feeling over all of this.

I am fine though and looking forward to Stephen being here again! More later.

Love,

February 13, Monday

Happy Valentine's Day to you and Jack!!!

I hope you get nice, sexy things from Jack and lots of love. Of course, as usual, you didn't leave him room for surprises from Victoria Secrets!

Stephen just called. He wanted to make sure that my Valentine flowers arrived okay. He got confused, since I'm home today because of the Presidents holiday. Originally, the flowers were coming here and then to work—the florist was confused and tried to deliver them to my work address, but instead of Santa Ana—they were looking for it in Huntington Beach. They called me to see where I was. They were delivered a couple of hours ago. Once again, he has out done himself. I took a picture so that you and he can see this gorgeous bouquet. Tamsin and I were just oohing and aahing over it. It is not only beautiful, but also smells incredible too.

Well, I've been busy and have made my plane reservations for San Francisco. I will enclose my flight schedule. Your turn now! I talked with Bud and he said that the week of Memorial Day is fine. He put us on the townhouse calendar. Bud also stressed for you to bring Jack. He wants to meet both of you. Stephen also would like to meet Jack.

I have so much to write you that I think this one letter is probably going to be book length in itself. But, you have to admit that you have been getting off easy lately—or your mailman has anyway.

First, I have to say that I have worked on accepting whatever happens with my job. I believe that no matter the outcome, it will be for the best. Sometimes, I forget what I believe in my heart. One of our former ministers used to remind us—during times like this—to ask ourselves, "When did God die and leave me in charge?" I don't know why I work myself up over these happenings. It's best if I just sit back and enjoy the "ride."

Tomorrow is my blood test and I see my oncologist on Thursday. Hopefully, my counts will be up and then we can get on with it! Oh, and the other good news…I weigh 110 pounds as of this morning. All the truffles Stephen keeps giving me have helped me reach this goal!

We have a joke going about truffles. I love See's truffles. He sent me some kind of gourmet truffles from San Francisco a few weeks ago. They were delicious, but I told him that I still liked See's the best. Then when he unpacked on Friday he gave me a box of Godiva truffles. Naturally, Tamsin and I went right into them. On Saturday, he gave me a box of See's. This is like the ultimate taste test!!! I told him that maybe I don't have a gourmet's palate, but I do know what I like…See's is the winner!

Thursday night, I was like on over drive after work: grocery shopping, doing laundry and cleaning house. Eric and Bridget came over with Tyler and I was rocking him and then I'd jump up and do some more dusting—then grab him back from Tamsin,—rock and play with him—then give him back, while I ran down to the garage to do laundry. I was very manic. In a way it was good, because I was so excited about Stephen coming that having so much to do kept me occupied.

Friday morning, I actually did some errands before going to the airport. I wore a dress, since he'd only seen me in jeans. I cannot tell you how it feels to see him coming off that plane. It's like one big sigh…

We came back to the apartment for lunch and I gave him his birthday and Valentine gifts. I think he liked them. Then he spent the afternoon working on my computer. He installed the tape back up peripheral, which he'd sent earlier. (I have no clue about these things, but I did know that I had wanted one.)

Friday night, we walked around South Coast Plaza as we had time to kill before our dinner reservations. He's so funny. Maybe this was one of those "had to be there" items, but Tamsin and I cracked up. I had put on my very short, black leather skirt and matching leather jacket with my white dancing boots. Normally, I wouldn't wear something like that in public. They were in the kitchen and I came in and said to Tamsin, "Do you think that people at South Coast Plaza will think I'm a hooker?" (I mean these are okay for dance clothes, but nowhere else.) Stephen says, "Only if I hang a camera around my neck." Are we bad?

Anyway, Stephen said he enjoyed the Crazy Horse. Tell Jack that at least Stephen has some taste! (Just kidding Jack—I guess you just have to like country to like the Crazy Horse.) After dinner we went into the saloon and listened to the band and watched the dancers. It was really too crowded for any good dancing though.

Saturday, I fixed breakfast—and Stephen did the dishes. I forgot to tell you that he did them when he was down in December too. He just jumps right in, even though I try to say that I will do them. Then he gave me two more Valentine cards…funny ones of course. He also gave me the See's and Tamsin a bag of gourmet jelly beans. He is so good, this man of mine!

We went to the Price Club, in search of more earthquake supplies for the apartment. I am now all prepared, other than the dehydrated food which he is out shopping for in Tahoe as I type. (I told him that I do appreciate all this, but I hope to never have to use them.) Stephen also got me a water purifier. This past year I stopped drinking the tap water at home and started buying bottled water.

Saturday afternoon, we checked in to the Hilton which is right on the beach. It was cool, but pleasant weather. We went walking on the boardwalk as the sun was setting. (Very romantic)

In the evening, we "dressed up" for the AOL party which was in one of the Clubs at the Hotel. Stephen looked great. He wore a sports jacket and tie and I was so proud to be with him. I had on my black silk Jessica McClintock... and a pair of very fancy black leather shoes, which are too big for me. I kept walking out of them all night!

We were some of the first people to arrive, so we got a table near the buffet and dance floor and I pigged out totally. The food was delicious. I was drinking champagne and there were these huge, sweet strawberries, which I went back for about six times through out the night. I was in heaven!

This party was very different than any I have ever been to. There were about five men to every female present. The men were all dressed up in suits and they were mostly younger guys too. I kept telling Stephen that if my friend Chris didn't show up soon I was calling her house to tell her to get on over to the party.

First Don showed up. I really didn't think he'd come, since this is not his scene at all. I introduced him to Stephen and we all ate together. (Later Stephen said that Don seemed like a really nice guy.) Then Chris showed up. She looked great in a fancy black top. So there were four of us at our table and we were the old folks there! The music was like the 70's replayed. It all sounded like disco to me anyway. Eventually, there was one song that was West Coast Swing and Don and I got up to dance, except I walked out of one of my shoes. Then between the three glasses of champagne, and my big shoes, I almost fell over when he put me in a spin. (And here I wanted Stephen to be impressed with my dancing abilities!)

Don left early so that he could dance at a country western club. Stephen, Chris and I stayed at the party until about midnight. They had a lot of raffle prizes and Chris won a copy of the video, "Mask" which made her night worthwhile.

I really did have fun at the party, but I think it was because I was with Stephen. Normally, this type of get together would bore me, but he is fun no matter what we are doing.

Sunday, we had a delicious breakfast in one of the Hotel's restaurants and then I took him to the airport. This is not my most favorite moment of the weekend. He got on the plane and I felt like a part of me was missing. Once again, I had to go through the withdrawal of not having him here.

It was a wonderful weekend. I wore your Valentine's "flamboyant" blazer, over the blue silk blouse you sent me, with jeans on Saturday. Thank you again.

I think because Stephen and I do not have a lot of routine time together that when we do get the occasional weekend to be with one another it is just so appreciated that we completely enjoy every second of it. It is very hard to be away from him, but then on the other hand our time together is always quality time. I cannot complain about our relationship being not enough, because I am so happy with the way it is. Does this make any sense at all?

Well, I have odds and ends to catch up on here. I'm glad I had today off so that I could get them done before going back to work tomorrow. Call me if you have any questions about May.

Love you lots,

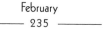

February 15, Wednesday

Yoo Hoo It's Me…

My name is Pinky Lee. (Bet you haven't heard that song in a long time!) I'm just being silly. Tonight is my usual babysitting night while Tamsin has her night class, but when I got home at six Nick was sound asleep on the couch. I took his tennies off and just poured him into bed. So now, I'm getting the opportunity to write you and then Stephen.

How are you doing??? Do I dare say that you haven't written for awhile? I know what happened the last time I said, "Write."

I am doing wonderful here. Every week I see myself as becoming stronger and more energetic. My hair is getting thicker and longer. I even called Regina today to schedule a hair coloring appointment. I think it's safe to do that again.

Do you remember the man that I met on my birthday? Warren? He called tonight to see how I was. He is such a nice man. He's the one who sings in the Barber Shop Quartet. Anyway, he said that his group does singing telegrams on Valentine's Day for charity and he had thought about them coming by my work yesterday to sing to me. Nice, huh? But, it was raining and they were all over the county for about twelve hours. Since he had been thinking about me he decided to call. It was great talking to him. I told him to let me know when he is performing somewhere locally and one of these days I will come by to hear him sing.

Sharon sent me e-mail tonight. Her surgery appears to be a success. For the first time since she got her expander put in, I can "read" that she is optimistic about her arm. She still has daily physical therapy to go to for it and will be off work for two weeks, but she sounded pleased.

I have so much to do lately when I get home from work that I try to run through my mind all the stuff I want to write to you about. Duh!

Work is fine. I really feel okay regarding myself and what will be will be. But, I did go through the job bulletins that our Human Resources staff have been putting in our lunch room. I'm not in any position right now to make a big job change, but there was one flyer that caught my eye. It is for a Program Manager position in Lake County. It sounds like the job is similar to what I was doing at the Work Program. I meet the Minimum Qualifications anyway. I made a copy and then asked Chris where Lake County was. She said it's just above Sonoma and is really pretty there. I called Sacramento and asked them to send me a job application. I might apply just for the heck of it. Why not?

I haven't heard more from Wendy since I last wrote you. I know that she has a lot going on right now. She is always in my thoughts though. I would love to go to New York and meet her in person.

Yesterday, Jessica and I were talking at work about the usual. She has an interesting theory. She said that she is starting to think that most of the breast cancer women fit a certain "A" type profile. (I told you we are always questioning what could be the common denominator here.) Well, I started listing my breast cancer sisters on my fingers. As I did this I was doing a mental inventory of our personalities. You know what? We are all over achievers. That's scary. Rita...slow down and everyday remember to smell the roses—just in case!

Also, tell Jack that yes, I started taking Beta Carotene and Vitamin E supplements daily along with everything else I've been taking since last June. I can't quite bring myself to do the garlic pills yet. But, I did see the odorless ones so they will probably be next.

Okay—now it's time for Stephen to get his nightly letter.

Love you,

February 17, Friday

Rita—

Hi. I'm at work and on break... a much needed break as I am almost in tears again. I hate these HMO disappointments. I called Dr. Trung's office yesterday to get the surgery scheduled, and they took a message to have his scheduling clerk call me back. (Yesterday, my oncologist said I was fine for the surgery.) When I didn't hear back from her by this morning I called again.

She said she had me down for the surgery to be done in April. I tried to explain to her that Dr. Trung and I had discussed my having it done as soon as my counts were up. She didn't seem to care, and said that she can only do what she was last instructed, which was from the October appointment I had with him. I could not convince her that in December he and I agreed otherwise. I was almost crying talking to her. Why do these people keep getting their lines of communication broken? To them it's just all in a day's work. For the patients—we are at their whim and screw ups! I hate this!!!

I asked her if I could see another plastic surgeon or discuss this with anyone else and she said, "No." This has been a whole year of having practically no control of my life and plans, and it is wearing me down.

The new plan is that if they get a last minute cancellation in March, then she will call me. At this rate, I may not be done with my surgeries by the time our vacation gets here. I am so frustrated I could scream!!!

Damn... I really don't like this and being at the mercy of others and their forgetfulness and misunderstandings.

I will calm done eventually, but right now I am not a happy camper. I will be glad when this is over. Yuck and double yuck!

Okay, I'm sitting here telling myself over and over that everything happens for a purpose and it will work out. I will overcome yet another disappointment and come out smiling again.

Sorry about all this once more.

Ray called last night and I invited him over for dinner Saturday before we go dancing. We will go to "Denim and Diamonds" for a change. On Sunday, I am meeting with the women from Southern California who are in my online support group. We are going to have brunch. This will be our first in person get together. I hope it won't be the last.

Thanks for listening again.

Love,

February 17, Friday

Hi—

Letter number two for the day here. Just like old times, huh?

I am still pretty upset and writing always helps me work things out. I hadn't yet recovered from the disappointment with the plastic surgeon's office, when Bruce came into my office to discuss my request for time off Wednesday morning to have my teeth cleaned.

Rita, I think I am having a nervous break down or something. I am so emotional right now. You know how sensitive I am about things. Well, it seems like lately everything is piling up on me. Help!!!

I called my dentist's office this morning, as I am anxious to get my teeth cleaned, since I couldn't have it done while on chemo. I asked them if they had any appointments for a Saturday, flex day Friday, or in the morning on my short day. Nada. So finally I just asked for their next available appointment. It was for Wednesday morning. I thought, "No problem." I knew that our monthly Sysco meeting was at the same time, but everyone else misses these meetings once in a while.

I put in my time off request to Bruce and he comes into my office and tells me that he doesn't know about approving it, because it might be a problem for the Manager if I miss her meeting. I was flabbergasted that he would even think this might be a conflict. Naturally, I started complaining, and he started back pedaling and said that it's not really a problem. I responded by saying that it must have seemed like a problem if he brought it up. He countered that he was just checking to be sure that I was aware that it was the same time as the meeting.

Bruce said he's not trying to come across as a "heavy" and I said, "Well you sure are lately." It did not go well.

I think I am becoming a basket case. Right now, I hate my job. Even when I worked at the Work Program I didn't dislike it so much as not wanting to go in to work.

I'll calm down eventually, but right now I am not so happy.

I will write again…hopefully when I am "up" once more.

Love,

February 20, Monday

Hello!

Am I driving you nuts with these up, down, up, down letters? Sorry. I debated whether to even mail the two from Friday or not. Friday night, I spent a long time on the phone talking with first Chris and then Jessica. Chris made one comment which has stuck with me. You know how you can capture certain phrases that stay awhile? Well, she reminded me that right now my body is going through hormonal changes, from the Tamoxifen, and this could be why I get so emotional at the drop of a hat. One thing I have to say about Chris is that she always hits the "nail on the head." So, now my new excuse for any bizarre behavior (or letters in your case) is "I'm menopausal." Sounds good to me!

Actually, I am doing much, much better than I was on Friday. I needed to vent by talking and writing it out. (I was also online with Stephen Friday night.) By Saturday morning, I was recovered and ready to get on with things. Friends are good therapy.

My long three day weekend has been wonderful so far. Saturday morning, Regina colored my hair and did a very light trimming. It looks great. Then when I got home, I babysat Tyler while Bridget did some heavy duty house work. He was precious. He also was good therapy for my raging hormones. How can anyone be upset when holding and rocking a baby?

Saturday night, Ray came over for dinner. It turned out okay, considering how little I cook anymore. After dinner, we went to "Denim and Diamonds" and danced for a couple of hours. He is sooooo good!

Sunday was an extra special day. I met some of the Southern California women from my online support group. I'm still up from that event. I got to the Red Lion Inn early and when I walked into the bar area I immediately recognized Bonnie from the collage, which Mike had put online. She lives up in the valley and drove down with her girlfriend Joyce. Awesome! Then Jacqui, my friend from work, arrived and we were all hugging and talking at once, and I turned around and saw a lady coming down the steps with her arms full of pink carnation bouquets. (Pink, as you know by now, is the breast cancer awareness color.) It was Peggy, who I've talked to on the phone, but hadn't met in person yet. What a day!

Bonnie and Peggy are the same personalities as they are online. It is amazing that we can come across the way we are "live," just by typing lines each Monday night. We ate and talked for about three hours. There was a delicious brunch buffet and guess who ate the most? (El

Piggo!) But, Bonnie talked more than me!!! I bet you find that hard to believe, huh?

Peggy gave us each a bouquet and she also had printed copies of the collage on 8 x 11 glossies for us. My copy is now framed and on my workstation, along with the picture of you and I, and also another picture of Stephen. Since you are the ones I write to the most on my PC, I just love having you all smiling at me as I type.

They all want to meet Stephen, since he is part of our group. Bonnie said that one weekend when Stephen is down she will host a pool party at her house. The other option is for all of us, with our significant others, to meet for dinner at the Disneyland Hotel and then be entertained by Peggy's friend, who sings country western there. Do you remember the night that we went there when you and Jack came out? Peggy and I think that is her friend. She said he has been there that long.

After the brunch, I went over to the Cowboy and still got a couple of hours of dancing in.

So, as you can see, my holiday weekend has been filled with lots of fun things and my mood is now back to where it should be—which is UP. Once more, I'm appreciating every beautiful day that comes along.

Speaking of beautiful days…our weather has been in the 90's. This is record breaking. I have shorts on and I should be at the beach—but not until I have two boobs please!

Hug for Jack.

Love you,

February 21, Tuesday

Rita,

I got your long letter today—and don't worry about writing. Your studying is important and I understand. Ace it!!! I know you will do great on the test. You are really dedicated to learning the language.

Me on the other hand... I have so much to write to you that this is going to be a lengthy and a jump around type letter again. I think you can handle it though.

Are you ready? I just finished printing out the new book. I mean, I am going to proof read it one more time and then pass it on to Tamsin, so she can critique it. I love it, but I have no idea if anyone else will. Shall I send you a copy? Maybe we better wait until after the Spanish test! I just e-mailed the man in my support group who does cartoons, to see if he was serious about doing illustrations for it. Cross your fingers!

Speaking of writing... Tamsin has a school project where she has to interview two to three people who are in a career that she aspires to. Well, since she doesn't know any "Cultural Anthropologists" she decided on her second wish—that of being a writer. I am honored that she wants to interview me! Then, she is going to ask Grace and Lillie if she can interview them online, and possibly one other writer that I met through AOL. When she explained to her teacher that she would be doing online interviews her teacher didn't even know what she was talking about. Tamsin had to explain how it works to the teacher.

Our weather is just so bizarre lately. We had hot beach type temperatures all weekend and yesterday. Last night, it got windy and cold and has been raining on and off ever since. I can't understand it. Tamsin tells me it is earthquake weather. When I told Stephen he said, "No way." (He hasn't sent down the food for the earthquake supplies yet.)

He also told me that he is sending down more See's truffles. I am going to get obese if he keeps this up. But, do you hear me protesting? Oh, you know See's. I've sent you some for the holidays in the past. They are a West Coast candy, which is very popular here. I'll have to send you more one of these days and let you do a taste test.

Stephen called me at work today. Unfortunately, I was not at my desk and so he left a message... something about Friday being my flex day. I don't know if he is teasing me or not. He has been saying that he is going to come down again one day, without warning me ahead of time and just surprise me. Any time would be fine with me!

Yes, I am incredibly happy with him. I love the time we have together. He is so good. I like where we are right now and I'm not in any rush to know where it is going. I'm just enjoying this to the max!

Stephen still comes to group as my support person on Monday nights. Last night, as they always do, everyone was teasing us. When he came into the room, I typed him the symbol of a hug... then my next line was, "I'd send you a kiss too, but everyone would see us!" They all cracked up over that. It was fun. I love this group so much, I cannot express it in words. I look forward to meeting my Northern California online friends when we are in Sonoma. I think you will enjoy them too.

Wendy wasn't in group last night. She has not responded to any of my e-mail this week. I called her today, but got her answering machine. I fear she may be in the hospital again. We are all concerned and I know you and Jack are too. If I don't hear from her soon I may call the hospital. Want to go to New York and visit her for all of us? Sharon wrote me a long letter tonight and she is doing much better. Her arm is improving finally. Geez, what we all have to go through is just amazing!

Yesterday, I called Aunt Dot to check on how she was doing. She said that she was glad I called because she had been thinking about me a lot and had wanted to tell me about her niece in Colorado. When I was diagnosed last May, Aunt Dot told me about her niece (on her side of the family) who is an OB/GYN doctor and how she was diagnosed with breast cancer a couple of years ago. Aunt Dot was encouraging me by telling me that she went through her surgery and chemo and was healthy and doing fine. Well, as it turns out she had a double mastectomy performed today. She is in her early forties and chose a lumpectomy the last time. They found a recurrence in the same breast. I am so saddened to hear this.

Aunt Dot said that she is so glad that I chose to have the mastectomy. I told her I was glad too. At the time I didn't know what to do. Now I have no regrets about my decision. The Physician's Assistant told me that either choice would be just as safe as the other.

Over the past year, I have met and talked with a lot of breast cancer sisters. Everyone that I have met who has had a recurrence chose the lumpectomy with their first diagnosis. I know the statistics say otherwise, but for me, and my peace of mind, the mastectomy was my best choice.

It seems like we get more bad news daily about the county's financial situation and how it will affect our jobs. The new CEO, which the county has brought on board, has decided to do away with our flex days. He announced it in the newspaper, and said that it would take effect in March. Naturally, employees are upset. I don't know how the public feels, but it could affect the longer hours that county offices are open. I know that people like being able to take care of business before or after work. Only time will tell what our working hours will be.

I filled out the job application for the position in Lake County. Once I read the supplemental questions I realized that I am most likely not qualified for it, but it's good practice in completing an application. Also, Stephen says that Lake County is depressed, but he also said that it is a tourist attraction. (?) Maybe because of the lake there. I had never heard of it before. He says it's inland and therefore very hot in the summer and cold in the winter, and it's also a rural area.

I have no clue where I will be working by the time we meet in San Francisco. I was worried that my second surgery would be during that time, but as lopsided as I might be by the end of May, I will just postpone it, and we can have a "come as you are" vacation.

Lillie's pin is a gift from me. I ordered one for the both of us. Mine is hanging on the wall over my desk at work... the memento collage. She has another design in the works and I'm a little confused as to if it is a butterfly pin or artwork. I so admire all that Lillie is doing and wanted to support her new group for the mothers.

Well, I've been typing away and it is getting late.

Study hard and do "A" work on your Spanish exam.

Love,

February 23, Thursday

Hi again,

This is just a short note to let you know that Stephen is flying down tonight and staying until Saturday. Now I'm feeling guilty about all the money he is spending on airfares too. Sheesh! I'm picking him up at the airport at 10:30, so I won't be writing for a few days either.

I dropped off the manuscript for "Love and Laughter" this morning on the way to work to have some Xerox copies made. Let me know if you want me to send you a copy.

Also, yesterday at our monthly meeting we mainly talked about all the changes coming down due to the financial crisis. Things do not look good at all. All of us are pretty much expecting "pink slips" around April 1st. We will get them with a note stating that if we want to use our bumping rights to demote to the next level below us, then we have to contact Personnel within twenty-four hours. I've never received a pink slip before. It sounds depressing.

After a rough guess at all the Program Assistants' hire-in dates, it looks like I will be demoted to Eligibility Supervisor…where I was four years ago! Oh well,—such is life in the big "O."

That's it until after Stephen's visit. (Now I need to find a stamp somewhere.)

Love,

February 25, Saturday

Good Evening!

I miss our phone calls, but I don't dare call lately. I have to start being conservative with money soon. Oh what the heck! Why worry about the future, right?

Tamsin and Nick just went to Teharu's. Stephen left a couple of hours ago. I'm "Home Alone"—and no dancing tonight. I got a funny video that one of the guys at work recommended, "Ruthless People." After I write you, I'm curling up on the couch and becoming a non-thinking, non-moving couch potato.

But, since I will probably be going every minute tomorrow, I decided I'd better write you NOW!

I love the white blouse. Your package came yesterday. I opened it and immediately tried the blouse on. It will go perfect with one of my short black dance skirts. Thank you. Tamsin spied the burgundy top and said, "That has to be mine cause it matches my hair!" She cracked me up. The psychic here! And Nick has already used his note pad and hung the kitten calendar over his bed.

I'm tired Rita. This has been another very busy past few days… busy, but so much fun. I love being with Stephen. When he goes I miss him terribly. Tonight, Tamsin told me that she feels he is the best of all the men I've dated in a long, long time. I told her that I think this is the best relationship I've ever been in. I am completely spoiled by him. He is so good and kindhearted.

Last night, it hit me as we were leaving Knottsberry Farm… Stephen reminds me of someone with what I have come to call, a "Cancer personality." What I mean by this, is that he does things in the now. Why put off until tomorrow what you can do, and enjoy, today? I know that my personality has changed somewhat in this way over the past year. Here I go again, off on one of my many tangents. I'll just shut up.

Anyway, he brought me two more boxes of See's truffles and a box of the Joseph Schmidt truffles. (I am going to the Mall soon to send you some.) Stephen knows that I lost a couple of pounds last week when I let myself become stressed out. I swear he thinks it's his mission in life to keep me at a stable 110. We are always eating and munching. I may not be all that big, but I sure enjoy food. I am so glad that he does too.

We spent the whole day from opening time to closing time at Knottsberry Farm yesterday. The shows were great, including a new one, which I knew that Tamsin would like… it's called "Mystery Lodge." The story is about Indian mysticism. We went on a few rides, but I do not do the scary ones! Today, Tamsin and Bridget asked me what rides I went on, and if I went on any of the wild ones. I said, "Well, yeah— sort of." They pressured me into naming it… The soap box derby race. When I said that they both started laughing and teasing me. Tamsin said, "Mom, that's a little kids ride." (For me it was daring enough.)

We had dinner at the Mrs. Knotts' Chicken Restaurant. Yum. Stephen also bought out the bakery as we were leaving. He got Nick a bag full of decorated sugar cookies, sticky buns which we had with breakfast this morning, and the most sinful chocolate cake which we ate after coming back home from a morning walk on the Huntington Beach Pier.

Nick went with us to the airport. He wants so bad to go for an airplane ride. I said, "When you are older we will go somewhere, someday." On the way home though he was quite the little man. We stopped at a flower shop and he picked out a beautiful bouquet for his Mom, and he "wrote" her a little card. He was so cute bringing it in and presenting it to her...for doing so well at school. She found out yesterday that to date she has all A's. She is studying constantly. (This pleases me immensely.)

I'm happy Rita. Just, really happy. Life is good. It has it's ups and downs and little surprises, but I'm pleased with it overall.

Love you,

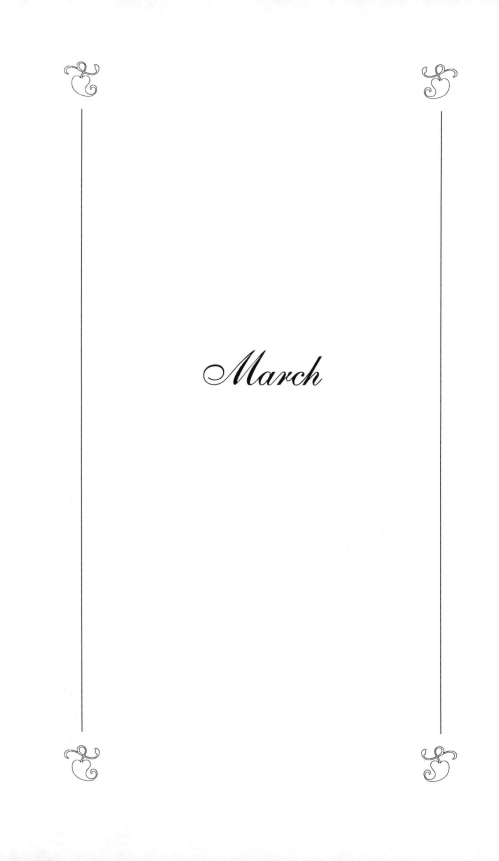

March

March 1, Wednesday

Hi—

I haven't been in much of a letter writing mood lately myself. All is okay, but there is just the continuous dark cloud hanging over our heads about our jobs. Last night, I watched the televised Board Hearing. The new County CEO, William Popejoy, spoke about the crisis and how it is affecting so many innocent people, including the county employees, who will be laid off. I don't know how closely you are following all this, but it's in our papers daily and of course we cannot stop talking about it at work. The waiting is the hard part. Here we stayed on with the county because of the security. Well, the joke was on us.

Personally, after hearing Mr. Popejoy speak, I am quite impressed with the man. He has volunteered to take this challenge for six months... without pay. It is quite an endeavor and so I can't help but admire and respect him. When he spoke it came across as sincere and honest. As a citizen, I think he is the right man for the job. As a County employee, I am of course concerned for my own financial welfare, that of fellow employees and for the public we serve.

No one has heard from Wendy. I sent Amy, her friend in New York, e-mail asking if she knew what was going on, but I haven't heard from her either. Stephen and I are hoping that Wendy is out of reach because she has gone somewhere to get treatment. It is not like Wendy to lose touch with all of us.

Did you get the book and the See's? Are you having your own taste test there? I brought in some of my various truffles from Stephen to share with my co-workers. We are all gorging ourselves on chocolates and sweets these days. (Stress)

When I went to the Cowboy on Sunday, I wore the new white blouse which you sent. It looked good and was very comfortable to dance in. It's great to be able to dance with lots of energy again.

Yesterday, my HMO's Member Services person called me, as I had written them asking if there was anything they could do to help me get scheduled for reconstruction sooner than April. The lady was very nice, but all she can do is let me know if there is a cancellation.

Nick keeps coming out with the cutest, funniest things. I tell myself I have to remember them to share with you, but I usually forget. This morning, Tamsin told me that when Nick saw the huge satellite dish over the campus yesterday he said, "Mom that thing's there so we can listen to aliens talking." (Too much TV???) He keeps me laughing. I love the spontaneous and innocent things he comes out with.

Before I forget…Stephen said to say "Hi" to you and Jack.
Love you,

$\mathcal{M}$arch 2, Thursday

Howdy—

Did you get an "A" on your test? And, how is your knee? Guess you won't be two stepping for awhile. Thank you for the card. (Cute) Yes, I was surprised to hear from you. I'm glad you wrote because— I just like knowing what's going on.

Please, tell Jack that I can truly empathize with him regarding all the layoffs going on at Polaroid. What type of early retirement package are they offering him? What will he do next? Unfortunately, I still have another year and a half to go before I can retire. I'm kind of stuck.

Things are just very much in limbo at work. It's hard to concentrate on anything. Also, we are all constantly talking about it. We say "Enough"— but, then we just keep on talking about it. It's maddening to not have any idea as to where we stand. The sad thing is that Social Services is going to lose some incredibly talented and experienced people. Employees are looking elsewhere already. I personally feel that we have some of the brightest, hardest working employees and they will either be laid off, resign or in some cases retire early. Other counties are going to make out from Orange County's loss.

My friend Rick said that he will just take the lay off instead of going back to being a line worker. He has eleven years with the county and doesn't expect that to be enough to keep him from bumping down three levels to where he was years ago. Rick is so smart and knowledgeable, and the thought of him leaving Orange County is painful.

This whole process is painful. I told my Manager today that a lot of us have grown up professionally together. (Look at Chris and I. We were in our early twenties when we first met at the Sheriff's Department as clerk typists. She and I have known each other for twenty-five years. She, fortunately, stayed on all those years. Me— because I left and came back twice, my seniority only goes back to my last hire in date, on Halloween in 1980. Chris will do okay, as she has enough years in.) Anyway, as I was saying— even though we don't think about it on a daily basis— over the years we have become like family. We may not work together for a few years, but eventually our paths cross and recross again. I feel like someone is tearing our family apart and it hurts.

Shoot. Listen to me. If I don't have one thing to worry about, I have to go and find something else. I have to stop this. It'll all work out in the end.

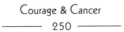
I keep forgetting to tell you that Arthur is in love. Yes, he's head over heels in love. He usually doesn't show his emotions if he can help it, but he can't stop talking about this girl. I look forward to meeting her. And, I am very happy for him. He deserves someone as wonderful as she sounds. Tomorrow night, he is coming over so that we can make lasagna together. They are going up to the mountains with a bunch of friends for the weekend. He wants to take it up already prepared for baking.

Did I tell you that Reid is moving in with his girlfriend, so Arthur is moving on the first of April? He is going to rent a studio apartment in Huntington Beach and will be living alone. The funny thing is that his girlfriend is moving two weeks later, and they will be living across the street from each other. This wasn't planned. They both found their new apartments at different times. (How convenient.) Oh, she has a three year old daughter and when Arthur has Dani on the weekends the four of them do things together.

You mentioned tax refunds. Well, yesterday I got mine from the state. It was a check for $9.39 and an explanation that I had miscalculated. (Wrong.) I think they are in error. Even though I filed as Head of Household, since Arthur was with me for over six months, they disallowed it. Of course, I wrote them asking for more of an explanation. (Bummer.)

Okay. I am glad that Jack knows that he is welcome to join us. I can truly understand why he can't make it. Tell him that next time we'll be sure to do it when he can come too.

Stephen just called. He cracks me up. He was calling long distance, from his cellular phone, as he was driving back to Tahoe from Reno. I miss him so much! Last night, we went online to talk, and we still e-mail each other daily. Stephen is so understanding and he always lifts me up when I am down. Somehow he seems to know the perfect things to say, and do to make me feel better no matter what it is I might be grumbling about.

Did I tell you that I lost my dance partner? Ray didn't call last week. That was fine, since Stephen was here through Saturday. When I saw Ray on Sunday at the Cowboy I asked him about it. He said that he was too tired. I haven't heard from him this week either. (Maybe he didn't like my cooking?) Oh well, it was fun while it lasted.

The kitchen is calling my name. I think I'll go and get a snack. At the rate I am eating lately I will probably be ten pounds over weight by the time we go on vacation.

Love,

*M*arch 3, Friday

Rita,

If it wasn't so late your time I would call. I just heard from Wendy's friend that Wendy is not doing so good. She has been slipping in and out of a coma. Her friends in New York fear that she is not going to make it. They will let me know tomorrow, when they have more information. I am so upset, that I am having a hard time typing, and the tears just keep flowing.

Why is this happening? Wendy is young, and beautiful, and she has given so much of herself to all of us. Why? I have no answers or guesses tonight, but I wanted to write so I could mail this first thing in the morning. I know that you and Jack have been concerned for her.

I will write or call you as soon as I know any more.

This is it for tonight.

Love you much,

*M*arch 4, Saturday

Hi,

I'm in a much better emotional state today than I was last night. There's no further news about Wendy. We are all waiting to hear what is going on. Naturally all the breast cancer sisters, and Stephen too, are distressed. She is a very special lady. I will call when I know anything more.

Lillie's artwork for the fund raising arrived. The artist signed them. I've ordered one for me. I didn't order one for you, because I didn't think you would have use for it.

Let's see— I got two very long letters from you today. So both of us claim to be busy, or not in a letter writing mood, and here we are writing more than ever. That's just us being us.

You and Jack both sound like you are falling apart back there. What am I going to do with you? Take care of all your ailments and be healthy. And yes, I am very glad you are scheduling another mammogram. I didn't want to bring it up again. Actually, I have my next one in May, and I was going to ask you to go then too. Let me know the results as soon as you get them.

What else? Yes, I've thought about calling off our vacation. It is a bad time for me to be taking it. (And, to add to all this I got a jury duty summons today for April 12th. Enough already.) Anyway, I really need this vacation and I've decided that I'm going to take it. When we meet it'll be almost two years since my last real vacation. What with all that has been happening these past two years, I desperately need some rest and relaxation. Bud's townhouse in Sonoma is the perfect place to do this. It's like going back in time, because of the slower pace. There is a sense of tranquility there, and I'm up for that big time.

I want to spend the week talking with you, reading, eating, and doing lots of sleeping. Will this be too boring for you??? Of course, we will do the sights and vineyards also. How could we go there and not do that?

Keep writing to me about how cold the winter is there, just in case I get a longing to move to Lake Tahoe, or something crazy like that. I don't think I could handle freezing winters again.

You can return the manuscript to me. Ken e-mailed me that he liked the book a lot and he is forwarding his copy to Jane. Oh—an after thought here. Do you want to send it to Mike for me? That would help. I'll enclose the note from the publisher, so that you can see his suggestions regarding the cartoons from Ken.

I don't think you look like Denise Brown. You are much prettier than she. But, then Tamsin tells me that I look like Bonnie Rait (sp?), and I don't see a resemblance there either. (She says that I look like her when my hair is long and curly.)

I'm also enclosing one note that I got today from Stephen. I've never shared any of his love letters with you, but this one is special. Ignore the typos and absorb the content.

Stephen suggested that I call Ray in case he was ill or working this past week. Well, I finally called him this afternoon and he has been down with a head cold. I told him that I was meeting Karen and Bob at In Cahoots tonight for a couple of hours of dancing. Ray said that if he felt healthy and rested he might show up.

And to keep you up to date— I got a note from Don. He and his girlfriend are back together again. Poor man. I wrote and told him to just go ahead and marry her and get it over with. (Teasing)

Today, I took Nick to the "haircut store" and then we did the usual buying of new shoes afterwards. When we came home, he and I watched "The Lion King" video. It was great. Have you seen it yet?

Talk to you soon.

Love,

March 5, Sunday

Rita,

Thank you again. You are a big help. Being there when I need you—to talk to and to cry with is tremendous support. I knew you and Jack would want to know right away. I beeped Stephen, but he must not be able to call right now. I called Wendy's friend in New York to thank her for letting me know.

We all knew it was coming, but I guess we didn't expect it to be so soon. Or, maybe I was hoping for a miracle cure for Wendy. She fought so hard since her first diagnosis, and when she was healthy, she put her energies into giving the rest of us so much love and support. I am glad I met her. My regret is that I didn't just get on a plane and fly back there to meet her in person.

Sharon said that Wendy had invited her and her husband to New York to show them the sights. That was last fall. Sharon's husband was ready to go right then and there. Sharon wanted to wait until the spring. She said that this experience has taught her a lesson about not putting things off. I guess we all have our regrets.

I am okay now. Well, I mean I have stopped crying. Now I am angry all over again that this should be happening. Why can't someone find a cure? I understand better Lillie's urgency to educate people about breast cancer. Someone, somewhere has to do something. Too many women are dying from this disease. (I'm just venting.)

Wendy and her love and support to so many of us will not ever be forgotten.

Our minister made the comment once that she believes that, "We are all here to learn a lesson and to give a gift." I do not know what my purpose is, but I do know that I have learned some valuable lessons this past year, and I vow to give back to the Universe in some way.

Please give Jack a hug for me. And, ask him to give you one back from me.

Love you both,

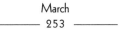

March 7, Tuesday

Hi—

I just got off the phone with D.D. (Danielle). I told her I had to go if I was ever going to get this letter written to you tonight. She is so good Rita. Danielle is always a "pick me upper." I'd really like for the two of you to meet. Geez—I was telling Jessica and Chris yesterday that maybe you should come to Orange County on vacation after all so that you and everyone down here can meet. But, maybe we should save that for another time.

First—Congratulations on getting an "A." That is wonderful. Yay!!!

Okay—there's lots of news here. Do you want to hear the good news or the bad news first? Let's start with the good news. Hopefully by the time I get to the not so good news it won't sound too bad.

Yesterday I received—delivered to work—a big vase with a humongous bouquet of white and purple lilacs. They are awesome. Chris immediately jumps up and says, "Oh those are my favorite flower." I said, "Me too." Then Chris told me that in order to keep them fresh I needed to hammer the stems so the water can get through all the wood. She and I went out on the cement staircase with a hammer. Actually,—she did all the work while I got fresh water and I could hear her hammering all over the building. I put them on the table that is between our desks so we can both enjoy them. She told me to tell Stephen thank you from her too.

I asked him how he ever got lilacs when they aren't in season. The florist who does all his bouquets for me recognized who he was, and remembered all the business he has been giving them. They made a special trip to Los Angeles to get them. Impressed? I am.

When I got home from work last night Tamsin said that my HMO had called. (I have no idea why they didn't call me at work.) So, I called them back this morning and it took about six long distance calls with my calling card to finally get through to them. They had forgotten to undo their answering machine when their office opened. I finally called their emergency number.

Anyway, there is good news here. I am scheduled for the reconstruction on March 28th. I am beyond excited over this. Rita, I knew I would be happy to have this surgery, but I didn't realize just how much I wanted it until the date was set. I was beaming the rest of the morning... and telling everyone whether they cared or not! My pre-op will be in the morning and the surgery in the afternoon. YES!!!

Well, you know how life is. We take the good with the bad. Fifteen minutes before I left work today, we were informed of the proposed budget cuts. It is not good. Out of all the county layoffs our agency is being hit the hardest. We will lose 725 employees and close down four of our financial assistance offices.

We all thought we were prepared since rumors had been flying. Nothing prepared us for this though. I know my face looked as shocked as the ones I was looking into. I was numb and unbelieving. I was sick.

I am distraught over the people who will lose their jobs. I am upset because now I am pretty certain that I will be offered a demotion. How far down I will be demoted I don't know at this point. One Program Assistant told me, as we were leaving the building, that she will quit before she goes back out as a line supervisor again.

It will be years before Orange County recovers from this blow. Mr. Popejoy is in Sacramento looking for bail-out monies for some bonds. The thought hit me that maybe this is just a scare tactic for the state, in an attempt to get the money there. Someone else said he thought we were getting the brunt of this, because of Welfare Reform. All I know is that there are many employees who are devastated tonight over this announcement.

I asked D.D. tonight if she is going to retire. She might consider it if they offer her some compensation for doing it early.

Man—I just keep sitting here staring off into space. I don't think it has really sunk in yet.

My emotional state is about the same as our weather lately. Sun, rain, sun, rain. Actually, considering everything, I am doing okay. I just count my blessings when I think things are getting too low—and I still have plenty to be thankful for.

Time for bed.

Love you,

March 8, Wednesday

Rita— Hi...

Daily letters here? I'll make this one quick, because I'm all letter written out. I just answered quite a few online letters from old friends, and a new cancer survivor friend. There's not much left in me for tonight.

I wanted to tell you though, I had a long talk with myself today at lunch time. By the time I got through, I had a whole new attitude on this job thing. And you know what? It worked. I really am okay and at peace over what is happening at work. But, I still feel for my co-workers. Phu didn't find out until this morning. He said that he almost got sick to his stomach when he heard what was going on. I tried to reassure him that he was in initial shock, like I was last night, and that it will past. Jessica called in sick today. I talked to her on the phone and she said that she caused herself to become sick and couldn't sleep last night. It is pretty traumatic for some, and understandably so.

My new perspective is to look at this as another great challenge. I will grow from this experience and learn a lot. It will give me the opportunity to become a better money manager. Also, I've been wanting to relearn the Financial Assistance programs and now I will have the chance. I am one of the fortunate ones. It's not like I will be without a job, and I will continue to have a roof over my head and food for my tummy. The luxuries that I have grown fond of will just be set aside for awhile.

I think I've had my share of bad news for the year. My quota's been met and possibly exceeded, but on the other hand... I have had many wonderful things happening in my life at the same time. Enough said here.

The future from here looks very positive to me. I can't complain about the past. I'm still happy and feeling lucky. And that's all she wrote for this one.

Good night. Love you,

⏃

March 11, Saturday

Hi,

I can't believe I am sitting here writing to you. I just wrote so many e-mail notes to people online, that I feel like there can't be much more "talk" left in me. I thought about calling, but I am determined to have a low amount on my next phone bill. I don't remember the last time I had a normal sounding bill.

I just wrote Lillie, Sharon, Paul, Stephen, and my new cancer survivor friend. When are you coming online with us?

This weekend has been very quiet so far for me and I like it. Yesterday was my last county flex day and I hustled to get lots of things done. I also hustled on the errand circuit because of the storm predicted, which did show up last night. It was heavy duty with wind, rain, thunder, and lightning. Anyway, I went to the Auto Club and got maps on how to get to Sonoma from the San Francisco airport. (You know how I get lost so easily. Well, I didn't want to take any chances.) Then I also got a book on the vineyards. Of course, after yesterday's storm in Sonoma and Napa let's hope that there are vineyards left by the end of May. They have really been hit hard this past year.

Tamsin's birthday, her 24th, is Monday. She had asked if she could borrow some money to go out and party with her friends. I gave her a card with $25 in it, and babysat Nick for the night. Oh, we also had a chocolate and whipped cream cake. (Yum.) Since Nick got me up so early this morning, I have already taken a nap. I was beat.

When I woke up from my nap, Bridget and Tyler were here. He is so cute— and so huge. At four months he weighs twenty pounds. I told Nick he had better treat his little cousin really good, because someday Tyler is going to be bigger than him.

Nick can read his name. I was typing a note to Paul...and was writing him that I was having a hard time typing because Nick was on my lap. Nick points to his name on the screen and says, "That's my name." Smart. Oh, and here's another cute saying from Nick. Yesterday, we were in the bathroom and he says, "Grandma—why do you have an operation box?" I looked at Tamsin for an interpretation. She said, "I have no idea what he means." So I asked him to explain. He opened the cupboard door and pointed to my first aid kit under the sink. (Got it!)

I am going to order a signed copy of Lillie's book for you. It should be out any day. Also, she said that a friend of hers in Virginia has just opened a bookstore and she has asked her to carry my book. With Lillie all things are possible. Did I tell you that she wrote a short piece for Woman's Day magazine, regarding her mother's support group? She wrote it under her mother's name, since her mother will be leading the group. They called and said it will be in the Mother's Day issue. She has added software to her PC for accessing the full Internet, and has made numerous contacts for the group. I am in awe of her and her energy and resourcefulness.

Sharon said that her arm is better and she can now move it 120 degrees. She is still getting physical therapy three times a week. Also, in April she will get her implant put in. I will beat her after all. My doctor has assured me that I don't need the expander and the gradual fill ups like she and Sue have been getting. He says I have plenty of skin for the implant.

Do you remember Cheryl, my online friend in Atlanta, who we thought would meet us on Club Dance? (By the way, they never returned my calls or fax, so I've given up on hoping to go back there.) She is the ballet mistress. Well, Cheryl has been having problems with weight loss and a recurring back ache. This week, she had x-rays and an MRI. Please, pray that they come back okay. Naturally, she is even more concerned because of the way things went for Wendy.

I don't mean to be getting paranoid, but my back has been aching since Thursday. Actually, I know I'm okay and it is just strained, but hearing about Cheryl's problem and tests kind of made me get a little seed of concern in my mind for myself. I am staying in tonight and resting so that it will be all healed by tomorrow, and then I can go dancing.

I guess I did have a few words left in me.

Hi to Jack, and please thank him for his caring.

Love,

March 14, Tuesday

Hi—

This has been a long night of typing already. I just finished writing answers to questions for Tamsin's interview of me, for her counseling class. Then I wrote to some friends on AOL, and of course, a long letter to Stephen.

I had to get it all in to him tonight. Tomorrow, he will be in a dormitory situation without phones, as he gets some refresher training for his job. As soon as he finishes that on Friday, he and his best friend are heading for Las Vegas for a "guy thing" type of weekend . It is his friend's birthday celebration. So Stephen will be out of reach for almost a week.

He will be coming down on the day before my surgery and staying through that week. He says he plans on cooking and pampering me while he's here. Sounds good to me. I'm anxious to try some of his delicious cooking, that I've heard so much about. Also, he and Danielle will get to know each other, as they make that drive back and forth to the hospital. They are both so loveable that I know they will hit it off. I will be sure to have one of them call you the night of the surgery. I know I won't be in any shape to do it.

Right now, I am concerned about catching a bug from Tamsin and/or Nick. She is so sick with a terrible fever and sore throat. She is sneezing and wheezing. And today she had two asthma attacks. Then Nick's nose is runny and he's coughing. I feel so bad for them, but I am also trying to avoid being around them. I do not want to catch anything now that I have a surgery date. Also, I got the pre-op packet yesterday and it said not to take any aspirin type products for the next two weeks. Think healthy and positive thoughts for me!

Yesterday was Tamsin's birthday and last night the whole family was here. It was great, except for Tamsin feeling so miserable.

Also, yesterday afternoon the mail clerk called me and said that a package had been delivered. It was huge. We opened it and it was from Stephen. There was a card that read, "For you and your co-workers as you go through nutty times." It was a giant tray with seven sections filled with the most delicious assortment of gourmet nuts. Everyone raved about the nuts— and Stephen. Marvette asked me if we could clone Stephen, cause she wants one of him too. He just tickles me with all the thoughtful things he does.

Hopefully, we will hear more tomorrow about the job situation. We were told that there would be another meeting in the afternoon, and there should be more information for us by then. The latest rumor is that of the 725 layoffs only 200 will be from the services programs and the other 525 will be from Financial Assistance. I guess this is why we are closing down some of our offices, but the other programs aren't.

Oh, I almost forgot. I got the artwork from Lillie today. It is the one that you saw, where it started with the Breast cancer symbol of a pink ribbon and becomes a butterfly. The print is called, "Transformation." It is so beautiful and delicate. The artist lives in Amherst, Massachusetts and she signed the print. I really like it.

Last night, while we were in our support group, the other members were teasing Stephen and I so much that I couldn't stop laughing. I was so hysterical that I could hardly type. I had tears in my eyes and a pain in my side. It was a wonder I didn't fall out of my seat. That is one chat log I ought to copy and send you. I told Jessica I would bring it to work for her to read.

Hey—I passed up $125 in cash, in order to babysit Nick tomorrow night. I got a call at work today from a Marketing and Survey company. Chris had given me a card to fill out for them a couple of months ago. They wanted me to spend two hours tomorrow night testing, and answering questions about, a new Window's based software. I am committed to babysitting Nick on Wednesday nights, so I turned the phone over to Chris. She is thrilled. Not only is it profitable, but it sounds like fun too. We were speculating that it might be the new Windows 95 that everyone's been waiting for. (I know— you have no clue as to what I am rambling on about and you could care less. I'll just shut up then!)

There's gotta be more, but my fingers are tired...too much typing here.

Love you,

*M*arch 15, Wednesday

Hi there.

I could not believe it this morning when I signed on and there you were. E-mail from Rita. Of course, I did not recognize who the screen name was that you were using. I checked for a profile, but there wasn't one. I assume it was your sister's, since you mentioned that she uses a computer for musical compositions. That was so cool. I loved getting it. Honest, it was like "you were right here." Now I am really going to bug you about getting a PC and coming online with us. What did you think about AOL?

Stephen is not available and this is the first time in six months that he has not written me at least one daily letter. I'm still writing him while he's away. By the time he gets back there will be a ton of notes waiting for him.

Rita, I have some sad news again. Cheryl met with her oncologist today. The cancer is back and is now in the bones of her vertebra and on a rib. She is starting radiation next week, and then will go on chemotherapy. She is very determined to beat it and has an excellent attitude. I am so impressed by the way she is handling this news. This was so unexpected. And just for the record, this blows my theory about a lumpectomy versus a mastectomy regarding recurrences. She had a mastectomy. I think it was about two or three years ago. Dang!!!

Danielle and I have been in touch daily lately. We've decided that Stephen and I will drive up to Los Angeles on the morning of my surgery. I will get my doctor's appointment and pre-op stuff done and get admitted into the hospital. Danielle will come up around noon, with lunch for she and Stephen. Then she will hang around with him, while I am being operated on. Stephen insists that he be there with me before and after. I love so much the caring that he shows me.

Today, I talked with Bud to let him know when I will be arriving at the San Francisco airport. He will pick me up that Saturday and I will stay overnight with him and Lynn. On Sunday, he will take me back to the airport to get you. Bud did say that maybe we can go out to eat when you arrive... if you are hungry. Also, he hopes that we will be able to get together one night for dinner. I hope it's when Stephen can come.

Today, we were told a little bit more about what will be coming in the way of downsizing. I still anticipate a pink slip and the chance to demote. There won't be many people left in the Systems division.

When my old boss, John, was in our office yesterday, I asked him how his staff was handling all this. He said, "Well, put it this way. We are having a St. Patrick's Day potluck on Friday and they are calling it 'The Last Supper'." I cracked up. It's good to know that employees are retaining a sense of humor.

Tomorrow, I have to call the scheduling clerk again at the HMO. I was talking to Chris and Jessica today, and I mentioned that I could not eat after midnight prior to the surgery. (The surgery is in the afternoon.) I am concerned that I will start feeling faint and shaky by ten in the morning. They both said that must not be right. They think I should be able to have at least a small bowl of cereal before I go in. So, I guess I should check this out. My body is so used to being fed, and refueled constantly throughout the day, that I don't handle fasting so good.

I didn't expect to be writing again—and writing you so much, but some things just don't change.

Love,

March 16, Thursday (AOL E-mail)

Stephen -

I just got off the phone with Rita. I had called and left a message earlier tonight, because she had her mammogram on Friday. I didn't know when I called her, that today was another doctor's appointment regarding her mammogram. She returned my call and, as usual, we talked for a long time.

Rita said that her mammogram showed that the "cyst" had grown by six millimeters, since it was last checked. Because I have bugged her, and because of all that has occurred with me this past year, she decided to have it aspirated again.

Once more, no fluid came out. She has had four doctors tell her that it is only a cyst. I am so proud of her, because this time she is pursuing it further. Next Tuesday, they will use an ultrasound to break it up and again aspirate it, in order to do a biopsy of the fluid.

Rita feels very sure that it truly is a cyst. Since I have nagged her so much, and since she has heard my stories about the women I have met this past year, she will finally get some tests done to put our minds at ease. She said she will call me Tuesday night with the results.

I know she is going to be okay, but I want to hear it and then I can stop worrying about her. She understands where I am coming from. The fact that she is not just taking an opinion from any of the doctors, and insisting that they go in and remove it, is a good sign.

I framed and hung up the "Transformations" breast cancer awareness print from Lillie. You'll see it when you come down, because I have hung it on the wall over my work-station. I told Lillie that just looking at it makes me feel good. It is so inspirational. There are twelve stages beginning with a pink ribbon, which progressively unfolds and transforms into a beautiful butterfly imprinted over a sketch of a ladies face.

That's it for tonight. Sleep well. I love you.

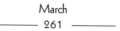

March 18, Saturday

Hi Rita—

I am so glad we got to talk the other night. And I am anxiously waiting to hear the results from next Tuesdays doctor's visit. How is Jack? When he goes for the surgery on his ankle be sure to baby him.

The circulation problem that you mentioned—I forget the name— is what Rob told me it sounded like you had four or five years ago. What do you plan on doing as treatment?

Well, I'm sick. The sore throat and runny nose and fever that Tamsin and Nick have been battling finally got hold of me. I'm bummed. I hope it comes and goes quick. If I have to reschedule this surgery, I am not going to be too happy. I want to get this show on the road.

Yesterday, I talked with Dr. Trung's nurse. She said that I will be fine going without food, as even though the surgery isn't until 12:30 or

1:00 o'clock they will probably start an IV with glucose at about 10:30 or 11:00. Also, I will be in the operating room for about two hours and I will be discharged the next day.

Stephen is in Las Vegas this weekend with his friend, and he has been able to hook his notebook up to a modem in the Hotel. I had written and told him that he didn't have to do all the cooking that week. He is still insistent that he wants to do it, even if it gets frozen for later.

The situation at work sounds like it might not be as bad as proposed. The Board of Supervisors has vetoed the plan to have our Agency take the brunt of the layoffs. We are talking about 725 people, while the Sheriff's Department is crying over six positions. So, they are looking for more money from other agencies to help ours. This would be wonderful for us, and the public who relies on our help.

I started my new hours yesterday. Flex days are a thing of the past. I now work Monday to Friday, 8:30—5:30 with an hour for lunch. When I go out to the districts to work it may change again.

Last night, I composed a note and questionnaire to e-mail to almost 100 people, who are in the "Love and Laughter" book. Rita, I am just in awe of these people. They are so inspirational. The response is very much in favor of having this book done, and they are encouraging me to continue with it. But, what is touching are the beautiful comments they are writing regarding their cancers, or loved one's cancers, and also how incredibly supportive the online group has been for them. So far, only one ex-member has asked me not to quote her, as she values her privacy. I understand and told her "no problem." So I have my work cut out for me on that book in the near future.

Stephen is pleased that you and Jack will be online soon too. He said that people who don't use e-mail for their correspondence just don't realize how much more efficient and less costly it is than postal mail. I think you and I are going to love this new mode of communication.

Take care. I will be thinking about you lots over the next few days.

Love,

P.S. I'm enclosing a copy of a short story, which Wendy wrote and also a poem that an online friend of hers wrote for her, when she was in the hospital for her BMT (bone marrow transplant). Please return both to me.

March 20, Monday

Hi—

It's Monday morning and I'm home from work. I debated long and hard with myself over whether I should go in or not. I think I need to rest and get this sickness out of me.

Yesterday morning, I went to Urgent Care and got a prescription for antibiotics and some cough syrup. Since I was already out, I had my blood lab work done for next week. I had a feeling I wouldn't be up to doing it today. Actually, I'm feeling much better than I was feeling Saturday night and yesterday. The doctor says it's bronchitis and I was also running a fever. Let's hope it's gone by the 28th. I think it will be.

So I have reasoned that it's better that I take off one precious sick day, in order to get rest, instead of being sick next week and having my surgery canceled. I'm glad I chose to stay home.

There was no church or dancing this weekend. I mostly slept, read and tried to relax.

Time for me to go back on the couch.

Love,

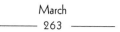

*M*arch 21, Tuesday

Dear Wendy's family:

I received your addresses last night from Amy. She has been sharing with me what has been happening in New York with memorials and gatherings in Wendy's honor. Since I am not able to come back there right now to participate, I wanted to write to you so that you know Wendy has touched many lives throughout the United States.

I met Wendy in September, when I joined the AOL online Cancer Survivors support group. She had been a member for some time. We instantly had a rapport and exchanged pictures and phone calls. I have a sweet picture of Wendy and her Mom together. When I got that picture, I immediately told Wendy that I thought she and I even looked alike.

We had much in common. One thing was that we had both recently met new men and were in the process of starting new relationships. The both of us teased each other and our online breast cancer sisters teased us, by saying that they were going to throw a double online wedding ceremony for us. (Of course, we didn't let the men know this. It was going to be their surprise!)

I loved Wendy very much. She was in my life for only a short time, but I will never forget her. I cannot say enough good things about her. Wendy was just a very special person.

Wendy may have shared with you that I will have a book published in October regarding my breast cancer. She was pleased to know that I was dedicating the book to her. It is really not just my story, but has the stories of quite a few breast cancer sisters in it also. Wendy, of course, is in the book as a key person. When the book is published I would like to send you a copy for your family.

I wish I could have been there to meet Wendy in person. She will always be in my thoughts, and I wanted you to know that myself and many other online friends of Wendy miss her and share in your sorrow.

Much love,

March 21, Tuesday (AOL E-mail)

Stephen—

I just got off the phone from talking with Rita. She is A-Okay. It was a cyst. She was there for an hour - without any local anaesthesia. They had to keep using bigger and bigger needles to go in and break it up… but finally fluid came out. I am so relieved for her. This has been on my mind for almost a year now. She is very sore tonight, but I think the soreness is worth it.

Oh, you had asked me about Jack's retirement. Yes, he is taking an early retirement. His last day is March 31st and it is also the day that he is having surgery on his ankle. Rita said that Jack is going into the same type of business that you have thought about. He is very handy, and already does some general construction type jobs. Now, he can do it full time. He is excited because this is what he has always wanted to do.

I'm out of here to have dinner. I wanted to share the good news with you.

I love you.

March 23, Thursday

Hi—

I keep thinking about what you went through, but I am so glad that you did it. I shared with Jessica and she thinks that you did the right thing too. Oh, she said she had a needle biopsy done once—long before her diagnosis—and she had the same thing happen with the needle hitting her bone. Jessica said it didn't hurt, but just hearing it hit was nerve wracking. Yuck.

Stephen is snow bound in Tahoe. All the roads are closed. He can't even get to work. He's hoping he can get through to get to the airport on Monday. I think he should be okay by then. Their lines might be down or something too, because I just logged on to see if there was a daily note from him and "nada." This happened once before.

Today, I called the lady that I spoke to in December, and who is also an implant patient of Dr. Trung's. Since she works at the hospital where I will be having the surgery, she told me to call her when I had it scheduled and she would come by to see me. Her name is Mary Beth and she is so nice, Rita. Anyway, I was especially glad that I called her, because she said that the pain wasn't that bad. I was getting somewhat anxious every time I thought about it. Now I don't dread it quite as much. Mary Beth did say that she was out of work for four weeks though. I told her I couldn't afford to do that, since I don't have that much time on the books. But, I had been thinking that maybe I could return to work after one week. Now it looks like I will be using the whole two weeks, which I had originally requested.

Mary Beth said that she would come by to see me some time on Tuesday. I am looking forward to meeting her in person.

Today, I saw one of our personnel people in the elevator. I asked her if they were really busy these days and she said, "Yes." It turns out that over 100 people have resigned because they have already accepted positions elsewhere. Between that, the early retirements, and the re-searching for more funds for our agency— maybe there won't be any layoffs. (Wishful thinking here.)

I have a lot to do this weekend...I'll try to write one more time before I go in to the hospital. If not, then you know there will be a lot of letters once I'm home.

Love,

March 26, Sunday

Another Beautiful Sunday Here!

Your note card and the pamphlet for the Caribbean came yester-day. Also, thank you for sharing Linda's sister's story with me. It was very sad. Yes, it was heavy on the religious aspect, but it was very touch-ing. I thought the article was well done.

I'll show Stephen the brochure about the vacation while he is here this week. The problem with his job is that he never knows in advance when he can get the time off. But it's a year away, so we have plenty of time to work on it.

Now your "Stress Diet" is definitely my kind of diet. I especially like, "The foods used for medicinal purposes never count...Sara Lee Cheesecake." Hmmm. I think I'll go defrost one right now for later today.

Actually, I'm typing this on the fly. I have been on over-drive this weekend. I miss my flex day. I had to cram all the things I usually do on Fridays into Saturday's chores and errands. And since I know I'm going to the hospital Tuesday, I am like a pregnant woman about to deliver. Everything has to be clean and caught up, or in my compulsive state—more like ahead of schedule even. I cleaned out my clothes closet. By the time I got through organizing it, I had two hours worth of summer clothing to be ironed. Naturally, I did that too.

Finally, I crashed late last night and over slept this morning, so church was out of the question. Now I am going out to look for some new tennis shoes, and then I plan to dance for one last time this afternoon. I know it will probably be months before I am able to dance again. My dance outfits are set to the back of my closet, so as not to torment me. (Didn't I already do this not too long ago?)

Tamsin and Nick have been at Teharu's for the weekend. This is why I have been able to accomplish so much without running interference with the little man. But yesterday Bridget and Tyler stopped by for about thirty minutes. Rita, he is so precious. He's got Eric's blue eyes and he knows how to use them on his Grandma. What a little flirt. I talk to him and he "talks" back, and he grins at me from one chubby cheek to the other. I think I am in love again!

Well, I doubt I will be writing you between now and when I get home on Wednesday—and then, too, it may be a few days after that. All will be fine.

Love you,

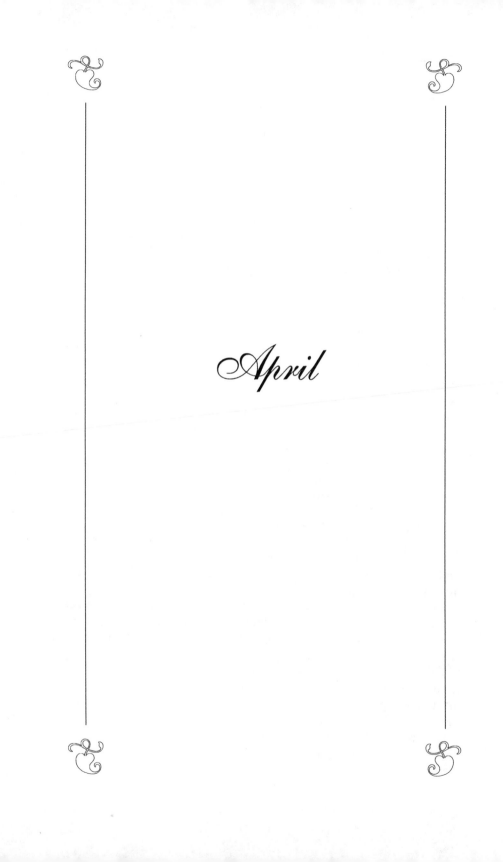

April

HAKUNA MATATA — which means "no worries"
(My new motto—from "The Lion King")

March 29, Tuesday— *April* 1, Saturday

Hi—

This one letter is probably going to take me days, and many stages to write. Please just bear with me. Hopefully, in the end I will have remembered everything that I want to write to you about. This is slow going, because I am making so many typos. I guess I can clean it up later. I am doing pretty good here. Actually, I am doing better than I had anticipated. Of course, right now is a good moment, so that's the place that I am coming from.

Monday night—or afternoon—I got to the airport, and are you ready? I came within one to two inches of being run over by a speeding car. I've never experienced anything quite like that before in my life. It was a car that ran the light at the airport crosswalk. He slammed on his brakes, skidded—and came to a halt right at my knees. I was pretty shook up and so was the driver, but I figured it just wasn't my time. When I got into the airport I told Stephen that I think I have a little angel perched on my left shoulder. How else could I have come that close, and yet not be touched by his car? (Tamsin later said, it's a "Wendy angel" watching over me.)

Stephen and I went out to dinner. Then we came home and went online to join the support group. We were late entering the room. Stephen made up a new screen name for the two of us to use. It was a joke, based on the night they were teasing us about his police handcuffs. We were called "Handcuffs." At first, our friends were treating us like a new member by welcoming us and all. We were giving them a rough time, teasing them, and getting them confused as to how we knew things about them. When it came time to switch to the new, larger room—and Jane said something about making the jump—I typed, "I need keys first." Eventually, we were found out. It was a pretty good joke.

Oh, and that day your large envelope with a zillion pictures came. I truly like the ones of you. You look like a model. In each picture you have on a different winter jacket. I'm jealous! And Nick liked the duck pictures. He's still showing them to everyone who comes over. I will return your pictures, along with a copy of the Cancer Survivors collage, which Stephen printed for you. (If I ever get this letter finished that is.)

Tuesday morning, we were up early and on the road at an indecent hour. We got to Dr. Trung's office a half-hour early. When I went into the exam room, I asked Stephen to come with me. Dr. Trung took a lot of "before" pictures. I'll enclose the one he gave me for a souvenir. While he was drawing lines on my left chest for the surgery, he asked me if I wanted him to "lift" the right breast at the same time. (As you can see from the picture, it was pretty droopy.) I told him "Sure."

We next went to the hospital, where we met D.D. True to her word, she had bags, baskets, and a cooler chest filled with food for Stephen's and her lunch.

I did my pre-op stuff and then they let Stephen come into the room, where I would be given the IV, and would be waiting for my turn to go into the operating room. While we were there Mary Beth, who I had talked to on the phone, came by. It was great to meet her in person. She is very pretty and, as I had suspected, also very friendly. Mary Beth was so encouraging and the timing for her visit was perfect, because it was right about then that I was getting nervous. I was like "Motor Mouth" and couldn't shut up.

Then D.D. came in and we three waited, and waited. Eventually, I conked out. I know I gained consciousness as we were going into the operating room and the nurse was putting a cap on my head, but I remember nothing else until I came to in my room later that evening. And, when I opened my eyes—there in the dark, sitting in the corner was Stephen...keeping his vigil. It was wonderful to see him there!

To be continued later...

Where was I? Since I left this letter, I got your card, note and the two packages of Sky Bars! Muchas Gracias!!! I haven't gotten into them yet, but Tamsin has. Maybe tonight I will be more up to it. Actually, my "mad chef" is at it again. Stephen is out grocery shopping right now.

Now, you are having surgery on your knee on April 5th? (That is when I go back for my Plastic Surgeon's follow up appointment.) Will you be getting it as an in, or out, patient? What actually will they be doing to you? I'll have to call you between now and then, because I want to know more about what is going on. I can't believe that all of us are having surgeries like this...one after the other.

Oh, and Jack's antique mirrors sound wonderful. I am excited for him, that he is getting into all these new things. How fun for him and yes, I hope it will be profitable too.

Okay, now I have to figure out where I was before I left this...

Dinner Tuesday night, after my surgery, consisted of three items that I normally detest... but, they tasted delicious. (A cup of beef bouillon, lime Jell-O and some grape juice.)

I slept fitfully, naturally, on Tuesday night. I could only sleep sitting up. I was also so thirsty that I drank, what seemed like, gallons of fluids. The IV had continuous antibiotics going through it, and I am still on a pill form of the same, now at home. They are to prevent an infection from all the stitches and the implant.

Stephen came by in the morning. Then Dr. Trung came to change my dressings. That was when I got my first look, and it's not a pretty sight. I am rather grotesque looking. I suggested that Stephen not look, because I didn't want him to get turned off! I know it will heal and I will have young and perky boobs, eventually. Right now I am stitched everywhere.

Mary Beth came by to see me again before I was discharged. That was nice. She said for me to stay in touch. Finally, I got to come home. This was such a big difference from after the mastectomy, when I didn't even want to leave the hospital. I was more than ready this time.

The only uncomfortable part, really is what I had anticipated. Where the muscle is pulled over the implant I feel some pain. I can't stretch out my left arm again, without the muscle being pulled, and sleeping flat on my back is out of the question. (I am still sleeping sitting straight up.) But, it's not too bad because I know it is only temporary, and pretty soon I will be healed and the muscle will have stretched out.

Wednesday night, Bonnie, from my support group, and her friend Joyce came down from the Valley. I appreciate their making that drive, and especially since it was during rush hour traffic. Bonnie and I met at the brunch about a month ago. She and Stephen still wanted to meet. Joyce is her girlfriend and both times she came down with Bonnie to keep her company for the long drive. Bonnie gave me a funny card and a small, pretty vase. Since Stephen had given me another mixed bouquet, and in it were some more lilacs, I removed the lilacs from the bigger bouquet and now have the small vase filled with the lilacs.

Stephen outdid himself Wednesday night. He prepared a delicious spaghetti dinner with vegetables, Italian sausages, salad, and bread. We also had fresh strawberries for dessert. (Yum.) He went shopping and then just went to "it" in the kitchen. By the time Bonnie and Joyce arrived dinner was about ready. I had no problem eating my first night at home!

Tired again…I will add more to this later.

One of these days I am going to finish this letter. It's now Friday morning. Yesterday, Stephen started coming down with another cold, or sinus infection. Both of us slept on and off for most of Thursday. The way I deal with pain is to sleep and escape it. But, I also realize that sleeping is great for healing.

As sick as he was, Stephen still cooked a big stew and corn muffin dinner for all of us last night. I am feeling guilty, so I told him that I will do the cooking tonight. Trust me, there has been no lack of eating here lately.

Eric, Bridget, and Tyler came over last night and brought me another gorgeous bouquet. Eric and Stephen each sat at opposite ends of the couch... They were both so tired that they barely said two words all night. And you know that is not like Eric, who is always joking and teasing everyone. I couldn't lift or hold Tyler, but I did help bottle feed him while he was propped up on the couch, and later I spoon fed him some green beans while he was in his car seat. (Cute.)

I gave each of the kids a Sky Bar...I will get to them today. That is a promise.

This week is flying by. I've gotten lots of phone calls and e-mail with good wishes. I am enclosing the one from Lillie, as she sent it to my "new breast." Funny, huh? I also called Jessica yesterday, to assure her that my reconstruction has not been that bad. I think I was expecting really horrible pain, but it's not happening. Nights are somewhat uncomfortable, because of the muscle in my chest, but I know this is temporary.

I'm just babbling so it must be time for me to quit this once more.

It's now Friday night, and Stephen and I just got back from a walk on the beach...to watch the sunset. I am so glad you called today, because I feel like this particular letter is never going to be finished.

Earlier today, Stephen and I went to the book store. I had ordered the book, *Answer Cancer—Answers For Living*, by Stephen Parkhill, my new online friend. I was hoping to be able to start reading it tonight. (But, we'll see. If I can't seem to find the energy and the time to write, how am I ever going to read a book?) After picking up the book we went down to the pier and walked a little, until I said, "I'm ready to go home for a nap." It's nice...sleeping, eating, and being still and quiet. I really do think that I am healing quickly, because of all this rest. After my nap, I was so energized that I cooked dinner. (Stephen is still not feeling so great. I think he is run down from all the back and forth traveling he does to here, there, and everywhere.) Then after dinner, he suggested the sunset walk.

I'm still not making a whole lot of progress on this letter, because now Nick is in my room and he is somewhat distracting.

Even though both of my boobs look ghastly at the moment, I can see that in the end they are going to be better looking than what I originally started out with. The thing is, I need to get used to the feeling of having a "basketball" on my left chest.

Nick is now playing "gopher" (his word—not mine) under my bedding. I think this is as far as I am going for tonight...

I bet you think this is never going to end. Well, April Fool's on you. My goal this morning is to finish this letter, and put it in the mail before I do another thing, and it's only 7:30 right now.

I continue to feel better each day. It's now Saturday and I can't believe how fast I am bouncing back. Being able to take showers right away has helped. Having Stephen here with me has been a real boost... and the pain has not nearly been what I had expected. (I've only used two of the pain pills since coming home.) I am finally sleeping soundly at night. Quite frankly, I feel on top of the world.

Stephen leaves tomorrow. I will probably start my usual daily letters to you then. Have you missed them?

Sorry if this is confusing. I should try to sort it out before I mail it, but forget that.

Love,

April 2, Sunday

Dear Rita—

How is your knee? I know that by the time this letter reaches you your surgery will be completed. I will call to see how you are doing. I hope that it is not very painful for you and that you have a speedy recovery. So, how soon do you think it'll be before you want to go two stepping? (Just teasing)

You know I mailed you a five page letter yesterday, but I have no idea what I put in it. It was a little bit hectic here for writing. I mean—not crazy, but just that I was having a hard time staying focused on letter writing. Sorry.

Today I can start fresh though, okay? Actually, I am waiting for a call from Grace. She said that she would call today around two o'clock my time. It is two-fifteen now, and I am hoping that she does get the chance, as this will be the first time that we have talked on the phone. And while I am thinking about special friends...yes, please send me Maria's address. I would love to send her some See's truffles. It would be my pleasure.

Well, my honey left this morning. I took him to the airport. This was my first day driving and it felt good. It did not feel so good to have him leaving again though.

But, time for some "true confessions" here? I was talking to him before he left and I said, "I think we should get married while Rita is out here on vacation." (It sounded like a good idea to me anyway.)

Stephen just looked at me like I was nuts (Hmmm) and said, "Do you ever want to see me again?" I guess that was a "No," huh? You can't blame me for trying. Now I know you won't be any big help in this department, and neither is Danielle. She is as confirmed a bachelorette as Stephen is a bachelor. What's with these Asian friends of mine??? (Ray is a confirmed bachelor too.)

Enough of that...

I am doing fantastic!!! I can now sleep on my back and on my left side. I am doing more and more every day. I'm not quite ready to go dancing (joke)—but soon. And, this may sound strange, but my new boob talks to me. I mean it gurgles every once in awhile. I can feel it and hear it... you know how a tummy sometimes gurgles? Well, now my chest does it too! The first time it happened I was freaked. Now I am getting used to it. Both breasts are healing nicely and someday they won't look so ugly.

Now the inside of my skin itches like crazy. When I told Stephen this, he said that maybe I was getting my sensation back on my left side. I said, "I don't think so." I don't think it's infected because I am taking the antibiotics and I have no fever, but it is so itchy, I feel like just scratching hard and yanking this basketball off of me. Instead, I just grit my teeth and try to ignore it. I hope this goes away soon.

When I can start wearing bras, without the surgical dressings, I am going to Victoria's Secret and buy the sexiest, prettiest, laciest bras there. Of course, I have no idea what size I will be wearing in the future, but this is the plan as of today. Then, when Jessica gets her reconstruction done, she and I want to have a bras burning party.... mastectomy bras that is. Want to come to this little party? Maybe we should invite Chris too. I told Chris on Monday that we ought to make her an Honorary Breast Cancer Sister, since she has been listening to Jessica and I talk on this subject for months now.

Honestly, I do feel wonderful. My boobs are eventually going to be better looking than a year ago. My weight is—(are you ready?)—drum roll here...110 pounds!!! Now, I think I may even consider getting a light perm soon. I know. My hair is still too short, but it is straight and I want some curls again. What I am trying to say here is that each day I am feeling more and more like the me that I used to be, before all this happened. (Actually, I think that I am a better me, but that's just my opinion.)

You will be in my thoughts on Wednesday. Take good care of you and Jack.

Love,

April 3, Monday

Hi—

How are you feeling? I hope by the time this reaches you, that you are out running a mile. Well, at least that you are able to be up and moving some. Today, I sent you a small package to give you something to do while you're recuperating with your leg propped up.

And, how is Jack? Shall we send future mail c/o your local Old Folks Home? (I know, I am one to tease, right?)

I just came out of group. Those people are so wonderful Rita. I love them a whole lot. No matter what is going on—and Lord knows there is much that each is dealing with in his or her fight with Cancer—they remain so up and cheerful. They give me so much inspiration. Cheryl was there, and she was her usual positive, happy self. Each person in the group is special. Oh, they all got their See's truffles from Stephen and were so appreciative.

It is so neat to be able to go online with all my new questions regarding the reconstruction. I have been bugging Mary daily. She is the lady from my group who finished chemo the same day as me. Mary got her implant done about three weeks ago. Even though she is in Virginia—there has been constant contact. This whole online experience has been the best thing. I send her e-mail in the morning with the questions of the day and she responds by afternoon. Is this great?

Today, I feel even better than yesterday. I feel so good that when I see Dr. Trung on Wednesday, I am going to ask him if I can return to work on Friday. I think that if I work the full day, and then have the weekend off to recover, I'll be fine. There is very little pain and discomfort left. And I feel so stupid. I figured out what was causing the intense itching that I had. The skin over the implant is super sensitive right now, because of the stretching going on. Even though I am numb in that area, it was still reacting to the nylon on the inside of my mastectomy bra. As soon as I added more gauze dressing to the area where I was being bothered, the itching stopped. (Live and learn here.)

When I talked to Jessica today, I told her about my wonder boob that "talks" to me. She said that she had heard that this can happen from the saline implants. I guess it's normal for it to swish around and gurgle some. So, I guess it's okay if I get talked to by my new "breast" friend, as Lillie calls it.

Speaking of Lillie, I got the funniest card from her today. I've gotten quite a few good ones, but this one is the best. I will enclose it for you to read.

Today, I got out and ran errands in the morning. No, I didn't get my hair permed. It really is too short,- but I will when it gets long again. Anyway, I am pretty tired tonight, but I don't think I over did it. Tomorrow, I am finally getting my teeth cleaned. I called my dentist and they had a cancellation. I'd much rather do it at noon tomorrow, than at 7:30 on Saturday morning!

Oh, Stephen Parkhill, who wrote the cancer book that I mentioned, is going to be on TV Thursday morning. I'm glad that I will be home so that I can watch it. He sounds so interesting. He is a Hypnotherapist. Grace does Hypnosis also. I have put them in touch with each other. (This online networking just amazes me.)

Grace did call yesterday. Rita, she is such a beautiful person. I have to admit that I did most of the talking, but I could feel very positive vibes from her across the phone lines. She said that she will call again, Wednesday night, to see how my doctor's appointment goes.

I want to meet all these people in person. Some day, maybe—I hope.

When Stephen was here, I asked him if he would like to play Tour Guide in June. Since he knows San Francisco, and you cannot come all the way to Northern California without seeing parts of the Bay Area. I suggested that we use the days that he is able to visit us to do those sights. He agreed. This will also work out well, because then we can plan to meet with our online friends while in the city. I know they would like to meet Stephen too.

Jessica told me today, that it looks like any Program Assistants who get layoff notices, and who choose to bump down, can go into the Social Worker II classification, if they meet the Minimum Requirements, instead of to a line supervisor position. (SWII pay is higher than supervisor in Financial Assistance.) I would love to be a Social Worker again. So the way I see it, no matter what happens to me—either staying as a PA or demoting—will be fine.

I will call Wednesday night to check up on you.

Love,

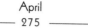

April 5, Wednesday

Hi there—

I want to call you, but I know it is too early your time. You are probably just getting home and I think you will be wanting a nap right off. Anesthesia does that to me anyway. So, I will wait until later this afternoon. I have been thinking about you lots, since the moment I got up this morning.

Well, I am out of here in a little bit. Regina is coloring my hair today. Stephen says he can't trust me being home from work. I get my oil changed, teeth cleaned, hair colored, and a new boob job. What next?

I had my follow up appointment today, and Dr. Trung released me to return to work on Friday. Yippee! He said, "Usually patients want me to give them an extension for more time off work." I go back to see him on the 13th, and he will remove the stitches at that time. Today, he just looked them over and took more pictures. Speaking of which—I will enclose the one he gave me.

Does it gross you out? Actually, the underside of the right breast is where the majority of the stitches are. You can see that it also looks like he removed it's nipple and sewed it back on after doing the lift. Now though—what do you think of the new boob? It's still swollen and sore looking, but it's coming along nicely. I am pleased. And check out the cleavage!!! Can you tell that I am proud? I guess this is the real reason that reconstructed women don't mind showing off their new boobs. I'll have to tell Jessica that my perception on this question has changed.

Ray called last night to see how I was doing. That made me feel good. He really is a sweetheart. I told him I was doing great, but I wasn't ready to go out dancing just yet. I hope that when I am, he will still meet me once in awhile on Saturday nights. I love dancing with him.

Tonight's my babysitting night. I stayed up late last night working on books, and then when I got into bed I turned the wrong way and thought I'd ripped out the stitches underneath my right boob. So I slept lousy and I then woke up super early this morning. Grrr.

That's it. I can't wait to talk to you.

Love,

April 5, Wednesday

Rita—

Here we go again. It's a two letter day and we just got through talking on the phone. At least we are consistent over the years. Do you remember years ago, when we would get off the phone, and then call each other right back? How did we ever afford those phone bills?

I am so pleased for you and Jack. You both sound like you are doing wonderful. That is great news.

Now, why am I writing again? Because I am home alone and cracking up—and I needed to share all this with you—and I know you are going back to sleep, so I didn't dare call again. Ready? I'm sitting here singing with Lillie. We are doing Patsy Cline songs. Lillie can sing. (I can't!)

The mailman came right after we got off the phone. There was a package from Lillie. It had a nice note and a great t-shirt. Over the right breast it says, "I was the Grand Prize Winner in the World Championship Wet T-shirt Contest ." Then over the left breast it says, "So was I." I'm hysterical over this.

There was also a smaller package and in it was a tape of Lillie singing Patsy Cline songs. I love it. She is too much. Didn't I tell you that she can do anything? So, I'm typing away and singing along with her... We could become a new country act. "The Boobsie Sisters"

Okay. No nap here after all. I have to get over to the college to pick up Tamsin and Nick.

I'm glad that you are doing so well, and that you got and like the book.

Love,

April 7, Friday

Good Morning!

Are you still bored? Shall I call you this time? Yesterday, when you called, I was still half asleep. I don't even know what we talked about. Well, I remember parts—like your being bored.

Yesterday was the pits. My throat was sore. My nose kept running and I was aching everywhere and going back and forth between fever and chills. Bruce called to see if I was going back to work today. I told him that I had wanted to, but it looked doubtful. Sometimes I just have to listen more to my body. This past year has taught me that anyway. I think that mentally I was ready, but physically I wasn't. When I was making plans to return early my body decided to teach me a lesson.

Today, I feel much better. I'm still sluggish, but I have managed to clean the apartment and water the patio plants and do laundry. Sometimes, I think I work harder when I stay home from work!

One of the members of our online group lives up in the mountains, where Arthur used to live. She had her reconstruction on the 31st. Jill had to have the TRAM. I called her yesterday, and she amazed me. Jill is up and doing as much as me, if not more. Her surgery is supposed to have her laid up for a much longer time than mine. Anyway, it was great to talk to her and she said that the next time the people from Southern California get together she wants to join us.

Last night, my friend, Warren, from Prodigy called. He is such a sweet man. He said he was just calling to keep in touch and see how I was doing. I still want to go to one of his Barber Shop Quartet performances one of these weekends. This coming weekend they are performing with Richard Simmons out in Palm Springs.

I am looking forward to going back to work on Monday. See, I really do understand about your boredom. We are so used to having a work routine that it seems strange to be home for so many days.

Keep healing. Love to Jack too.

Love you,

P.S. I forgot to tell you that I got excused from Jury Duty, and I also got notification of a panel interview up in Lake County on April 20th. But, I doubt I'll go to it.

April 9, Sunday

Hello again—

How are you doing now? Has the swelling gone down some? Are you ready to go back to work tomorrow? Last week, I thought I was ready until I got that sore throat. Now, I am just depleted of energy. I feel so lethargic. I hope I can handle a full week. That's partly why I'm writing today. If I am this tired during the coming week, then for sure, I won't be writing much when I get home in the evenings.

Nick is crashed out on the couch. It's tempting to join him. He and Tamsin had a very full day yesterday at Disneyland. They got there when the park opened and didn't come home until about 11:30 in the evening. It's no wonder he's taking a nap today. Oh and yes, he did get the post card which you had sent him. I just wasn't aware that it had come.

Well, I met Arthur's new girlfriend and her daughter today. He invited me over to his new place after church. I got there before Amanda and Caitlin. His studio apartment is a little beach cottage. It is very tiny actually, but Arthur is so organized and clean that it all somehow fits perfect. Also, he has good taste, so it's decorated really nice too. I am so happy for him. He is finally getting his life back together after his divorce.

Amanda is so sweet and very pretty. She has a natural beauty, and doesn't wear make-up. She doesn't need it! She's thin, the way Arthur likes, and again—I am happy for him. Amanda is very pleasant to be around. I like her. Caitlin just turned three, and she is probably Nick's size or bigger. She is a very active three too. It was nice to see Arthur enjoying himself with her and her Mom. He is such a family man, and it looks like Caitlin is helping to fill up the void of Dani's absence in his life.

This morning, our minister announced that our singer, and he's also the Church Musical Director, is dying from complications from AIDS. He has been there for the whole time I've been attending.

Everyone loves this man. The news was hard to deal with. The ushers were passing out boxes of Kleenex to the congregation. One of the members, who had seen him on Friday, told us that he has accepted his death and is dealing with it bravely and in a positive manner. We will miss him incredibly.

Are you ready for Easter? I got large, filled, chocolate eggs for each of the grandkids and one for Stephen, and had their names written on them. Naturally, Tyler won't be into his, but Eric and Bridget will enjoy it. Do you have any special plans? I am going to meet Laura for the Easter service, and then we might go out for brunch after.

Love for now,

April 11, Tuesday

Hi,

I have about ten minutes to write this and then I have to get to work. So here goes a quick one.

Yesterday, I found out that I will have a new assignment beginning next Monday. We will start training for it tomorrow. Actually, both Jessica and I will be on the new team along with five other Program Assistants. We spend Wednesday, Thursday, and Friday training at our Staff Development office. On Monday, we start the new assignment, which will last two weeks.

On Friday, about one hundred line workers will get layoff notices. But, they will still be employed for the next two weeks. The agency is concerned about sabotage and fraud through our computer systems. Our new team will be responsible for the security end. We will be monitoring and authorizing all the case actions. Pretty sad state of affairs, huh?

Anyway, Jessica says that because we were chosen to do this she doesn't think we will be demoted. Her reasoning is that, originally three temporary Program Assistants from Systems were going to be on the team. The Manager nixed that idea and said that since they were being demoted she didn't think it was a good idea. I guess this makes sense then, to conclude that Jessica and I will continue to be Program Assistants.

Also, Program Assistants will be the last ones getting notification of layoff or demotions. This probably won't take place until the end of May.

One last thing…As soon as you get your PC and know what programs are on it let me know. I can send you and Jack some of the books, which I had bought to help me. They are pretty basic books and easy to understand.

Hope your leg is okay. I'm off to work.

Love,

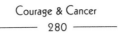

April 13, Thursday

Hi—

This has been a night of phone calls. Barbara called and left a message last night, so I finally returned her call. She made me feel good. She said that people at the Cowboy have been asking about me. Then Ann called to see how I was doing. I told the both of them what I am going to tell you right now...

My boobs hurt!!! (And notice that is a plural noun.) I went to see Dr. Trung this morning, to get my stitches removed. He didn't remove all of them. Most of them are out, but I go back next Tuesday to have the others removed. And, my breasts are so sore right now. As it turns out, I was supposed to have taken the antibiotics for two weeks. I didn't know to get a refill once I finished the first week. I'm now back on antibiotics, because the stitches in the implanted breast are a little infected. I'll also be using a hot compress on it at night, to draw the infection out. I went to work from his office. The pain wasn't unbearable—just more like very uncomfortable. (I exaggerate sometimes.)

Did you get Lillie's book? My copy arrived today and I plan on starting it tomorrow and reading it until I'm done. I can't wait.

This past year, three women employed in my agency have contacted me about themselves, or in one instant about a sister, finding lumps. Tuesday, the third lady called me at work. I've known her for years because she dances at the Cowboy. Anyway, she called me back today. In all three instances the lumps have turned out to be cysts, or some other type of lump, and not breast cancer. Whew.

Oh—I went to See's last night after work, and sent out the truffles to Maria. I wrote the note that you sent me, in Spanish. I hope she enjoys them.

Things are very busy at work. The first layoff notices were given out today. I started my new assignment right after they were given out. We are doing the Security checks on all the computer entries for the next two weeks.

Fortunately I won't even be demoted. But, the next round of layoffs have to be effective by May 25th. Then all the movement of the employees on my level should be in place by May 26th. As yet, I don't know where I will wind up. I just hope that our vacation doesn't get canceled because of all this. I will keep you posted.

Okay. I think this is enough damage for one night and I want to put the hot compress on my chest. I hope your knee is healing rapidly.

Love,

April 15, Saturday

Hi,

After so many long phone calls this week, I had no intention of writing you today, but Nick got his Easter card and he was thrilled with the "paper" money inside of it. He says it's to buy ice cream with. Okay. Why not? Thank you.

I did the hot compress again last night. Between that and the antibiotics I had no sign of infection this morning. And, my boobs are looking great—if I do say so myself. I even have on that tight, floral print t-shirt which you sent me awhile back. I think the top half of me looks better than it ever did!

But, speaking of top half—the bottom half is too big for a lot of my old clothes. The first two pair of jeans that I put on this morning I couldn't even zipper. Tamsin is making out from my weight gain. And I am not complaining. After this past year, and trying so hard to put on pounds, I don't think I will bitch over being a little heavier than usual. I mean, I am still on the skinny side, but fat for me. You know what I'm saying.

This is it. I just wanted to thank you for Nick and wish you, again, a Happy Easter tomorrow.

Love,

April 18, Tuesday

Hello—

This won't be a long one. At least, I don't think it will be. Today was my appointment with Dr. Trung, to get the last of the stitches out. He took more pictures and I wanted to send one to you. It's looking good! I showed Tamsin and she said, "Oh you have a 'Barbie doll' boob." I've been saying that the implanted breast looks "bald" without a nipple and areola, but I guess her new description for it is more like it.

I've decided that I am not in as big a rush to get the next surgery done. It's not that I'm not looking forward to it, but I really think my body is in need of some time to heal, rest, and repair. Originally, when Dr. Trung said it could be as soon as six weeks after the first one I was aiming for the six weeks. Now, if it's after our vacation that is just fine with me. I'd like to get stronger before I go under again. My body has been through so much this past year that waiting a couple more months sounds good.

The infection has healed, but I am still doing hot compresses at night and now I'm also putting Neosporin ointment on the areas where the stitches came out today. Dr. Trung opened and drained some cysts that had formed around the incision. When he removed the stitches under the good breast he had to cut it open. So, I am raw in some places, hence the ointment. Once the open areas are healed, then I can start using Vitamin E and cocoa butter lotion on the scars to lighten them up.

So, I'd say I'm really moving right along here. I'm not quite ready to go dancing as yet, but soon.

Stephen is coming down again on April 30th, and staying until May 2nd. I will be working, but at least we will have the evenings together. He said he would cook and clean for me while he's here and I'm at work. I told him that the cooking was okay, but I think he should go to the beach during the day and enjoy his days off. Honestly, I can't believe him.

He also said that he will try to spend Monday through Friday with us in Sonoma. I hope that's okay with you. Let me know how you feel about this.

The singer from my church passed away on Easter Sunday. He was so young, handsome, and talented. We will all miss him tremendously.

I guess this is getting longer than I expected. All's well here and I hope it's the same with you and Jack.

Love you,

April 20, Wednesday

Hi,

I take it back. I take it back. No matter what else happens in my life I will be at the San Francisco airport on Sunday, May 28th. (I got your message.) If I lose my job—well, that's okay. I'll come and live with you and Jack. No problem. (Just kidding) No one has said anything to me about canceling the vacation, so it must be all right.

Rita—I've never seen you looking "fat." What are you talking about? It sounds like we are both in agreement about eating. I'd prefer to eat our big meal, when we can, early in the day and snack at night.

Speaking of San Francisco... Stephen is there as I write. He was in Las Vegas on business when the bombing occurred in Oklahoma, but he got pulled to San Francisco. The Federal building in San Francisco had some bomb threats too. He is working long hours and is exhausted, but he assures me that he is fine.

My breast cancer sister, Deanna, works five miles from where the bombing took place. She said that she is okay, but it has devastated the city. I also wrote to Janette who works at the University of Oklahoma, but I haven't heard from her as yet. She is the one who wrote the Primate book.

Tamsin said she watched the news this morning and cried. What is happening to this world of ours?

I have an infection on the good breast. I'm not really worried about this though, as it should heal quickly. (Is all of this a pain in the butt or what?) Now I understand why Mary Beth thought I would need four weeks off work. It is taking that long for all of this to heal. But, I have set a new goal. My plan is to be able to go dancing on Mother's Day. Let's see if I can reach it. (I will. I know me.)

A friend of mine heard about my transfer request. There will be an opening in her district because of a demotion from the cut backs. She asked me if I was interested. I said, "yes." She is going to put in a good word for me, with her Manager. I warned her about the week's vacation, that I had two more surgeries coming up, and also about my lack of Financial Assistance knowledge. Keep your fingers crossed for me.

I guess this is one of those, "this and that" letters.

Bye. Love,

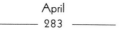

April 22, Saturday

Hello again,

Every time I think I'm done writing you stuff, I come up with more. Poor you.

I held a very private fashion show this morning in my bedroom. After my shower, I tried on all my bathing suits. Do you remember I bought them last year and didn't get to wear them? Well, they look great. I am so happy. By looking at me, you would never know what I went through this past year.

Today is as hot as summer. I told Nick that if it is like this tomorrow, I'll take him to my little beach for a while. He's excited, but I don't think he's got me beat.

My right breast is still sore and infected, but I am my usual weekend, braless self today. Last night was the first night in 3 ½ weeks that I went to bed without a bra on. It felt so good. I even slept a little on my stomach, and it didn't feel like I was on some rocky hill either. I'm healing and adjusting.

Last night, Grace held her monthly online Writer's Workshop. She invited me to it, since my publisher, Rich, was the guest speaker. I've never been to an online workshop before. It was fascinating. They have a formal protocol and Grace hosted, while Rich did the "talking" and informing. Members took turns asking him questions about how to get published. I was so proud of him. Once again, I really lucked out when I met him and the rest is history.

Mike, from the Cancer Survivors Group, just sent us all e-mail. *People* magazine is thinking of doing a piece about our group. So, Mike was asking who would be interested in being interviewed. I immediately answered in the positive. Sounds like a fun thing to do.

But, then I got to thinking that maybe it is time for Rich to look at the "Love and Laughter" book. He has a rough draft and we had agreed to wait awhile before he looked at it. I sent him e-mail and said I'm almost done with the final manuscript, so it's probably time for him to look over what he has, and give me his opinion. I'll let you know what happens.

All good things are happening here. Yesterday, I ran into one of my prior Managers. She, too, will have an opening for a Program Assistant in her district. She would like me to work for her again. So I might be going there. It's nice to know that I am wanted professionally.

I'm melting here at the keyboard. It's too hot to do anything. I'll write more later.

Love,

April 24, Monday

Hi,

We are almost there. One more month and four days. Now I sound like Stephen and I do when we are counting the days until he flies down here.

I have this philosophy that all things work out for the best at just the perfect time. Well, I had been thinking about volunteering my services to a breast cancer organization. I was waiting until I was finished with my own issues, and I was also trying to decide which group to contact. Yesterday a meeting was held by the Orange County Health Care Agency in the same building where I am currently assigned. It was for a newly funded program for a Breast Cancer Early Detection Partnership. Quite a few agencies, including the Susan Komen Foundation, are making a joint effort to educate women regarding the necessity of going for their mammograms. After talking with the coordinator for the group I signed on as a volunteer. This way I am going to be working with all the local breast cancer groups.

My next step is to donate my prosthesis to the American Cancer Society. I'm ready to let someone else receive the pleasure that I did right after my mastectomy. I remember how good it felt when I got it.

Today is my first day, since last June, to wear one of my regular bras. It feels great. I am obviously still the same size. Soon I am going on my shopping spree though to buy up a drawer full of fancier ones. (I've earned that splurge.)

My publisher doesn't feel that the chat log book is marketable based on the one line format of the conversations. But, I am not discouraged as I still believe in this book. I'll give it a try with some other publishers.

All's well. I'm happy.

Love,

April 27, Thursday

Hello,

I got "the" long letter from you today. My, my you are one busy lady. I was tired just reading your schedule for the week. Your leg must be feeling great if you are able to keep that up.

Things are happening here too. I have two dozen other things to do tonight—so of course I'm writing to you. Well, that's okay. Maybe I should get it all down tonight. Stephen is coming Sunday and you know I won't be writing while he's here. And, thank you for saying he could stay the whole week with us in Sonoma. Actually, now it looks like he'll only be with us for a few days.

Rita, I have to say my life is so fascinating for me lately. Everyday is special and I have this new and glorious attitude. It is as if I am standing here with my arms spread wide open and I'm saying, "Okay— now what is today going to bring?" And, I am ready, willing and able to embrace it all. I love life!

I was telling the above to Tamsin tonight, and I also added that sometimes there are good things in a day and sometimes there are not so good things. And, too, there are days where I get some of each. I know. I am just rambling again, but soon I will tell you what has been going on.

My poor publisher Rich—I think I must be giving him an ulcer. When he told me that he wasn't interested in the Love and Laughter book I accepted it. But, I wasn't giving up on it. The next day I had an e-mail note from Rich and he said that they still loved me, and just to prove it he wanted me to know that he'd also read the book of prose that I wrote fifteen years ago when I was Agoraphobic. They are currently discussing marketing for that book as they are interested in it. He thinks it is a wonderful book. (And, no, you have not read that one. It was written for me. I kept it close to my chest for those fifteen years and now I'm ready to let it go.) I was in a state of shock. I wrote him back and said, "Rich, you only love my neurotic side." (He has a wonderful sense of humor.)

So, I put together twenty query letters to send out to other publishers and I let my online friends know that the Love and Laughter book was rejected. My author friend in Florida wrote back and told me to send him a copy of the manuscript as his publisher might be interested in it and he would hand deliver it to him. Well, his publisher currently has the #1 best seller on the market. It is the book which I sent to my boss Bruce when he was having his brain surgery. (Chicken Soup for the Soul)

I dropped off the manuscript at Kinko's this morning for Xeroxing. On the way home from work I picked it up and then I got a box to send it Priority Mail. But, this morning before I went to work I sent Rich another e-mail and told him the above and mentioned that one of his other authors, who I have become friends with, had read "Love and Laughter" and that she liked it too. I asked him, "Are you sure you don't want this book?"

When I got in tonight he had answered and was teasing me that I'd only sent him the rough draft and to send him the cleaned up copy. He did say that he is still reluctant since it is in the transcript style. Tomorrow I'm sending him the final version. Wish me luck!.

I finished my special assignment as of today. Tomorrow I am back at Systems. Today 96 line workers worked their last day for Social Services.

The sad piece of news I received tonight was about one of our members. You will remember her from the "Love and Laughter" book. She and Wendy were very close. Wendy had sent her some posters for the hospital ceiling as she was going through her Bone Marrow Transplant. Her husband found her in a coma a few mornings ago. Things do not look good. I am very saddened to hear that she is not doing well. (She is the one who was originally diagnosed with less breast cancer than me.)

There must be more, but my energy is slowly running down.

Love,

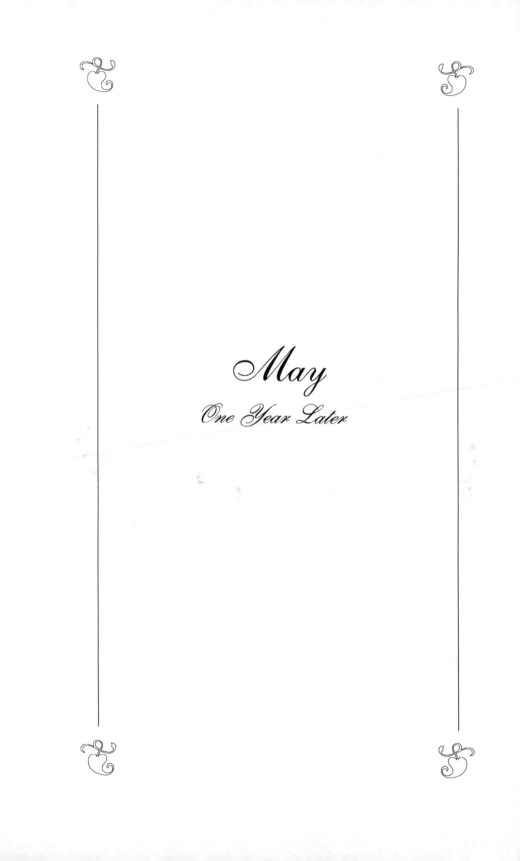

May

One Year Later

May 1, Monday

Happy May Day!

I said I wouldn't be writing while Stephen is here, but I lied again. Actually, it's lunch time and since I can't be home with Stephen I'm going to pick on you. I called him once this morning to see what he was up to. I thought he'd be relaxing or doing something fun. Well, he says that what he's doing is fun and relaxing for him. He went grocery shopping and he's making all kinds of food and putting it in the freezer for me. When I told this to Ann, she asked me if I ever get tired of him—could she have him? I told her, "Never."

My weight is now 112 pounds. I've gained ten pounds since I went off of chemo. Stephen also brought me another pound of See's truffles. Help! My pants are all too tight. I'm still skinny, and I like the weight that I have right now—but, I told him that I do not want another ten pounds added on here.

The real reason I'm writing is so that I can enclose a couple of pictures, which Stephen took in December. They were taken at Disneyland. I really like the one of him and me with Santa Claus.

Stephen and I were talking last night. Now, he too is getting into the questioning of why so many women are getting breast cancer. His thought is that maybe it has to do with our bras. He says that is one common denominator, and then if women are wearing under-wire bras, maybe the wire is acting as an antenna to pick up Electro Magnetic Radiation from computers and microwaves. I just looked at him dumbfounded. While he kept on talking, I walked over to my dresser drawer, pulled out all my old bras and showed them to him. They are all under-wire.

When I got to work today, I asked Jessica if she wore under-wire bras before her diagnosis. She said, "Yes." Now I'm waiting for an answer from Bev. Also, tonight in group, I'm going to take a survey there. It's an interesting theory anyway.

Last night, we went out to dinner and when we got home we watched "Forrest Gump." I finally got to see that great movie. I cried at the end. Have you seen it yet?

Our car rental reservations for Sonoma are made. Stephen will join us from Wednesday night until Saturday night. Hopefully, we can get together on Saturday with Bud and Lynn, so that they can meet Stephen too.

When we talked on the phone Saturday, while I was babysitting Tyler, did I tell you that he was sick? The kids told me that he was just teething, but I said I thought he had a cold or something else too. He was really hot and was going back and forth between fever and chills. Yesterday, when Bridget's Mom babysat him, she took his temperature and it was over 102. She couldn't get him to keep any food or fluids down.

Bridget took him to the Emergency Room last night. His fever was almost 105. They told her she brought him in just in time. He was dehydrated too. They gave him a cool bath, a shot of antibiotics and an IV to get fluid into him. He's home and doing fine now, but that's pretty scary.

I need to start dancing again, because I need the exercise. I hope I haven't forgotten how.

Thank you again, for my "Happy Boob Day" card and gifts. You are too much.

Love,

May 4, Thursday

Hi,

It's lunch time again and I thought I would have news by now, as to where I'm going next as a Program Assistant. Our Manager told us yesterday that we would all know today what our future will be. It looks like we will be told this afternoon. I'll hold this letter and add to it later. No matter where I wind up, I will be happy there.

I do know that I'll be going on that special assignment again on the 11th, when the largest volume of layoff notices go out. The same team that did the security checks will be doing these, but we'll be using a different approach. I'm looking forward to having something new to work on.

Lunch was left over steamed vegetables. How is your diet going? I would like to lose two pounds before we go on vacation. My pants and shorts are all too tight, and I know I won't be getting new clothes between now and then.

Finally, I called the State Franchise Tax Board, as they never responded to my letter questioning the error about my refund. The lady was very helpful and said that I had filled out the wrong form. She will send me the correct form and I can have my filing amended, and then I will get the big refund that I thought I was getting a couple of months ago.

I wrote to a group in San Francisco called "Breast Cancer Action." They are involved with environmental issues relating to breast cancer. I've asked them if they had ever heard of any studies or research into Stephen's theory, regarding the under-wire bras.

Jessica told me that she saw a show on TV last night, that said a research group has identified "Cancer Types." She said it concluded that we are people who are anxious, worriers, and also we keep things bottled up inside us. I told her I meet the first two, but I don't hold things in too often. Someday this puzzle will be solved.

After work tonight, I go for my annual mammogram of my right breast. It's healed enough, and I need to have it done before I meet with Dr. Gruber next Tuesday. It's been just about one year from the last one.

I'm also going to stop at a store and buy a vegetable steamer to take to Bud and Lynn. It's always difficult deciding what to get them. I figure, if they already have one then maybe they can use it at the Townhouse.

Stephen has been offered a new position as a permanent, full time employee with the Federal Government. He has until the middle of the month to decide. I'll tell you more about it if he accepts.

Tyler is better and eating lots again. Tamsin and Nick finish school in a couple of weeks. Now she is preparing for her finals.

All's well in this neck of the woods.

Love,

P.S. I just found out that I will remain in Systems, but I will be transferring to the mainframe group. I'll write more later.

$\mathcal{M}$ay 4, Thursday

Hello -

Another two letter day and it's late, but I wanted to let you know about this afternoon. We had a brief meeting. It was sort of anti-climatic after the months of waiting and wondering. I will be taking over my friend Rick's job. In a way, I am glad it worked out this way, because I don't feel like I am bumping someone out of a job. I mean he wants the layoff, so I won't be dealing with feelings of guilt. Rick's last day will be May 25th. I asked him if I could sit with him tomorrow, to get an idea of what it is that he does. I feel like a weight has been lifted off of my shoulders, now that I know where I will be. This position is actually less stressful than if I went out to one of our districts. I feel fortunate once again.

After work, I got the mammogram done. When the technician put them up against the light, I looked closely at them and they looked clear to me. Of course, I am no radiologist, but after last year I sort of have an idea as to what to look for.

You're going to hate me for this, but I lost one pound already. (Only one more to go.) This is how my body reacts to stress, and today was stressful for me. I can't take credit for being disciplined. As a matter of fact, tomorrow twelve of us are going out to a Mexican restaurant to celebrate Cinco de Mayo. You know I will be pigging out for that.

Tonight, I went clothes shopping for Nick and Tyler. I got them each two shorts outfits. Now I have to think of something for Dani. That'll be this weekend.

I'm out of here again for tonight.

Love,

May 6, Saturday

Hi,

It's been a full day here and I still have the weekend ironing to do, but I just felt like writing to you—not that there's much to say. I got your letter and laughed about your fruit and vegetable diet. That's how I eat most of the time, along with grains and yogurt. Of course, I splurge some times, but I like fruits and vegetables a lot.

Guess what??? I have "curly" hair again and we are talking "very" curly hair here. It's short, but I like it. Next week, I go back to have it colored. I might ask Regina to trim my bangs, as they are almost in my eyes, but other than that I am pleased. It feels great. I think I am meant to have curly hair.

And, I went to Victoria's Secret today. I got two bras and another lace teddy. My choice in bras was limited, as almost all of them had under-wire. Since I don't need the under-wire to lift me up anymore, and I'm still thinking about what Stephen said, I got them without.

I also found the funniest birthday card to give to Jessica. It has all types of cartoon boobs on the front of the card and inside it says, "Have your breast birthday." I don't know when her birthday is, but it's got to be about now, since she is a Taurus.

Arthur took Dani, Nick, and Caitlin for the whole day. They went to a dinosaur show at the Fairgrounds and then to a playground. It sounds like they had fun. I took some pictures of the three of them before they left. The pictures should come out cute. The kids are like little stepping stones. In one, I had Nick cover his eyes, Dani cover her ears, and Caitlin cover her mouth.

I feel so good lately that I am ready to go dancing. Unless anything unexpected comes up, I will be at the Cowboy tomorrow. Yea!!!

Okay—the ironing is giving me a guilty conscience. Gotta go.

Love,

*M*ay 8, Monday

Rita,

CURLY HAIR IS EVERYTHING! I am so happy and I feel so good. Not only do I have two boobs again, but I have curly hair once more. I love it. After playing with it a bit, I've decided I don't even want my bangs cut. It looks terrific with it going to the side, instead of all on my forehead. I am getting a swelled head from all the compliments I'm getting. And you thought you were the only one with great hair! Ha. Last night at the Cowboy, one of my dance partners said, "You look so cute I just want to kiss you." I told him he'd better not because I have a boyfriend and he is married. He laughed.

I wore a romper that is v-neck, with a large white collar. Between the style of the clothing and my curly top—I walked into the living room and said to Tamsin, "Do I look like Little Orphan Annie or what?" She cracked up.

Dancing was wonderful. I missed it so much. No one knew I was going. I didn't tell Ann or Barbara. I just showed up. They saw my car pull into the parking lot and started grinning. I ran over to give them one huge, group hug and said, "She's baaackk!!!"

And all good things continue to happen to me. Stephen, my love and my hero, is reconsidering the possibility of our getting married, "maybe" "someday." This is a big step for him. He said not to go around shouting it out and I won't, but he didn't say I couldn't write and tell you. It'll happen. I know it will. I cannot imagine my future life without him in it. He is becoming my other best friend and that's that.

Also, I had a great idea last night. When I get back from our vacation, I want to start another book, "Seeking Self-Empowerment." Now that it's hit me, I am anxious to start it. Whether it ever becomes a real book or not, I will still benefit from the way I plan to write it. Life is being so good to me and I just embrace all of it.

Oh, and I lost the other pound. I knew it would happen when I started dancing. Ever since I became a dancer, I don't have much of a problem with gaining weight no matter how much I eat. I dance it off and have fun doing it.

So now that I really can wear a bathing suit in public—are we taking them on vacation? There's a pool at the townhouse. What are you bringing for clothing? When we go into the city you might want warmer clothes, as it tends to be cool there even in the summer. Let me know what you are bringing. I sort of have an idea of what I am going to take. I can't wait!!!

Bye. Love,

Rita -

No cancer! No cancer! No cancer! I feel like calling you. I'm jumping with joy. Today was my round of doctor's appointments. Dr. Gruber's was this afternoon. She walked in grinning and said, "Well?" I flashed her with the hospital gown and said, "I've got two!!!" She and I both started laughing. Then she said, "Your mammo was clear." I almost cried. (Happy tears this time.) She looked over the new "parts" and said, "Nice work." I told her they were the best. (Dr. Trung "done" good!)

We caught up on what's been happening. And, we hugged twice. She is a wonderful lady, Rita. She said that my positive attitude made her day, because she has been feeling down lately. There have been so many mastectomies. Dr. Gruber got serious and said, "One in eight." And all I could say was, "I know." I told her that she could give my name and phone number to any new breast cancer sisters, who might need someone to talk to. She was pleased and said that she did a mastectomy this morning on a patient who was only forty-two years old. The lady is very despondent. She asked if I was sure about wanting to talk to her. I said "Yes. It's my turn to give back."

This morning, I saw Dr. Trung. He was pleased and said that I have healed nicely. I also told him that he can use me as a reference for his patients, because I think he did a remarkable job. The "decorations" will be done next month after we get back from our vacation. He won't be able to graft from the good nipple, since so much work was done on it when he lifted that breast. Instead, he will use skin from my inner thigh. Dr. Trung said that he can also graft some skin over parts of the mastectomy scar. I'm thrilled with all this.

Then I talked with Bud today. He told me that he is proud of me. That made me feel great, and I told him that I was proud of me too. I'm excited about seeing Bud and Lynn again. They have invited the three of us to their house for dinner on the Friday night of our vacation. Then Stephen and they can meet too. I'll enclose the address and phone number of the townhouse, in case Jack wants it.

All my work buddies were in my office this afternoon, after I returned from the doctor appointments, and they got caught up in my excitement and happiness. I told them this year really has many happy endings for me. I've got the man. I've almost sold two books. I've got two boobs. I've got curly hair. Then I looked at Rick and said, "And I've got your job too!" We all went hysterical. (He really wants his "vacation" bad.)

Seriously though—Rita, a year ago I felt like I was falling through the looking glass. And, you know what? I came out the right side. We have gone full circle on this. Although, I wouldn't have chosen for this to happen, I still feel that I have come out ahead. I thank you again, and again—with all my heart for helping me when I needed you.

I've been thinking about a bumper sticker, which I saw in the church bookstore last Sunday. It said, "Life's a dance—if you just take the steps." We did take the steps, little by little, day by day, and week by week— and I do believe we won the grand championship.

Love you lots,

May

Dear Reader,

If you are not a breast cancer sister, I cannot emphasize enough how important it is to do self breast exams, and to stay on top of your mammogram schedules. I admit that I was not doing this and that I have my General Practitioner, Dr. Elizabeth Tioleco-Cheng to thank for always remembering to send me for a bi-annual mammogram. I went on these referrals, not because I was concerned that anything would be found, but because it is my nature to "follow through" on things. I knew very little about breast cancer, other than it existed—for other women I thought—but never for me.

If you have been diagnosed with breast cancer, it is your responsibility to do your own research. Read books and ask questions. I would also recommend that you talk to other women who have been through this experience. Accept all the love and support which is offered from family, friends, and even strangers. Nurture and love yourself.

I was very fortunate this past year, in that I always had Rita to talk to as I was going through my diagnosis, surgeries and treatments. At the same time, my world continued to expand when I went online and met so many wonderful people—from my breast cancer sisters, to my publisher and of course, to Stephen. There have been so many blessings in what could have been a negative experience. For me, personally, cancer taught me to live. Each day has become precious. I appreciate what I do have so much more.

It is devastating to hear that you have breast cancer, but it is not the end of the world. Learn and grow from this challenge. I wish for you a healthy recovery and I want you to know that you are not alone.

Much love,

M

To the Reader

We hope that you have enjoyed reading this book. Marilyn is busy working on her prequel and sequel to *Courage & Cancer.*

To recieve information about these and other titles by Marilyn Moody, or about titles by our other authors, please send your name and mailing address to:

Rhache Publishers, Ltd.
9 Orchard Drive, Gardiner, NY 12525–5710
(914) 883–5884, (914) 883–7169
e-mail: Rhache Pub@aol.com

Writing to Marilyn

Marilyn would love to hear from you.
She may be reached through the Internet at:

DncrLady@aol.com

or by writing her in care of Rhache Publishers.